Language Intervention
for School-Age Students
Setting Goals for Academic Success

Language Intervention
for School-Age Students
Setting Goals for Academic Success

Geraldine P. Wallach, PhD
Associate Professor
Department of Communicative Disorders
California Sate University, Long Beach
Long Beach, California

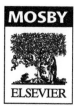

MOSBY
ELSEVIER

MOSBY
ELSEVIER

11830 Westline Industrial Drive
St. Louis, Missouri 63146

ISBN-13: 978-0-323-04033-4

Vice President and Publisher: Linda Duncan
Senior Editor: Kathy Falk
Managing Editor: Kristin Hebberd
Publishing Services Manager: Julie Eddy
Project Manager: Andrea Campbell
Cover Design Direction: Paula Catalano
Interior Designer: Paula Catalano
Chapter-opening photos: Copyright 2007 JupiterImages Corporation

Printed and bound by CPI Group (UK) Ltd, Croydon, CR0 4YY

Dedication

To Dr. Joel Stark

Joel brought me into the "LLD" world, and I have, happily, never looked back. He taught me many things along the way both professionally and personally—especially to "let that river flow." Joel influenced many of his students and made us rebels for the kids (and future students) in our care. He is surely the Wizard himself, but behind the curtain is knowledge, logic, and love that guide all of us who were lucky enough to be influenced by his vivacious, and sometimes beautifully outrageous, style. Lucky us! And lucky children and adolescents with language learning disabilities who are helped by Joel everyday, through his continued teaching and through us.

GPW

Foreword

It may be difficult for some of the readers of this text to imagine what it was like in the early days of the "language-learning disabilities" movement, as we youngsters in speech and language pathology in the early 1970s and 1980s, liked to call it. Others, like myself and the author, do remember those times when language disorders and learning disabilities were farther apart than they are today. (See *Topics in Language Disorders*, [2005]* for a review.) We were there when many concepts in the forefront of theory and practice today, were being launched. For example, it was not common practice in the early 1970s to work with adolescents with language disorders, and in truth, school-age language disorders were not widely understood. The core idea that the majority of *learning* disabilities are *language* disorders that have changed over time (see Chapter 2 in this text) was considered as crazy as saying that reading was not a visual process. Likewise, concepts like "curriculum-based" and "strategic-focused" intervention were rarely mentioned or operationalized in practice. It was also an innovative notion 30 years ago to say that oral and written language were reciprocal systems, and it was even more controversial to suggest that speech-language pathologists (SLPs) had a role in literacy.

At what our mentors might say was the dawn of our careers, the author and I joined the language-based learning disabilities "cause" (including what the role of SLPs might be in "learning" disabilities) and began a professional partnership and personal friendship that has endured over time. Through the years, we have had long conversations about many of the themes that are explored in this text. We have written and presented both together and separately and have tried to create frameworks that fuse theory and practice. We see ourselves as committed to school-based professionals and issues. We understand the challenges facing SLPs and their colleagues in that setting but we also believe, as Wallach notes in her final chapter, that we can do better for the children and adolescents in our care. This text reflects that "do-better" concept directly in the last chapter but provides readers with an arsenal of information that may help them "get there" in the chapters that precede the last one. The "getting there" may not be to Nirvana (or "perfection"), as also noted in the final chapter of the text, but it may include being better equipped to create and deliver language intervention programs that are relevant and effective.

There are many aspects of this text that resonate with me. Although there is much I might say about each chapter, I will only highlight some key points at this time. Thanks to my colleague, readers can evaluate for themselves my thinking about this subject in a number of the chapters that follow. To start, I appreciate the way the author has organized the text so that it moves readers

---

*Butler, K.G., & Nelson, N.W. Editors: Wallach, G.P. Issue Editor (2005). Language disorders and learning disabilities: A look across 25 years. *Topics in Language Disorders*, 25(4), 287-336.

between conceptual (theoretically focused) and practical (intervention focused) frameworks with relative ease. Wallach uses "real-life" examples from students with language learning disabilities throughout the text to put a spotlight on many of the things we actually do with them in classrooms and clinic rooms everyday. The theoretical underpinnings are discussed within this context— that is, the "what we do with students." The question that follows, ala Wallach, is: Does "what we do" make sense? The principles delineated in Chapter 1, through the use of visual images and metaphors (including a multilayered cake to represent basic and "meta" levels of language), set the tone for the text and lets readers know from the start that some of our beliefs about what language intervention might "look like" at school-age levels (and other levels) require further scrutiny (to put it mildly).

I also like the way the author weaves curricular materials and examples from textbooks throughout the book. Even when talking about early literacy in Chapter 6, the author includes a section at the end of the chapter that uses a Grade 5 social studies excerpt to remind readers to keep their eyes on the horizon of language change and curricula demands. As an avid basketball fan, in contrast to the author as baseball aficionado, I really enjoyed the sports topics woven throughout the text. Being a strong advocate of using curriculum-based materials as a backdrop or context for language intervention, I appreciate the author's suggestion that practitioners consider using familiar topics with students as a way to help them make transitions to curricular content. As emphasized throughout the text, SLPs and content-area teachers have complementary (not duplicative) roles to play in the education of students with language learning disabilities. Wallach covers the challenges of SLPs falling into the "tutor trap" and makes a number of important points about complementary roles and responsibilities in language and academic learning. My colleague captures my notion of "language underpinnings" and the consequent role of SLPs in many excellent examples of students and curricular requirements.

Chapter 5 is "classic Wallach." She tackles the central auditory processing (CAP) issue with examples from second language learning and other processing scenarios that should help readers consider viewing these problems from a broader, linguistic perspective. The self-questioning outline at the end of the chapter that asks readers to form a dialogue with themselves and colleagues is particularly helpful. It asks professionals to consider internal, external, and metalinguistic factors when making assessment and intervention decisions and pulls the chapter together. Chapters 9 and 10, mentioned below, are also noteworthy for their presentation of language intervention missteps and alternatives, following up on many concepts raised in Chapter 5.

The text takes a "where we are," "where we've been," and "where we might be going" approach to language intervention at school-age levels. I think that readers will appreciate the way Wallach asks her readers to keep questioning the conventional wisdom of the day, including hers. The language intervention excerpts, cases, and scenarios that encourage readers to form discussion groups bring theoretical, practical, and collaborative components together. Chapters 9 and 10 are especially useful because they present to readers actual cases and scenarios and then outline what we might do—or not do—with these students.

As we look back and look ahead, we can say that we are fortunate to live in an era in which so much information is available and accessible so quickly. There is more "coming together" of professionals from speech-language pathology, literacy, and curricular arenas, among others. Wallach highlights some of this joint thinking in the text. Responsiveness-to-Intervention (RTI) models, such as the evolving one presented by Nicky Nelson and myself (see Figure 2-2, p. 34) offer additional promise in this post-millennium era. Thus, although better understood than they were 30 years ago, there is still more to learn about the connections among language, learning, and literacy and the disorders therein. Likewise, the notion that the majority of learning disabilities are language-based is still a work-in-progress.

Wallach's text brings many of the pieces of this complex puzzle together and encourages readers to consider the possibilities that are in our midst. I know I can speak for my colleague and myself when I say that we hope we continue this conversation for many years to come. After all, we are only in the half-time (or fifth inning?) of our search for answers to the following questions:

■ What should language intervention look like at school age levels?
■ How can I begin to create and deliver language intervention goals and objectives to students that are curriculum-relevant and strategic?

Barbara J. Ehren, EdD
Professor and Director
Doctoral Program in Language and Literacy
Department of Communication Sciences and Disorders
University of Central Florida

Preface

Audience and Purpose

The text is intended to be a working manual for practitioners from diverse fields who work with students experiencing language learning disabilities. Although it takes a strong language/language disorders perspective, it also should be useful to teachers and other specialists who share with their school-based speech-language pathologists (SLPs) in the education of students with academic difficulties. The text takes a positive tone, demonstrating how professionals have unique roles to play that complement, not duplicate, services.

Background

This text began as a result of my return to full-time teaching after several, sometimes painful years, in higher education administration. It started as a look back and a look forward as I prepared syllabi, readings, and assignments for my new courses in child and school-age language disorders. It is interesting to note that when one takes a fresh look at the field of language disorders and learning disabilities, it is true that while some things change, others remain the same.

As I returned to clinical supervision and field visits to school-based settings within and outside of California, I was interested in what seasoned and newly graduated practitioners had to say about the state of language intervention. What I found interesting was that many of the concepts of the 1960s and 1970s were alive and well in the clinic and resource rooms across the country. For example, there was still a tendency toward looking at children as being either "visual" or "auditory learners." Some practitioners were focused on working on what we might call "discrete skills"—skills like auditory and visual sequencing—and the like. On several Individualized Education Plans (IEPs) for children with language disorders, I observed "is...verbing" as an objective across Grades 1 through 3. Another trend that remained popular was to label seemingly every other child with an academic problem as having a "central auditory processing disorder" (CAPD) and/or an "attention deficit disorder" (ADD).

Unique Contribution to the Language Learning Disabilities Community

No doubt, I have exercised some hyperbole in these examples. Nonetheless, although there are many excellent resources available today—suggesting that a number of the above-mentioned concepts require re-evaluation—the theory-to-practice gap is alive and well. Moreover, "older" theories about language learning and language disorders are pervasive in practice. This text examines some of the popular practices that exist today with an eye toward suggesting ways to make realistic modifications within the context of having too many children with diverse problems on professionals' caseloads and too little time. The text asks readers to ask themselves a number of questions including:

- Where does a goal or activity "come from?" Is it theory-based? Data-based? Intuitive?
- What are the differences between language intervention (or therapy) and language arts instruction?

■ How does intervention outside the classroom connect with what's going on inside the classroom?
■ What are some of the barriers to successful programming for students with language learning disabilities?
■ What are approaches to overcoming these barriers?

Text Goals

The text has four major goals as follows:
1. To encourage readers to evaluate past and current clinical and educational practices in language intervention at school-age levels
2. To present intervention goals and activities that are theoretically-sound but may require further research scrutiny
3. To explore aspects of curriculum-relevant language intervention for students with language learning disabilities
4. To provide guidelines for school-based practitioners that clarify how professionals with diverse backgrounds and roles share responsibility in language, literacy, and academic programming.

Organization

The four sections of the text build upon one another. Key questions and a summary statement are used at the beginning of each chapter to guide readers through the information presented in the chapter. The text also has many sample forms, outlines, visual maps and other supportive materials that are easily reproduced. Parts I and II present strong conceptual and practical frameworks. Chapters 1 through 4 present the building blocks for intervention across the grades. Chapters 1 and 2 are broader in the sense that both chapters provide the macrostructure, or overarching themes, that pull the forthcoming chapters together. Readers are challenged in Chapters 1 and 2 to explore what they think the term "language disorders" means, among other popular definitions. The chapters ask tough questions about the things we do to help children within school settings. Readers will recognize many of the challenges presented. A continuum of language learning and language disorders is presented that links preschool and school-age issues. Metaphors and visual images are used in Chapter 1 to highlight some of the ways in which learners comprehend and retain information. The metaphors and visual images also serve to pull together key ideas about school-age language intervention. Chapters 3 and 4 ask readers to "look at" language disorders and intervention more critically. Readers are encouraged to ask themselves a basic question: Is what I'm doing in my speech-language or resource room relevant to the classroom? Follow-up questions include: How do I make language intervention "curriculum relevant"? How do I make the time to observe in the classroom or talk with teachers when there is no time? Suggestions are presented and shared in this section of the text.

Part III marries conceptual and practical frameworks. A discussion of a very misunderstood relationship—that of language disorders and central auditory processing disorders—is presented in Chapter 5. A series of scenarios that relate to comprehending language in "real" situations is used to make processing–comprehending connections more explicit. Examples of second language learning are used to highlight some of the symptoms we see in students with language learning disabilities. Readers are asked to explore possible alternatives to the "processing" diagnosis. A checklist is provided at the end of the chapter that takes readers through a series of question related to developing a shared responsibility in language and literacy. Chapter 6 takes us back to some of the preschool milestones in literacy that are connected to academic success. The chapter asks readers to look at early language intervention from within a literature-based framework. The continuum is revisited with a focus on connecting early and later literacy experiences. In both chapters, we look back at both theory and practice as well as look ahead to the curriculum and the changes that face our preschoolers with language disorders as they grow up to face the demands of an ever-changing and challenging curriculum. Chapters 7 and 8 present a thorough discussion of the interactions among connected discourse, including narrative and expository discourse, content knowledge, and sentence- and word-level skills. A discourse protocol is presented in Chapter 7 that includes conversational, narrative, and expository text components. Excerpts from average achieving students and students with language learning disabilities are presented to complement the discussion. An example from the science curriculum brings the pieces of discourse together. Chapter 8 continues the themes of Chapter 7. Chapter 8 outlines the differences between foundational and derivational literacies and reminds readers that many popular reading comprehension strategies must be viewed from within a prism of the language skills and abilities that underlie the strategies. Activities that demonstrate both macro (connected text structure and content) and micro (sentence- and word-level components) elements of language are presented with an eye toward how they relate to the science and social studies curricula. Examples from the curriculum across a number of grade levels are weaved throughout the text's chapters.

Part IV moves toward a summary of key concepts discussed throughout the text. Chapter 9 reminds readers to keep language intervention relevant and functional. State standards are presented as a way to create language intervention goals and objectives within the context of grade-level expectations. Because vocabulary and word-finding issues are so pervasive in the language learning disabled population and because they intersect with decoding issues, "word learning" is also included as a route to curriculum-relevant and authentic language intervention. An exploration of selected intervention activities ends the chapter. Readers are asked to consider the reasons why an activity might be chosen as a review of some of the ideas presented in previous chapters. Chapter 10 continues to move toward closure. A series of abbreviated scenarios that include assessment and intervention challenges are presented. Readers are encouraged to consider alternatives to the conclusions reached in the scenarios and to open a dialogue with their colleagues about other ways to interpret student, material, and clinician choices. Both chapters in the summary section use mini cases and scenarios as tools for encouraging conversations among colleagues who share students with language learning disabilities. As the text closes, some positive thoughts are expressed about finding "enlightenment" in schools and looking toward a better future for students with language learning and academic difficulties. The text leaves readers with a positive message about how much information is available currently and expresses the view that we can "do it"; we can move to more innovative practices in language intervention that are both curriculum-relevant and strategy-focused.

Learning Aids and Features

- **A Summary Statement** begins each chapter, providing readers with an overview of the chapter discussion and goals.
- A listing of **Key Questions** focuses the chapter's goals for readers and encourages them to read the information with an eye toward answering the queries presented.
- Chapter text begins with **Introductory Thoughts,** a section of text that helps set the stage for each topic, covering its history and current state and outlining where practitioners want to be in the future.
- **Marginal notes** throughout each chapter pull out key questions, interesting facts and points of view, and new terminology from the main chapter discussion.
- Chapter discussions are organized in a **question format,** with key queries mixed throughout the chapters to encourage readers to critically evaluate the origin and purpose of various treatment strategies and techniques.
- **Case scenarios** are mixed throughout the chapters, bringing the text discussions to life with real-world examples of intervention.
- **Curriculum excerpts** and **sample forms and paperwork** help readers see the challenges students with language learning disabilities face and provide them with practical classroom-relevant ways to help them.

Geraldine P. Wallach

Acknowledgments

There are always so many people who make the completion of a text possible. I have many to thank from the different corners of my life. A number of my wonderful speech and language colleagues have influenced my thinking throughout the years, as reflected in this text. Dr. Barbara (Angelina) Ehren has taught me what excellent language intervention should be and what collaboration is all about. Her ideas appear throughout this text. Barbara's ideas have helped us become better practitioners and thinkers and have changed the way we look at the things we do with the students in our care. Dr. Anthony Bashir has had a life-long influence on my work, as evidenced by his words that are woven throughout this text. A magician with both words and recipes, Antonio is my guardian angel and an ongoing inspiration. My radical and forward-thinking partners-in-crime from the "Divas Plus One Players": Dr. Kenn (Brad) Apel, Dr. Bonnie (Michelle) Singer, and Dr. Kathleen (Zelda) Whitmire (along with Dr. Ehren, already mentioned) make the world a more tolerable place for students with language learning disabilities. The "Players" are a joy to work with as we try to find new ways to change the world of schools, or a little piece of it. Dr. Katharine Butler, known to me as the "Goddess of Language" (and many other things), has always been there with steadfast encouragement and wisdom. I would not be writing if it weren't for Kay's encouragement, generosity, and love. She taught me how to put a book together and, more importantly, showed me that it is possible to be a "Supreme Language Diva" and a spectacular human being at the same time. Many mentors taught me everything I know about language learning disabilities and brought me to the point where I was willing to take risks. Along with "Goddess" Kay are Dr. Margaret (Peg) Lahey, Dr. Norma Rees, and Dr. Sylvia Richardson. Dr. Peg Lahey has influenced the way I view language disorders and has shown me time and again what a consummate, class-personified professional should be. She's also a great friend and a wonderful kayaking partner. Dr. Rees was there when I became a true professional during my doctoral studies at the Graduate School & University Center of the City University of New York. I lived (and still live) by her article on auditory processing, "The View from Procrustes' Bed." She continues to have an influence on my thinking, and I use many of her writings in my classes today. Dr. Sylvia Richardson, my soul mate, my "Mama Syl," my Dr. Occhella, enriches my life and always moves my thinking in innovative directions. Dr. "Occh" has also taught me to embrace my Italian heritage and bring passion, art, and humor to the world of language learning disabilities (LLD) and to life in general. And, as mentioned in the dedication of this text, Dr. Joel Stark got me into the "LLD arena." He taught me how to cut through all the noise to hear what's really important about helping kids in trouble. Joel has always been there to calm the rough waters both professionally and personally. They are all here on the pages of this text.

A most incredible friend and colleague, Dr. Carolyn Conway Madding, Chair of the Department of Communicative Disorders at the California State

University at Long Beach in Long Beach, California, makes coming to work each day an absolute joy. She is what leadership is all about. This book would not exist without her help and continued encouragement and the space she gave me to write it. She always understood when I couldn't volunteer for a committee or have a report completed because "the book wasn't ready yet." She is my "myth-busting" partner in language intervention and one of the field's most innovative thinkers in cultural and linguistic diversity. I also owe much to my graduate and undergraduate students in the Department of Communicative Disorders at Long Beach. They teach me so much each time I walk into a classroom or clinic room. I thank them for their patience and understanding and for pushing me to answer the question: "But what do I *do* with these children?" Along with my Long Beach family are the parents of the children and adolescents who attend the Speech-Language-Hearing Clinic on campus. They teach me so much about courage and grace every day.

My cousin Carol, the world's greatest fifth-grade teacher whose classroom is a collage of joy, was always there to provide insights into the curriculum. She shared many textbooks and examples with me from her class and from her own children. And to Carol's children—my little cousins Danielle, Matthew, Michael, and Sydney: each day is brightened by their presence and their accomplishments that help me understand what I need to do for students with LLD.

To a most wonderful editor, Kathy Falk from Elsevier, who has the patience of a saint and who really knew how to keep me on track. She made writing this book less painful than it might have been and encouraged me to take on this project when I wasn't sure I was up to the challenge. I am so glad I took her advice to jump into the pool. And to two other superb professionals from the Elsevier family, Kristin Hebberd, Managing Editor, and Andrea Campbell, Production Editor, I thank them for working so fast and with such enthusiasm to put together a final product that worked for me and for our readers. Their creativity and ongoing support was so needed, especially as the proverbial light at the end of a long tunnel came into view.

And finally, and most importantly, a huge thanks to my husband, Walter, who endured so much during the various phases of giving birth to this text. He has always been there to support the craziest of my schemes and dreams, and this project was no exception. He would stop whatever he was doing, except maybe playing golf, to help me over a barrier I couldn't seem to surmount like facing a blank computer screen and wanting to give up. Life continues to be one fabulous narrative with him at my side.

Contents

Part I **A Conceptual Framework** **1**
  1 Innovative Language Intervention at School-Age Levels: *What It Takes to Get There* 3
  2 Language Learning Disabilities: *Where Are We?* 22

Part II **A Practical Framework** **43**
  3 What Language Intervention "Looks Like" at School-Age Levels 45
  4 Creating "Curriculum-Relevant" Therapy: *Making the Tough Choices* 79

Part III **A Marriage of Conceptual and Practical Frameworks** **103**
  5 Successful Language Literacy Intervention: *A Look Back to Look Ahead* 105
  6 Integrating Spoken and Written Language: *An Eye Toward Becoming Literate* 136
  7 Seeing the World Through Connected Text: *Bringing Structure and Content, Macro and Micro Pieces Together: Part 1* 170
  8 Seeing the World Through Connected Text: *Bringing Structure and Content, Macro and Micro Pieces Together: Part 2* 213

Part IV **Toward a Summary** **267**
  9 Back into the Field: *Starting to Pull the Missing Pieces Together* 269
  10 The End Becomes a New Beginning: *Coming Full Circle* 317

Appendix A **Examples of Scripts at Each Level Using the Book-Sharing Intervention** **337**

Appendix B **Suggested Sequence of Literature-Based Intervention Activities** **339**

Appendix C **Eliciting Conversation, Narrative, and Expository Samples of Connected Speech and Eliciting Story Retelling/Generation** **341**

Appendix D **List of Connecting Words and Their Definitions and Words with Similar Meanings** **347**

Bibliography **349**

Index **367**

Language Intervention *for* School-Age Students

Setting Goals for Academic Success

Part I

A Conceptual Framework

PART OUTLINE

1   Innovative Language Intervention at School-Age Levels
    What It Takes to Get There

2   Language Learning Disabilities
    Where Are We?

Those who choose to use a new intervention tool because it is easier, faster, or more glamorous are in danger of losing their clinical creativity and scientific mind . . . . It puts them at risk of becoming a technician, not a scientist.

(Apel, 1999; quoting Aram, 1991)

1 Innovative Language Intervention at School-Age Levels

What It Takes to Get There

SUMMARY STATEMENT

Chapter 1 asks readers to reflect on a number of concepts that relate to creating more effective language intervention programs for school-age students with language learning disabilities (LLD). The introductory information presented sets a tone for the remainder of the text. Readers are encouraged to take a ride on the wave of change by asking themselves to engage in self-reflection about many long-held philosophies and practices. Among the chapter's suggestions to speech-language pathologists (SLPs) and their colleagues are the following:

1. Be willing to question the conventional wisdom of traditional language intervention practices.
2. Think of the metaphors and visual images used as scaffolds for comprehension and retention, and ask if their use is facilitative to learning—a question we should be asking about the techniques used to help students with academic difficulties.
3. Consider alternatives to some of the popular practices that are alive and well in language intervention circles such as focusing on small pieces of language behavior (e.g., the ever-persistent "is...verbing"), teaching the meanings of vocabulary words out of context, and working on various aspects of central auditory processing using nonlinguistic content, among others.

The format and content of this chapter draw their inspiration from information processing theory and constructive comprehension research, topics we will return to time and again in this text. Metaphors such as "focus on the forest, not the trees" and the "tip-of-the-iceberg" phenomenon serve as visual and verbal images to highlight past and future directions in both assessment and intervention.

KEY QUESTIONS ■■■■■

1. How does one's definition of language drive one's intervention practices?
2. Are we prepared to ask "where" language intervention ideas "come from"?
3. What concepts in language and literacy intervention require closer scrutiny as a result of our answer to question 2?
4. What are some of the principles that underlie the creation of more innovative language intervention approaches at school-age levels?

INTRODUCTORY THOUGHTS

What do I do with the students with language learning disabilities (LLD) in my classroom or clinic room on Monday morning?

There will never be a shortage of educational and clinical materials. Conferences at national, state, and local levels in the fields of speech and language pathology, education, psychology, reading, and related areas all include exhibit halls larger than most football fields. The halls are always packed with the newest and most alluring-looking tests and intervention tools. To most professionals, these are welcome additions to their therapy rooms and classrooms. Many of us leave conferences with bags of brochures, samples, and Web site numbers (if not the actual book, kit, or test) offering any number of ideas for reaching the children and adolescents with language and academic problems in our care. We often feel better knowing that we have made some progress in answering the following question: What do I do with the students with language learning disabilities (LLD) on my caseload or in my classroom on Monday morning?

But a more interesting question that needs to be asked and answered remains: What creates this mismatch between what one sees in the exhibit hall and what one hears in lectures and workshops? A similar mismatch is reflected in the apparent gap that also exists between classrooms and clinic rooms in graduate programs across the country. Indeed, the gap between what one hears in an innovative workshop or lecture about curriculum-based assessment, integrating spoken and written language intervention, and connected discourse sampling and what one actually does with a student can be a relatively large one. In some cases, students' individualized education plans (IEPs) or their language therapy plans have little relevance to classroom and curricular demands. For example, it might be reasonable to teach an older student with LLD to comprehend figurative language forms; however, if the forms chosen have little or nothing to do with his or her comprehension of social studies or science, intervention loses its relevance. It might also be useful to have more precise (or grammatically perfect) syntactic forms when speaking, but if those structures practiced in an intervention session are too disconnected from classroom discourses and textbook language, they, too, become isolated paint chips on a complex canvas of language needs. To understate the obvious might be to say that while both frustrating and fascinating, the theory-to-practice gap has led us to a place where we, as practitioners, must recognize its causes, as well as discover some much-needed solutions.

Kamhi (1999) is one of the research-based clinicians who has discussed the theory-to-practice gap in some detail. He has asked practitioners to ask themselves a number of questions about their clinical practices with children and adolescents, including the following:

■ Is the intervention method you used based on a theoretical principle?

■ Is it evidence based? Can you site studies that provide evidence?

■ What made you choose the approach you used?

Ehren (2006a) asked additional questions of clinicians who are working specifically with school-age students with LLD. She encouraged self-refection in this way:

■ Are your language intervention choices curriculum relevant?

■ Is your intervention strategically focused?

■ Do your activities integrate oral and written language systems?

And, reiterating Kamhi's (1999) points, she continues:

■ Is your language intervention based on current research? Are there data to support your approaches?

Practitioners who are in the business of helping children and adolescents with language, learning, and literacy problems talk to themselves quite often. Self-talk can be an excellent form of problem solving. It is a technique that clinicians use frequently with students who are receiving language intervention services. Asking two basic questions—"Why am I doing this?" and "Where does this technique or approach 'come from'"?—is a recommended strategy. Indeed, obtaining the answers to the "whys" and "wheres" of language intervention is a critical piece of the clinical and educational decision-making process. Self-questioning, along with an evaluation of the theoretical foundations that influence our intervention choices, helps us to put the "what to do now?" and "what to do next?" into a broader context.

> Self-talk can be an excellent way to help practitioners problem-solve difficulties in working with children and adolescents with language, learning, and literacy problems.

> **Forming a Framework for Language Intervention: Some Beginnings**

What Is Your Definition of Language? Of Literacy?

On Language. Where do professionals start? How do they begin to answer the questions asked in the previous section? They begin by asking themselves how they define language. Apel (1999) points out that one's definition of language should have a connection to what one "does" clinically and educationally. Not meant to be taken literally, the point Apel and others make is that practitioners should reflect on their philosophical views about language and language learning when creating and delivering language intervention programs for their students. If one views language from Bloom and Lahey's (1978) classic framework or Owens' (2004) updated version that describes the systemic and interactive nature of content-form-use, one would hope that intervention is driven in that direction—a direction that tries to integrate rather than separate semantic, syntactic (plus other form aspects), and pragmatic pieces. If one views language primarily as the production of grammatically correct sentences, one's intervention might be driven in that direction.

In her now-classic chapter, Friel-Patti (1994), like her colleagues Kamhi (1999) and Ehren (2006a), also encouraged her readers to answer a number of self-revealing questions. She focused on professionals' views of language learning theories, including nativist, environmentalist, and behaviorist theories, among others. She asked the following questions:

■ Are you a proponent of behaviorism as a theory of language learning?
■ Are you a Vygotskian theorist?
■ Do you believe language is innate or preprogrammed?

Taking a similar perspective as her colleagues, Friel-Patti (1994) reminded us that intervention approaches often evolve from the philosophical beliefs of clinicians. She wrote:

> Even the words used to describe the intervention process often disclose a theoretical bias: clinicians who portray their role as *language facilitator* are fundamentally different from those who are concerned with *teaching children to talk*. Whether or not they are acknowledged, such differences in theoretical underpinnings alter treatment options. (p. 374)

The answers to Friel-Patti's (1994) questions and others raised, in addition to one's definition of language, provide clinicians with a clearer understanding about "where" they are "coming from" as they sit down to work with students with LLD. Indeed, clinicians should continue to engage in self-reflection and bring their core beliefs and their clinical practices together. For example, is there a match or mismatch between core beliefs and what clinicians actually "do" with the children and adolescents in their clinics and classrooms? Do clinicians recognize that behaviorism falls very short as a theory of language learning even though its principles, including establishing all kinds of elaborate reward systems for "good talking," are quite prevalent in language intervention circles? As suggested earlier, we do many things that require a closer look. Is "good talking" defined by longer sentences and more grammatically precise syntax? Is the "is . . . verbing" goal alive and well? Are the "listening" drills we choose facilitating functional and constructive language comprehension? Are criterion-referenced statements such as "Billy will achieve a score of eight out of ten correct responses in the clinical setting" relevant measures of language growth (Wallach & Madding, 2006)?

> There is no agreed-on definition of *language* in the profession of speech and language pathology.

Apel (1999) points out that understanding language learning and language intervention choices is complicated even further because there is no agreed-on definition of language in the profession of speech and language pathology. The American Speech-Language-Hearing Association (ASHA) talks about language in the following way and provides us with some direction (italics added):

> Language is a *dynamic* system embedded in and influenced by a number of factors (e.g., social, cultural, cognitive). It is a rule-governed system involving the *integrated* use of its components, phonology, morphology, syntax, semantics, and pragmatics. *Proficient use* of language involves knowledge of human interaction and understanding the demands of the environment. Language is expressed in a number of modes including oral, written, and signed modes. (ASHA Committee on Language, 1983)

Using the ASHA definition as a starting point, one could ask whether intervention measures up. For example, do clinicians approach language intervention by setting goals that are truly integrated? Are oral and written modes seen as systemic and interactive?

On Literacy. Similar challenges face professionals and their definitions (or perceptions) about what it means to be "literate" or how one defines literacy. More narrow definitions propose that literacy is the acquisition of reading and writing (sometimes known as print literacy). Acquiring reading and writing is certainly a major piece of becoming literate. But current thinking broadens our views of literacy to include *spoken* as well as written language in definitions of literacy (Dickinson & Tabors, 2001; Silliman & Wilkinson, 1994; Tabors, 2001; Westby, 2005). From this broader perspective, preschool language learning experiences set the pace for the acquisition of print literacy. In addition, preliteracy and emergent literacy experiences that begin in the prechool period are better understood in terms of their influence on reading and writing in the early grades (Gillam & Ukrainetz, 2006; Roth & Troia, 2006). Expanded views of literacy also include consideration of the acquisitions and advancements in spoken language that reflect a move from informal to formal styles of language use. Informal language includes casual conversations; formal language includes giving presentations at conventions (Westby, 1994). When children use more formal styles of spoken language, their language includes "literate" or booklike structures such as embedded/relative clause sentences, and other complex structures. Within current contexts, these advances in spoken language are also considered advances in literacy. (See the discussion of the oral-to-literate continuum in Chapter 2, pp. 29–32.)

Westby (2005) takes the concept of expanded definitions of literacy even further. She talks about how our changing world has created the demand for several types of literacy. For example, critical literacy requires that people read between the lines (includes interpreting, analyzing, synthesizing, and explaining, among other abilities). Dynamic literacy involves mastering multiple texts, comparing and contrasting content, integrating ideas, and so on. Thus the reality of what it means to be literate in the twenty-first century goes well beyond what was defined as literacy even twenty years ago. Indeed, becoming computer literate is yet another example of this ever-changing concept.

> Our changing world has created the demand for several types of literacy, including critical, dynamic, and computer literacy.

Taking a look once again at ways in which one's definition influences practice, we might consider several examples to highlight this notion of expanded definitions of literacy, including ways we view reading and writing. For example, a special education teacher who views learning to read primarily as a visual process may create instructional activities that move in that direction (e.g., strengthening visual memory, visual sequencing, and similar skills). By contrast, a teacher who views reading as a linguistic process might move in another direction (e.g., learning the meanings of words before reading a story). The learning disabilities specialist who views children as "auditory" or "visual" learners may suggest remedial reading techniques that reflect these categorizations (e.g., the visual learners get a "whole word approach" to reading and the auditory learners get a "phonics approach"). The SLP who views literacy acquisition and its problems as areas that are separate from spoken language learning and disorders may see written language intervention as being outside of her scope of practice. Thus philosophy, training, and experience influence the choices clinicians and teachers make for their students. Awareness of "where we're coming from" is a step toward looking at alternatives if and when they are needed.

The Crux of the Matter: Can We Let Go of the Past?

In essence, although we have come a long way in our appreciation of language-literacy relations and preschool–school age intervention connections and disconnections, we are left with some interesting challenges. How do we begin to bridge some of these gaps between theory and practice, definitions and goals, philosophical and perceptual differences? And we must ask again: Where do some of the things we do with children "come from"? This is the core question we will be asking throughout this text.

The answer is complex. Some of the things we do are steeped in long-standing traditions. These traditions may be based on faulty or outdated models of language and language learning. We may not know the source of other traditions. For example, discrete skills approaches such as those that encourage working on "prerequisite" skills (e.g., auditory memory and auditory sequencing or categorizing children as "auditory or visual learners") appear to have grown out of practices based on the Illinois Test of Psycholinguistic Abilities (ITPA) models that were popular in the 1960s (Kirk et al., 1968). The "is… verbing" goals for syntactic proficiency may have morphed from Chomsky's transformational grammar models that had a tremendous influence on language learning theories (e.g., Chomsky, 1965). Likewise, the "pull out" model of service that takes students out of their classrooms into "speech" rooms for intervention sessions grew out of medical model and clinical orientations in "treatment" that left the unexplored opportunities within curricula and classrooms behind. (As noted in quotation marks, the terms "speech" room and "treatment" also require modification for educational settings.) Clearly, looking at the way we always did things has value. Traditions of the past provide us with frameworks that have many useful components. But, again, we must also look at what current research and practice says about modifications that are necessary to move forward. Further, in some cases, we may have to recognize that some of the procedures and approaches of the past are best left there.

Principles of Intervention to Consider: Visual Images and Metaphors to Set the Stage

This section uses visual imagery and metaphors as a way to introduce some principles that may provide a framework for critically evaluating a number of key concepts in language intervention. Readers should ask themselves if and when the visual images and metaphors are effective for their own comprehension and retention of information. This self-reflection may help us evaluate the choices made for children and adolescents with LLD.

Another Look at Language: The Definitional Issue Resurfaces

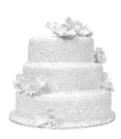

The definition of language presented earlier reminds professionals who are in the business of facilitating (and/or teaching) language to consider a number of its critical elements: language is dynamic, influenced by several variables, and embedded in context; language functions with a systemic connection among its components and presents itself across different modes, spoken, written, and signed. What might be added to this definition is the concept that language has the following two major *layers:*

1. The first layer is the "basic linguistic" layer.
2. The second layer is the "metalinguistic" layer.

This distinction between the two layers of language is probably among the most widely misunderstood ideas in clinical and educational practice.

Put simply, "metalinguistic abilities are evident when our awareness shifts from the meanings of our utterances to the utterances themselves" (McLaughlin, 2006, p. 366). The prefix "meta" means going beyond, or rising above (McLaughlin, 2006). Thus, when we talk about metalinguistic abilities in children and adolescents, we are talking about those advancing language skills that "go beyond" the ones learned for communication. When speakers and listeners are engaged in conversation, talking quickly and seemingly effortlessly, they are involved in the *spontaneous* use of language. They generally do not stop to think unless there is a problem or some distraction (e.g., a very thick accent). Speakers and listeners exchange messages in a back-and-forth partnership without analyzing what they are saying consciously or stopping to think about every sound, word, or sentence used. This spontaneous, message-driven type of communication involves the first layer of language.

As McLaughlin's (2006) quote suggests, when we communicate with one another, the focus is on the meaning. By contrast, when we stop to think about language, to reflect on language, to analyze language, and to make judgments about language, we have moved to the second layer of language, the *metalinguistic* layer (van Kleeck, 1994). Conscious awareness and analyses of language, that is, talking about language, are aspects of metalinguistic ability. (See van Kleeck [1994] for a classic and thorough discussion.) Examples in this chapter and future chapters cover this area in greater detail.

Indeed, the linguistic-metalinguistic distinction weaves its way through clinical and educational practice. Clinicians and teachers can disambiguate some of the confusion that exists in this arena of language study by considering the following clarifications. First, clinicians and teachers should evaluate their language learning goals and techniques by asking themselves the following three questions:

1. Is my focus to improve a child's performance on the first or second layer of language? Am I using second-layer/metalinguistic approaches to "get to" first-layer abilities?
2. Are the techniques and materials being used in my language intervention sessions appropriate or are they "too metalinguistically advanced" for the student?
3. Do standardized tests of language target the first or second layer of language?

Van Kleeck (1994) reminds practitioners to recognize that the road to metalinguistic awareness is a long and gradual one, starting with "glimmers" (early awareness) in the preschool period and advancing well into the later elementary and high school years. And while the distinctions between layers are not meant to be rigid and disconnected, some cautions underlie the questions raised in the previous paragraph. When we take language out of context and ask children to "do" something with it, to analyze it on a conscious level, or to pull it apart and put it back together again, we have stepped into metalinguistic territory. Thus asking Billy to "use his words," a basic reminder expressed by clinicians everywhere, encourages him to be a bit more "meta" about language. When we ask Tiffany to decide whether two words sound the same or different,

Stopping to think about, reflect on, analyze, or make judgments about language all involve the metalinguistic layer of language.

we have asked her to make a metalinguistic judgment about phonemic differences. When Sarah has to write a complete sentence for a list of words for homework, she is engaged in a metalinguistic activity. The sentence-writing activity calls on her ability to bring her syntactic knowledge "to the surface," and it assumes that Sarah can make a judgment about what "complete sentence" means.

Many tasks involve metalinguistic awareness with different degrees of difficulty. Pointing to a picture from a choice of four to demonstrate "receptive vocabulary" ability, identifying the first and last sounds of a word, deciding whether a sentence is grammatical, and correcting one's morphological omissions consciously, among other tasks, all reflect metalinguistic—or second language layer—activities. Much of classroom learning also falls within the metalinguistic domain. Thinking of another meaning for a word, finding an opposite meaning, and presenting a report to the class all involve metalinguistic ability. All standardized tests of language are, to a greater or lesser extent, metalinguistic in nature. Clearly, understanding the meta-link to language learning and learning in general, a theme we will return to many times in this text, is an important addition to our definition of language and to our assessment and intervention practices.

Metaphors and More: Toward an Exploration of Language Intervention Practices and Principles

We began the work of creating a framework for assessment and intervention by starting with the most basic of explorations: one's definition of language. We added a critical layer to our definition, the metalinguistic layer. "Meta" aspects of language learning and disorders are important to study and to understand because metalinguistic abilities influence and interact with the acquisition of literacy learning and school success. While other skills and abilities are also required for these acquisitions, developing a conscious awareness of language, including the ability to manipulate language on many levels (pragmatic, semantic, syntactic, etc.), is a necessity for advancing basic language learning, as well as academic learning.

As indicated previously, students with LLD are faced with activities that require making many different judgments about language in their classrooms every day. When they are tested by SLPs who use standardized instruments, they are being asked to engage in a metalinguistic activity, as noted earlier. In addition to recognizing all the meta tasks that students face daily, van Kleeck (1994) makes another point about the importance of advancing metalinguistic knowledge. She reminds us that metalinguistic abilities should not be thought of as "frosting on the cake" (continuing our cake image). Rather, says van Kleeck (1994), metalinguistic abilities should be recognized as part of children's expanding higher-order thinking and reasoning abilities.

Leaving our definitional issue behind for the moment, we now move to the question of how practitioners operationalize their views of language clinically and educationally. When things "go wrong" with language, then what? The next section uses three metaphors to demonstrate a number of widely held views about what symptoms of language disorders suggest about the children and adolescents who demonstrate these symptoms in their language processing and production. The three metaphors—(1) the forest-versus-tree metaphor, (2) the tip-of-the-iceberg phenomenon, and (3) the one-way mapping approach—start the discussion. A final section that covers a discussion of language disorders as being both "inside" and "outside" of children's heads leads us to a number of alternative interpretations that have the potential to take language intervention in a different, more innovative direction.

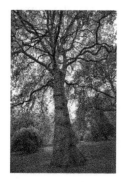

This visual image starts with a raging fire in the hills of California. How does one get control of hundreds of acres in trouble? Would one focus on an isolated tree in the forest, or one branch from that tree, to put out the fire? It would seem obvious that the narrow focus (on one tree or one branch) would be a less effective way to deal with this significant, more encompassing problem. Even if one could proceed from tree to tree and make some progress putting out the fire, one would have to ask about the overall success for the forest and the forest's future. Clearly, a broader approach is required to save the forest from total destruction.

The forest fire metaphor leads us to ask additional questions about language intervention choices. For example, is the choice to work on "is... verbing" and other specific syntactic or morphological forms similar to trying to put out the forest fire by starting with an individual tree? Do various "sequence" activities (defined differently by different people) and central auditory processing drills represent isolated branches? Can intervention that focuses on smaller pieces of language, sometimes known as discrete skills approaches to language intervention (mentioned earlier), have a positive impact on a child's/student's communication and academic performance? While it may be appropriate to focus on one component or one aspect of language at certain points in time, it helps to keep our eyes focused on the forest—stepping back to assess the way our day-to-day clinical and educational choices relate to where we really want to "go" with the children and adolescents in our care.

Are we sometimes too focused on the trees when we should be focused on the forest? If Billy is lost in his Grade 3 forest, we need to think about what language intervention should "look like" (see Chapter 3) to help him find his way out. If Kenn is lost in Yosemite (the curriculum-rich forest), it won't help if we look for him in Sequoia (the teach-to-language test results' forest). In brief: This forest/tree metaphor reminds practitioners to keep their eyes focused on the "bigger picture" and to keep asking themselves the following question: What are the significant language learning changes I hope to make for Billy, Kenn, and students like them (Wallach & Miller, 1988)? To be effective language facilitators and teachers, think about language intervention as being *direct, authentic,* and *real-world relevant* for our students. The metaphors that follow reiterate and complement this theme.

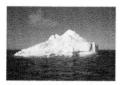

We all remember the story of the *Titanic*. Its tragedy made icebergs famous. The idea that only a small portion of an iceberg is visible because the bulk of its mass is underwater provokes some interesting questions about cause-and-effect factors and language intervention decisions. When we speak of "tip-of-the-iceberg" phenomena, we usually mean that there's more to the issue (or situation) than meets the eye (or ear). One has to delve deeper to get to the truth or to a complete understanding of something.

Symptoms of LLD often reveal only the tip of the iceberg.

This metaphor relates to language intervention because it asks clinicians to think about some of the symptoms of LLD as "tip-of-the-iceberg" phenomena. Consider the following cases:

■ Student no. 1 with perfect articulation fails an auditory discrimination test. He has trouble judging whether two words, such as *king-ring, leaf-thief,* and so on, are the same or different.

■ Student no. 2 performs poorly on a battery of central auditory processing tests demonstrating problem-sequencing phonemes, among other difficulties relating to sounds and their sequences.

■ Student no. 3 cannot follow a series of spoken instructions sometimes described as "having difficulty following two- and three-level commands."

■ Student no. 4 cannot sequence a series of pictures that represent a story.

Do these abbreviated examples suggest, for example, that we create auditory discrimination activities for student no. 1? Should we recommend a central auditory processing program for student no. 2? Does student no. 3 need to work on listening activities that become progressively more difficult—following "two-level" and then "three-level" commands (although it is unclear what is being counted for the two and three)? Should student no. 4 work on a variety of sequencing activities?

The metaphor suggests that there may be another way to consider these findings and, ultimately, the intervention programs that follow to help these students improve linguistically and academically. The metaphor suggests getting to a deeper understanding of these students' problems. For example, student no. 1's "failure" on the auditory discrimination tasks may be related to the metalinguistic nature of the task and the lexical knowledge the student brings to the task (see Chapter 9, page 279). Similarly, student no. 2's difficulty on central auditory processing (CAP) batteries maybe the *result of*, not the cause of, a broader, more overriding language problem (i.e., it is the forest, not the tree; see Chapter 5). Likewise, the difficulties reflected in the performances of student no. 3 and student no. 4 may need to be considered from a less narrow, symptom-specific perspective. Is there more to all these stories than the performances suggest? Should language intervention go in different directions, beyond the "tip-of-the-iceberg" phenomena, as the next metaphor also suggests?

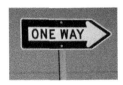

A "one-way only" traffic sign means that the driver must proceed in a specific direction. There are usually consequences to violating the agreed-on direction for a particular route. Unlike the one-way road map, the relations between and among language components and systems are more dynamic and reciprocal. Nonetheless, sometimes clinicians and teachers function in a "one-way only" approach to intervention. This notion can be broad, that is, there is only one way to do something, or it can be more specific. The more specific aspect of this topic is the focus of our discussion.

As noted earlier in this chapter, a clinician's theoretical and practical bent about cause-and-effect relations may set the stage for the intervention "steps" the clinician devises for his or her students. For example, if one believes that auditory processing is the *cause* of a language problem, intervention may proceed in that direction—that is, auditory processing training is the *foundation* for higher levels of language processing. The direction one follows on this one-way street is reflected in the notion that auditory processing work will "lead to" better language processing and comprehension. If one believes that spoken language *comes before* written language, intervention might proceed in that direction.

Likewise, relations such as receptive and expressive language, cognition and language, sequencing and narrative ability, and visual memory and reading may be viewed as a progression or a one-way mapping from one direction to another. By contrast, however, a number of these relations are closer to two-way streets than a first look might suggest. We are reminded of the complexity—the reciprocity—of these relations by many researchers and clinicians (e.g., Gillam et al., 2002). For example, Nittrouer (2002) talks about ways in which language knowledge "leads the way" to more efficient and accurate speech perception and auditory processing. She asks her readers to think about "how strongly language underlies other communicative and perceptual processes, affecting even the very reception of the acoustic speech signal" (p. 237). She goes on to suggest that various auditory processing difficulties may not be the cause but a result of language difficulties. Similarly, Catts and Kamhi (2005a) stress the reciprocity (or the two-way street dynamic) between spoken and written language and their disorders. They point out that language disorders are both the *cause* and the *result* of reading disabilities. Indeed, while spoken language leads the way to written language development at certain points in time, written language also influences spoken language development (Bashir et al., 1998; Wallach, 2004).

Catts and Kamhi (2005a) make another interesting point about the complex relations between the written and spoken word. Reiterating points made about expanded definitions of literacy, they note that many items on standardized language tests are closer to print than they are to speech. Hence, readers of a language tend to perform better on formal tests of spoken language than non-readers. Here again is another example of the intertwined, back-and-forth relationship between spoken and written language. It helps us realize that looking in only one direction limits the clinician's vision.

A Mini Summary. The three metaphors presented represent ways of looking at the symptoms of language disorders from a different perspective. They point out that some of the more traditional interpretations of language disorders failed to capture the dynamic and systemic nature of language (Box 1-1). In addition, the translation of theoretical information to clinical practice missed the mark in terms of accounting for how speakers and listeners (and readers and writers) function in the real world. For example, when studying models of processing that proposed a step-by-step progression from the ear to the brain, the notion that "levels" of processing (sound, syllable, word, sentence) occur simultaneously was often obscured. Nonetheless, the temptation clinically was to follow the step-by-step hierarchies from models even though the models are idealized and abstract views of complex behaviors, not replications of actual language performance. (Remember articulation therapy, which started with the phoneme and worked its way up to the sentence and text level?) Similarly, the idea that higher levels of processing (e.g., sentence and text levels) influence lower levels (e.g., phonemic levels) also got lost in translation (Gillam et al., 2002). And beyond looking at spoken and written

Language disorders can be both the cause and the result of reading disabilities.

language systems in a static way, intervention models of the past, especially for school-age students, remained somewhat isolated from the context and content of students' problems, the classroom, and the curriculum. The next visual image relates to this last point and highlights an idea that language disorders reside both within and outside of children's heads (Nelson, 2005; Wallach & Madding, 2006).

BOX 1-1   *Metaphors in Language Learning Disabilities*

1. *A tree with many branches:* Concentrating on one component or aspect of language can cause the clinician to miss the bigger picture. Keeping the forest in focus provides an overarching image that brings discrete skills into a broader perspective.
2. *An iceberg:* Clinicians might consider the possibility that many symptoms of LLD are like the proverbial tip of the iceberg, acknowledging that there may be more complex issues underneath the surface.
3. *A one-way street sign:* Assuming a direct, cause-and-effect relationship in intervention—for example, that intervention focused on central auditory processing will lead to better language comprehension and academic success—may cause a clinician to miss the two-way, reciprocal relationship among the different facets of language.

"It's in the Kid's Head" Phenomenon

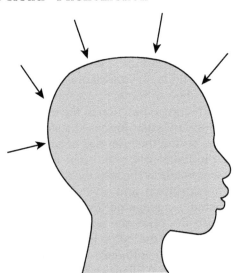

The chronic and pervasive nature of language disorders certainly suggests that a neurological base underlies LLD (or specific language impairment [SLI], as it is sometimes called) and its evolution across time (see Chapter 2). As a consequence of neurologically based models of LLD, logic indicates that we look *within* the child for answers about the type and severity of his or her LLD. Language assessments of past and current times typically include descriptions and/or quantitative profiles of the "gaps" that children demonstrate in various components and processing modalities. So far so good, but this piece of the assessment process, when it is focused on creating and delivering language intervention services, is only halfway there.

When the results of tests and language samples remain isolated from the classroom and the curriculum, the insights they can provide, which may offer some clues to the direction intervention might take, are limited in their scope. For example, when a student performs well (or not) on a subtest that involves processing complex syntactic forms, it is not only important to look at the pattern of correct responses and errors (as we will see in our "alternatives" section that follows), but it is also critical to connect these findings to processing classroom instructions and curricular materials. Moreover, the best one-on-one testing situation will always fail to replicate the instructional challenges that take place in a classroom of 30-plus students. Likewise, if a student performs poorly on test items that suggest difficulty with figurative language, developing intervention recommendations that "teach to the test" have little relevance, especially if the student never encounters the specific test stimuli in his or her books or classroom assignments. Thus one aspect of the "it's in the kid's head" phenomenon that improves significantly occurs when diagnosticians connect their test findings to the classroom and curricula demands.

Connecting test and assessment findings to school performance speaks to an understanding of external factors that may exacerbate LLD. Lahey and Bloom (1994) talk eloquently about the concept of competing resources; this concept relates to "what's going on" *outside* of a child's head that contributes to his or her *inside* struggle with language. In other words, children come to tasks with certain inherent abilities that include having (or not having) background knowledge and experience, as well as cognitive, linguistic, and metalinguistic abilities. These are "in the head" abilities.

> When inherent abilities are unstable or evolving or when tasks are difficult, resources compete for attention; and when contextual support is limited, resources can be stretched to the limit.

Lahey and Bloom (1994) talk about representations of people's inherent abilities as mental models. (See Chapters 3 and 5 for an in-depth discussion.) These inherent abilities (or what's in an individual's mental model) interface with task demands and the contextual supports available. When inherent abilities are less stable or evolving (like the language systems of students with LLD) and when tasks are difficult, resources compete for attention. In addition, when contextual support is limited (e.g., when one has to read a dense textbook without many pictures or other supports), resources may become stretched to the limit. For example, a competing resource scenario occurs when students are faced with new and unfamiliar content (e.g., the American Revolution) that is embedded in complex language (e.g., expository text) in a low-context or decontextualized situation (e.g., a language-heavy textbook). This triad of difficulties is faced by students with LLD every day. According to Lahey and Bloom (1994), the three aspects of the scenario (content-language-context) are competing for attention and, as a result, are putting students with LLD in an impossible situation.

Lahey and Bloom's (1994) work, among others' writings, suggests that clinicians should be sensitive to the external as well as internal factors in language disorders and apply this knowledge to their intervention decisions. They must understand, for example, that students with LLD have difficulty learning and using complex language when that language occurs within a complex task, involves unfamiliar information, and is surrounded by little or no contextual support. Thus speech-language clinicians must think about "freeing up" resources so that their students can focus on language learning. For example, providing more contextual support and using more familiar content "frees up" resources so that the student can focus on "the language." Higher context (e.g., using pictures and other supports), familiar content (e.g., discussing a topic the students knows), and a known routine (e.g., a particular game's rules) "frees up" resources because attention can go elsewhere, that is, to the hard piece, to the language (Lahey & Bloom, 1994). Clearly, school-age students with LLD have to learn to manage many things at the same time, and our role is to help them get there. And the "getting there" means looking for answers within and outside of students. This is a major theme of this text.

Where Do the Images and Metaphors Leave Us? The "So What?" Phenomenon

The major point being made that overrides the principles that follow is simple:

Paint your language intervention canvas with broad brush strokes.

Let's step back and keep the forest in focus. Let's keep the significant language learning and literacy-oriented behaviors in the forefront of our intervention planning endeavors. Let's learn from the past but look toward the future as we explore three overlapping principles. These principles highlight a number of ideas that are weaved together throughout this text, as follows:

■ Connect language intervention to the real world.
■ Recognize that things are not always what they seem.
■ Keep your eyes on the horizon.

Connecting Language Intervention to the Real World

SLPs must question not only the theoretical principles on which they operate but also whether those principles connect to the real world in which their students must learn.

As our self-reflection continues, we ask again: What do I really want to do to help children and adolescents "in trouble"? How can I help them succeed communicatively and academically? The quest to create and deliver effective language intervention programs begins and ends by testing one's own beliefs. As noted at the beginning of this chapter, practitioners must evaluate the theoretical principles that underlie their language intervention choices. Moreover, they must question whether those theoretical principles connect to the real world of their students. This text is focused on the real world of schools, the world of "Monday mornings in the classroom." It is also focused on helping students "take ownership" of the language and organization strategies that we introduce to them (Ehren, 2005b, 2006a). Clinicians should take a hard look at some of the tests and intervention activities that are popular and ask if they are too far removed from the contexts (e.g., the classroom) and the content (e.g., the curriculum) that their students must return to (from an isolated "speech" room?) each day.

In addition, when tests and intervention techniques are focused on "abstractions" of complex behaviors, they may have little impact on both social and academic language learning. For example, how do dichotic listening tasks relate to students' comprehension of Grade 4 science and social studies text? How does following commands, such as "Stand up, clap your hands three times, and then pick up the third picture on the desk," connect to classroom instructions? What does tracing letters in a sandbox have to do with learning to read? Is working on morphological endings in spoken language a broad enough goal for a fifth grader with LLD?

In her classic yet still current article, Lahey (1990) discussed the challenges involved in identifying children with language disorders. She made a number of important points about the goals of assessment. She also addressed the ways clinicians define language. One point that relates to the issue of the real world of children and their performances on tests (and in therapy situations) is expressed this way:

> The perspective taken here is that...identification of a language disorder should be based on differences in language behaviors (e.g., the production and comprehension of units of connected language) and not on inferences about the nature of the underlying system based on these performance variables. One reason to focus on performance is the practical consideration that there is no agreed-upon way to describe the underlying system and, thus, no way a description of the expected system could be used as a comparison. (Lahey, 1990, p. 613)

Norris (1997) moves us from the question of testing and teaching abstract behaviors (such as some of those behaviors in the auditory and visual areas) to the reality of school activities. She was forward-thinking a decade ago when she reminded clinicians about the linguistic demands that challenge our students on a daily basis. As Norris (1997) put it:

> Most school activities require the application of multiple types of language uses simultaneously. For example, taking notes in response to a lecture requires processing complex sentences to derive the meaning of new vocabulary or new concepts; translating this into written language during notetaking; imposing order and organization on the information in the form of topics, subtopics, and supporting ideas; following expected classroom rules for asking questions or contributing to the discussion; and associating new information with prior knowledge both in comprehending the lecture and taking the notes. (p. 50)

Norris (1997) took a strong language-based perspective to academic learning and pushed for the involvement of SLPs in curriculum-based assessment and intervention approaches. Ten years later, we can say with some confidence that progress has been made. Indeed, we know more about ways to create and implement language intervention programs for school-age students that are real-world focused, that is, that are connected to content area learning and classroom communication (e.g., DeKemel, 2003a; Ehren, 2000, 2005b; Nelson, 2005; Ukrainetz & Ross, 2006; Wallach, 2005a; Wallach & Ehren, 2004; Westby & Torres-Velasquez, 2000). Nonetheless, with all the progress that has been made, the resurgence in popularity of CAP programs and oral-motor training, as examples, remind us that there is still much work to be done. (See Chapters 2 and 5 for further discussion on this topic.)

Recognizing That Things Aren't Always What They Seem

A visual image one could use in this section would be the famous picture of President-elect Harry Truman holding up a newspaper (in the days well before computerized returns) with a headline that reads: DEWEY DEFEATS TRUMAN. This image reminds us that there is more to the story. What appears to be true may require further scrutiny. A number of points made at the beginning of this chapter can be reiterated here because these concepts set the tone for the chapters that follow (Box 1-2).

Recognizing the Metalinguistic Nature of Some Everyday Tasks. Asking children to make a judgment about whether a pair of rhyming words is the same or different is a metalinguistic task; it is not a simple task of auditory discrimination. Asking a student to move blocks around to demonstrate he has "heard" and "sequenced" a series of sounds, tasks that one might see on the Lindamood-like tests and programs (e.g., Lindamood & Lindamood, 1979; Lindamood Phoneme Sequencing Program [LiPS]) relate to phonemic awareness and word segmentation tasks. Many of these meta-tasks are closer to understanding writing conventions than they are to "auditory" processing abilities.

Reevaluating Concepts about the Nature of Tasks that Reflect Student Strengths and Weaknesses. The notion that children can be categorized as "auditory" or "visual" learners, a concept that is popular in general and special education settings, requires a closer look. There is little research to suggest that this notion is a viable one for educational programming and language intervention, especially when one looks at the knowledge and skills that are required for reading and spelling and other academic endeavors (Apel et al., 2004; Ehren, 2005b; Wallach, 2004). While people might have preferences, proficient learners tend to shift and modify the strategies they use to meet the needs of the situation (Ehren, 2006a; see Chapter 8). Moreover, many tasks have been mislabeled as "auditory" or "visual" when completion of the tasks requires a combination

---

BOX 1-2   *A Broader View of Language Intervention*

- Recognize the metalinguistic nature of some of the tasks used in daily practice and rethink conclusions reached about what children "can" and "cannot" do.
- Reevaluate some traditionally held concepts about the nature of tasks and go beyond popular labels used to categorize children, tests, and programs.
- Think of context, linguistic structure, and strategies available as intersecting variables and assess the possible factors that may influence a student's performance.

of processing efforts and background knowledge (Gillam et al., 2002; Lahey & Bloom, 1994). For example, adults tend to label items, using naming strategies, when asked to recall a series of visually presented stimuli. Many tests and programs (including those that require students to sequence blocks in a left-to-right arrangement or produce a spoken sentence for a given word) say less about auditory proficiency and more about an individual's reading and spelling ability, a point alluded to in the previous section and one that was also made by Catts and Kamhi (2005a). The progression across the oral-to-literate continuum of language learning from informal to formal aspects of language and from spoken to written language and back again reflects both stylistic and metalinguistic changes in ability that go far beyond moving from one modality (auditory) to another (visual) (Scott, 1994; Wallach, 2004; Westby, 1994, 2005; see Chapter 2).

Thinking of Context, Linguistic Structure, and Strategies as Intersecting Variables. Consider the following three sentences to begin the discussion:

1. Before picking up the red circle, touch the white square.
2. After picking up the green circle, touch the red square.
3. Feed the baby before putting her to bed.

The first two may look familiar since they are similar to stimuli that might appear on several standardized language tests that tap processing and comprehension. The first two sentences are somewhat different from the last sentence. Although one could make the case that testing (or teaching) sentences in isolation or out of context is limited, let us assume for the moment that this approach, that is, looking at individual sentence comprehension in a decontextualized format, has its merits (see Chapter 3). Getting beyond the contextual issues, we would consider the semantic constraints and real-world logic in sentence 3 as elements that facilitate comprehension. Sentences 1 and 2, on the other hand, lack semantic constraints; one cannot use real-world knowledge to comprehend the sentences.

Looking even further, we could consider the differences between sentences 1 and 2. Sentence 2 follows what linguists would call *order-of-mention*. Order-of-mention means that the word order follows the way the items must be sequenced (you pick up the green square first, then you touch the red square). A student who follows a "do it the way you hear it" strategy would respond to the item correctly. By contrast, sentence 1 violates the order-of-mention, which contributes to its potential difficulty. Clearly, there are many semantic and syntactic issues one could raise about the processing and comprehension of complex sentences, a topic for a later chapter in this text (see Chapter 8; see also Caccamise & Snyder, 2005; Gillam et al., 2002). Likewise, we could also raise the issue of keeping the interaction between macro (text) and micro (sentence) levels of processing in our frame of reference. Suffice it to say at this point that the statements made about what students can and cannot "process" require a closer look. A statement such as "Justin has difficulty following two-, three-, and four-step commands" is not only an inaccurate representation of syntactic processing, but also fails to capture the factors that influence comprehension.

Keeping Your Eyes on the Horizon

Another question that frames the creation of meaningful language intervention programs is, How will the choices I have made now for a student with LLD affect him or her in the future? In other words, does goal X or Y have relevance beyond this week or this cycle of therapy? Are some of my intervention goals too narrow or too focused on an immediate moment in time? Keeping one's eyes on the horizon is a final metaphor for consideration. It involves another round of self-questioning. Where am I going with Brad when I work on sequencing a series of pictures with him? Where do I think I am "taking" Sharon with the phonological awareness activities? Do my language intervention goals have any connection to grade level and teachers' instructional expectations as defined by state standards in English, or language arts, or social studies (Ehren, 2006a)? What are the long-term "payoffs" for students for any of the decisions I have made? While far from seeing into the future, the notion of looking ahead encourages clinicians to remind themselves to keep the proverbial forest in view and to avoid getting lost in "fixing" one tree or one branch. Viewing language goals and objectives from a broad-based vantage point that sees the challenges ahead underlies current practice with school-age students with language disorders.

> How will the choices SLPs make now for students with LLD affect these students in the future?

Fey and colleagues (1995) also encourage clinicians to focus on "what will be" for preschoolers with language disorders (see also Chapter 2). They talk about the significant connections between the preschool period and later language learning. These authors ask clinicians to be mindful of the ways that their language intervention choices in the preschool period can influence what children do when they reach school. Fey and colleagues (1995) point out that we have learned a great deal about the kinds of language intervention that may better prepare children with LLD for the academic challenges they will face later on. For example, the language-rich, shared literacy experiences that children have in their preschool years have a positive effect on the language and literacy skills they bring with them to school (see Chapter 6). In a most eloquent and meaningful discussion, Fey and colleagues (1995) said it perfectly as they reflected on the notion of keeping the horizon in our sights when they wrote that

> ...it may be far more productive to view language impairment (LI) in preschoolers not only for what it is at present, but also for what it is likely to become as the child grows older. (Fey et al., 1995, p. 3)

To Conclude and Move Forward

We will explore these and other concepts in the chapters that follow. Starting with an exploration of the state of the art in LLD, we will move toward additional analyses of the things we have done traditionally to help students with LLD and offer some alternatives to traditional practices. Practical applications of current theoretical constructs will be presented throughout the text. They represent an array of possibilities that help us pull many sources of information together. In the journey we will take together in the text, we will discover that there is both good and bad news to consider in the world of LLD

(Wallach, 2004; see Chapter 2). The strong research base that is available, coupled with some of the positive changes in professionals' roles and responsibilities, suggest that the time is ripe for creativity that is rooted in a sound theoretical and empirical base. This text invites readers to explore the many possibilities available to them and to become change-agents for the students in their care.

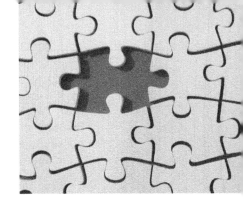

Are we speaking about a group of children, who by virtue of learning context, are called by different names, but who in reality evidence a continuum of deficits in language learning?
(Bashir et al., 1984, p. 99)

2 Language Learning Disabilities

Where Are We?

SUMMARY STATEMENT

Chapter 2 explores the state of the art in language learning disabilities (LLD). It covers the complex terrain expressed in the landmark quote that opens the chapter. The discussion continues with a look at the progress and roadblocks that exist in professionals' understanding of the pervasive and sometimes elusive nature of language disorders and their impact on academic success. The chapter also addresses current thinking about the ways we have classified and categorized students with LLD, including the use of labels such as "specific language impairment," "learning disabilities," "reading disabilities," and "dyslexia" that may or may not represent distinct populations. A continuum of language disorders and some of the language learning changes that occur across time are explored. An alternative model of assessment and identification is also presented in the form of responsiveness to intervention approaches that are set against changing federal mandates to "put reading first."

KEY QUESTIONS

1. What do current and frequently used labels say about the nature of children's language and academic difficulties?
2. What are the practical implications of viewing both language learning and language disorders on a continuum of change?
3. What should professionals know about the language and culture of schools?
4. What questions drive school-age language intervention?

INTRODUCTORY THOUGHTS

Professionals working in school settings face many challenges. There seem to be more students with and without language learning disabilities (LLD) who need help to survive and thrive in their classrooms and less time to meet their needs. Paperwork, new federal and state mandates, turf issues, and pressure by activist parents and others to adopt a new technique, program, or curriculum are only a few of the many challenges that school-based professionals face daily. Nonetheless, within the sometimes frenetic and fast-moving world of schools and their curricula is a belief that teachers and the specialists who collaborate with them can and will make a difference.

Clearly, there is much more useful and practical information available to practitioners today than there was even a decade ago, as mentioned in Chapter 1. Many excellent texts and resources are out there to help clinicians and teachers navigate the complexities of language learning and literacy (e.g., Catts & Kamhi, 2005a; DeKemel, 2003a; Silliman & Wilkinson, 2004a; Ogle & Blachowicz, 2005). A recent issue of *Topics in Language Disorders* (Wallach, 2005a) reflected on where we have been these last 25 years and where we might be going in our quest to understand students with LLD. A number of the authors who contributed to the issue noted that we are still struggling with the terminology used to describe these children. For example, students with language disorders at school-age levels appear under the guise of other labels, including "learning disabled," "reading disabled," "attention deficit disordered" (ADD), and "central auditory processing disordered (CAPD)," among others with or without any number of alphabetic variations (Wallach, 2004). In essence, however, the *Topics'* authors also noted that the majority of these disorders manifest themselves in spoken and/or written language difficulties. They recognized, too, that, as with all complex issues, there are no quick and easy solutions. As the contributors to the journal's twenty-fifth anniversary issue looked back 25 years and then looked ahead, they told their readers that while some things do indeed "stay the same," others, such as the focus on curriculum and strategic-based language intervention, offer opportunities for future success. Indeed, the state of the art in language assessment and intervention for students with LLD looks promising. The term *language learning disabilities* (LLD), which was also used in the *Topics* issue (Wallach, 2005a), is used in this text to refer to children and adolescents with school-age language disorders.

School-age students with language disorders have been labeled *learning disabled, reading disabled, attention-deficit disordered (ADD),* and *central auditory processing disordered (CAPD),* among others.

Learning from the Past

More than 25 years ago, Lahey (1980) (cited in Wallach & Butler, 1994a) presented her view at a conference about where we were in our understanding of some of the connections between *language* disorders and *learning* disabilities. Lahey (1980) used a wonderful visual image to summarize the then state of the art. She said that a learning disability was like a complex puzzle with hundreds of pieces that was missing the most important piece—the puzzle's box cover. Lahey believed that a framework or "big picture" was missing to guide us through the many possibilities and diverse directions taken by professionals from different camps in their attempts to help students who are in academic trouble. She went on to say that terms such as *learning disabled* are not necessarily useful because they fail to describe the students in question; in addition, many of the explanations about what learning disabilities appear to be are very circular. Lahey (1980) used the following dialogue to make her point:

Question: Why are these children with normal intelligence having difficulty learning to read?

Answer: Because they are "learning disabled."

Question: How do you know that?

Answer: Because they have normal intelligence and they are having difficulty learning to read.

(Wallach & Butler, 1994a, p. 19, quoting Lahey's unpublished presentation to the Language Learning Disabilities Conference at the Graduate School of the City University of New York, May 1980)

Lahey's words still resonate with us through the decades, although some alternative ways of understanding the children and adolescents "in trouble" in schools are finally here and will be discussed later in this chapter (see also Ehren & Nelson, 2005; Troia, 2005). Many researchers and practitioners now believe that relevant assessment and intervention approaches for language learning disabled students will not be found in new labels or new tests but in "finding better ways of observing the contexts, materials, and instructional patterns of classrooms and clinics as well as observing the linguistic...and academic patterns of children in those contexts" (Wallach & Butler, 1994a, p. 19). Snowling and Hayiou-Thomas (2006) agree that moving away from categorical diagnoses and looking toward children's responsiveness to intervention (RTI) will take us in a more meaningful direction. Categorical diagnoses may, in reality, be part of a hair-splitting endeavor, especially if we believe that children with language, learning, and reading disabilities are not necessarily individuals from *distinct* populations. But, clearly, future research will have to tell us more about the ebbs and flows of both spoken and written language disorders (Snowling & Hayiou-Thomas, 2006). This text focuses on the overlapping needs of children and adolescents with spoken and written problems and recognizes the influence of language on learning and other academic endeavors, as the next section demonstrates (Wallach, 2004; Wallach & Butler, 1994a).

> Many practitioners and researchers believe that relevant assessment and intervention comes not from new labels or new tests but instead from observing the contexts and actions of children and teachers inside classrooms.

Who Shall Be Called "Language Disordered"?

> **The Road to a Concept of Language-Based Learning and Reading Disabilities: Have We Come Far Enough?**

There is always an upside and a downside to changing theories, new research, and alternative approaches to any situation (Wallach, 2004). But as we navigate the roads we have taken or not taken, it may be useful to start by once again asking a basic question that was asked by Lahey (1990): Who shall be called "language disordered"? Still timely in its core concepts (as noted in Chapter 1), Lahey asked professionals to take a hard look at the way children are classified and, echoing Apel's (1999) thoughts, asked us to consider how definitions (and labels) influence what happens to children across time and learning tasks. Although focused on preschool language disorders, Lahey's points relate well to school-age language disorders.

In her provocative discussion of assessment and identification issues, Lahey (1990) encouraged readers to evaluate a number of practices, including the ways language is tested (using meaningful or nonmeaningful tasks) and the adequacy of language sampling (including the need to sample across different contexts and situations). From Lahey's perspective, looking at language performance as a closed or static system (and something that is mainly inside a child's head) misses observing the ways in which language performance is influenced by the demands placed on the system and the contexts in which performance has to be demonstrated. This was one of the main points made in Chapter 1. Lahey (1990) points out that "the criteria and procedures for identifying children with language disorders appear to vary widely among research and clinicians" (p. 612), which only adds to the confusion about who these children are. Offering some alternatives, including the ones mentioned earlier (understanding the ways language is tested and accounting for task demands and contexts), Lahey asked readers to evaluate critically the entire identification and assessment process, an issue that Ehren and Nelson (2005) and Troia (2005) also raised recently. Indeed, the question of who is language disordered and who is "something else" continues to present practitioners with a unique challenge, particularly as the boundaries between language, learning, and reading disabilities become somewhat "fuzzy" across time (Silliman et al., 2002).

Definitions Revisited

Language Disorders Over Time. In Chapter 1, Apel (1999) reminded readers to think about how their perceptions or definitions of language drive their intervention choices. The term *specific language impairment* (SLI) is used widely to refer to a group of children who show a discrepancy between nonverbal intelligence quotient (IQ) measures and performance on spoken language measures (Troia, 2005). This practice, sometimes called *cognitive referencing*, has also been used in learning disability and dyslexia circles and has been open to much scrutiny and criticism, especially lately, as we will discuss later in this chapter when we review definitions of language disorders, learning disabilities, and dyslexia (see the Bashir quote that follows; see pp. 28–29). Nonetheless, children with SLI have been viewed as having strengths in many aspects of development and growth except for language. Bashir (1989) took the longer view and offered a definition that considers language disorders as dynamic and ever-evolving, as follows:

Cognitive referencing is the practice used to compare IQ scores and language scores as factors to determine a child's eligibility for speech-language intervention.

> Language disorders is a term that represents a heterogeneous group of either developmental or acquired disabilities principally characterized by deficits in comprehension, production, and/or use of language. Language disorders are chronic and may persist across the lifetime of the individual. The symptoms, manifestations, effects and the severity of the problems change over time. The changes occur as a consequence of context, content, and learning tasks. (p. 181)

One of the significant concepts expressed in Bashir's definition and in the quote by Bashir and colleagues (1984) that opened this chapter is that language disorders are pervasive and changing in their form. These statements are as innovative now as they were at the time they were written. Although there is much more information now about the ways that language disorders change, this area of research is still a relatively new and complicated one. While there are no simple answers to what happens to preschoolers with language disorders when they reach school age, research has taught us many things.

Embracing the idea that there is a continuum of language change in which language disorders manifest themselves differently across time and contexts encourages practitioners to think along a number of lines. For example, taking a long-term view of language disorders means keeping the horizon in mind (see Chapter 1, p. 20; see also Chapter 10, p. 327). It also means looking at ways that preschool intervention can better prepare the preschooler with early language disorders for the changing demands of school, as noted in the statement by Fey and colleagues (1995) in Chapter 1 (see also Chapter 3).

Clearly, understanding the ways in which language disorders "play out" may provide clues for early identification and prevention of academic problems; it also might help children develop language and learning strategies that can facilitate literacy and other aspects of school learning. Consideration of changing contexts (e.g., school) and content (e.g., the curriculum) connects language and its disorders to authentic situations and tasks. Nelson (2005) would agree that looking at the role of changing contexts and topics across time advances professionals' understanding of school-age language disorders as an interaction of child/student abilities, the context in which language must be used, and tasks' demands. She continues to remind us, as demonstrated in Chapter 1, that language disorders occur both *within* and *outside of* a student's head (Nelson, 1998, 2005).

As mentioned previously, decades of research have contributed a great deal of information about ways in which language disabilities show themselves across time, contexts, and learning tasks; longitudinal research has contributed to our knowledge of the sometimes uneven ways in which oral and written language development and disorders change and intersect with one another as children move across the continuum of language learning (e.g., Aram & Hall, 1989; Bashir & Scavuzzo, 1992; Bishop & Adams, 1990; Boudreau & Hedberg, 1999; Catts et al., 1999; MacDonald & Cornwall, 1995; Scarborough, 2001; Snyder & Downey, 1997; Stothard et al., 1998; Tomblin et al., 1997; Westby, 2000a; Williams & Elbert, 2003). And while we still have much to learn about the evolution of early language disorders and their "metamorphosis" into different forms at school-age levels, we do know that some of the aspects of continuing language disorders include difficulties with spoken and written comprehension, figurative language, classroom instructions, written expression, and various aspects of metalinguistic and metacognitive processing (Merritt & Culatta, 1998; Nippold, 1998; Scott & Windsor, 2000; Singer & Bashir, 2004; Wallach & Butler, 1994a; Westby, 2005; Windsor et al., 2001).

Longitudinal research has begun to answer the question of what happens to preschoolers with language disorders. Research has also taught us about the importance of early literacy skills and reading abilities in the elementary grades. For example, Catts and colleagues (1999) found that young children with the most severe language disorders in the preschool period were the most at risk for reading failure. Taking more of a preventive approach, the follow-up study by Catts and colleagues (2001) looked at various language, literacy, and nonverbal cognitive factors at kindergarten levels and considered if and how these factors may be predictive of reading difficulties by Grade 2. Their findings suggested that letter identification, sentence imitation, phonological awareness, rapid naming, and mother's education predicted reading success in the second grade (Catts et al., 2001).

Other studies have shown that preschoolers who are identified early as having expressive phonological difficulties often continue to have language difficulties as they get older. Whereas their spoken language difficulties may seem improved and, in some cases, eliminated, they demonstrate difficulties with metalinguistic abilites such as segmenting sentences into words and words into their constituent sounds as they approach school age and the early elementary grades (e.g., Bird et al., 1995; van Kleeck, 1998; Wallach, 2004). Furthermore, a significant number of children who are identified as language delayed in the preschool period, manifesting both receptive and expressive language disorders, remain below their peers in written language acquisition in first and second grades (Fey et al., 1995).

Taking a slightly different route, Williams and Elbert (2003) studied the long-term outcomes for a group of preschoolers with specific phonological impairments. They found that outcomes for resolving these early-form impairments varied based on the initial pattern of phonological impairment. For example, children using phonological processes including the omissions of initial and final consonants and backing were more likely to persist with expressive language problems in schools when compared with children who had different error patterns. While not the focus of this text, the Williams and Elbert (2003) study adds to the body of research that looks at various aspects of language disorders, and the subgroups therein, across time.

Box 2-1 summarizes some of the longitudinal research in this area.

BOX 2-1   *Research Studies of Early Language and Literacy Skills and Subsequent Reading Abilities in the Elementary Grades*

- Young children with the most severe language disorders in preschool ages are most at risk for reading failure (Catts et al., 1999).
- Letter identification, sentence imitation, phonological awareness, rapid naming, and the mother's education can help predict reading success in the second grade (Catts et al., 2001).
- Preschoolers who are identified early as having expressive phonological difficulties often continue to have language difficulties as they get older (Bird et al., 1995; van Kleeck, 1998; Wallach, 2004).
- A significant number of children identified as language delayed in preschool remain below their peers in written language acquisition in first and second grades (Fey et al., 1995).
- Outcomes for resolving early-form impairments vary based on the initial pattern of phonological impairment (Williams & Elbert, 2003).

What Do Learning Disability and Dyslexia Definitions Say About Language?

Professionals from diverse fields who come to the table with different levels of training and different interests have different perceptions about the central role of language in learning and literacy (Roth & Troia, 2006; Silliman et al., 2002; Wallach & Ehren, 2004). As we look to definitions that have been used to talk about children and adolescents with language, learning, and reading disabilities, do we see similarities and differences among the Bashir, LD, and dyslexia approaches? Consider what the definitions of both "learning disabilities" and "dyslexia" suggest.

The National Joint Committee on Learning Disabilities (NJCLD) provides the following definition (italics added):

> Learning disabilities is a general term that refers to a *heterogeneous* group of disorders manifested by significant difficulties in the *acquisition and use of listening, speaking, reading, writing,* reasoning, or mathematical abilities. These disorders are *intrinsic to the individual,* presumed to be due to central nervous system dysfunction, and *may occur across the lifespan.* Problems in self-regulatory behaviors, social perception, and social interaction may exist with learning disabilities but do not themselves constitute a learning disability. Although learning disabilities may occur concomitantly with other handicapping conditions (for example, sensory impairment, mental retardation, serious emotional disturbance) or with extrinsic influences (such as cultural differences, insufficient or inappropriate instruction), they are not the result of those conditions or influences. (NJCLD, 1991, p. 19; see also *Learning Disabilities OnLine*, 2005.)

The International Dyslexia Association (IDA) defines *dyslexia* as follows (italics added):

> Dyslexia is a *specific learning disability* that is *neurobiological* in origin. It is characterized by difficulties with accurate and/or fluent word recognition and by poor spelling and decoding abilities. These difficulties typically result from a deficit in the *phonological component of language* that is often unexpected in relation to other cognitive abilities and the provision of effective classroom instruction. Secondary consequences may include problems in reading comprehension and reduced reading experience that can impede the growth of vocabulary and background knowledge. (Lyon et al., 2003, pp. 1–2)

In both the LD and dyslexia definitions one sees a recognition of language factors to greater and lesser degrees. In some ways, the definitions present overlapping concepts that relate to the three groups—language disabled, learning disabled, and reading disabled (dyslexic). The LD definition, created by an interdisciplinary group of researchers and clinicians, recognizes listening, speaking, reading, and writing in the mix, as well as the possible long-term nature of learning disabilities. The dyslexia definition makes the case for a language base to reading problems more specifically by isolating the role of the phonological component in the reading process. Both suggest a central nervous system base (intrinsic to the individual) without acknowledgment of the context-content factors that interact with an individual's inherent abilities (Nelson, 2005). The "exclusionary" approach to identifying these distinct groups (i.e., it is not cognition, it is not sensory impairment, it is not instructional impairment, etc.), as well as the use of cognitive referencing approaches mentioned earlier with SLI, are all being reevaluated today (see also Catts & Kamhi, 2005c; Catts & Kamhi, 2005e).

The definitions for both LD and dyslexia suggest a central nervous system base but do not acknowledge the context and content factors that interact with a child's abilities.

Clinicians, regular and special educators, and specialists in this postmillennium era are moving beyond definitions. Many recognize how controversial definitions and labels can be. Further, in some cases, there is no agreed-on, unified definition among professionals. This is the situation in the learning disability community (Graner et al., 2005; Proctor & Prevatt, 2003). Professionals are also reevaluating ways in which their roles and responsibilities are bound too tightly to one definition or another (e.g., Ehren & Nelson, 2005; Whitmire, 2005). Finally, clinicians and educators are looking to the research to learn more about the ways in which language, learning, and reading disabilities overlap, intersect, and separate (Sawyer, 2006; Snowling & Hayiou-Thomas, 2006).

Disorders Viewed on a Continuum of Change. To say that reading and writing are aspects of language development (Kamhi & Catts, 2005; van Kleeck, 1998; Wallach, 2004, 2005b) or that many early language disorders become school-age learning and reading disabilities as noted by Bashir and colleagues (1984) is to express concepts that are more accepted today due, in part, to advances in both research and practice (Silliman et al., 2002). But researchers such as Scarborough (2001) caution professionals to review how language changes are measured over time, how populations studied are defined, and the overall research methodology used in longitudinal studies. Further, Scarborough (2001) reiterates the finding that language changes occur in sometimes uneven and nonlinear ways, a concept mentioned earlier and one that Bashir (1989) also expressed in terms of "spurts" and "plateaus" in language learning.

Related to the issue of how language disorders change over time is an even more thought-provoking question: Do labels follow children across time or do they change along the way? Is it the case that some labels change, for example, from *specific language impairment* (or disorders) (SLI) to *learning disabilities,* as a child moves from preschool to school-age levels? The top portion of Figure 2-1 provides a visual image of possible label changes as seen on a continuum of changing language challenges that are shown at the bottom of the figure. We will return later to a discussion of the bottom of the figure.

Early on, Bashir and colleagues (1984) indicated that labels may change when children move from one context to another (home to school). In reality, however, their verbal-linguistic needs remain a priority even though these children (with ongoing language disorders) may be described as "learning" and/or "reading" disabled as mentioned earlier in this chapter. Silliman and colleagues (2002) agree with Bashir's notion, adding that labels can be misleading, especially when and if the direction and focus of intervention change because a label changes. Moreover, it is misguided to let labels dictate the direction of intervention, especially if children described as "learning" or "reading" disabled have ongoing language problems that may be obscured by inaccurately applied labels. Silliman and colleagues (2002) go on to say that "the overarching importance of language in the educational lives of children" should be kept in focus (p. 5). We will return to the issue of language and school success later in this chapter and throughout this text.

Professionals might ask whether rigid classifications of children lead them in the wrong direction. Do children and adolescents with language disabilities,

Do labels follow children across time, or do they change along the way?

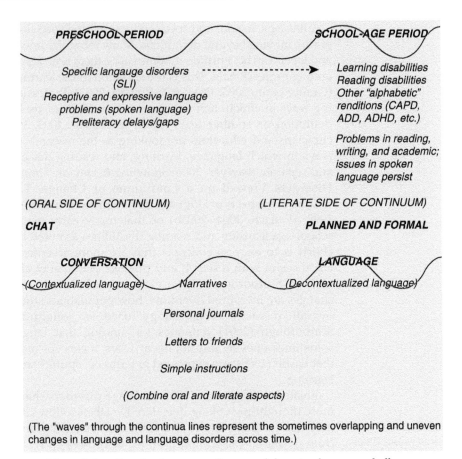

Figure 2-1 ■ Two tracks on a continuum of changing language challenges representing (1) language disorders changing over time and (2) language learning changes across time. *(Data from Scott, C. M. [1994]. A discourse continuum for school-age students: Impact of modality and genre. In G. P. Wallach & K. G. Butler [Eds.], Language learning disabilities in school-age children and adolescents: Some principles and applications [pp. 219–252]. Boston: Allyn & Bacon; Westby, C. E. [1984]. The development of narrative language ability. In G. P. Wallach, & K. G. Butler [Eds.], Language learning disabilities in school-age children [pp. 103–127]. Baltimore: Williams & Wilkins; and Westby, C. E. [1994]. The effects of culture on genre, structure, and style of oral and written texts. In G. P. Wallach & K. G. Butler [Eds.], Language learning disabilities in school-age children and adolescents [pp. 180–218]. Boston: Allyn & Bacon.)*

reading disabilities, and learning disabilities represent the same or distinct populations (Nation et al., 2004; Silliman et al., 2002; Wallach, 2004, 2005b; Wallach & Butler, 1994a)? Clearly, the heterogeneity within and among these groups, recognized in Bashir's definitions and the definitions that follow, suggests an overlapping relationship for at least some children, some of the time. The issue of "sameness" or "distinctness" among groups may not be the most useful one professionals could ask, especially if the answer to the question fails to move intervention for these students in innovative and appropriate ways. Catts and Kamhi (2005c) offer some provocative ways to look at language disorders and dyslexia, suggesting that evaluating listening comprehension differences, along with decoding and other reading measures, may provide insight into the groups' differences. They add, however, that there is often a fine line between language and dyslexia groups and point out that, regardless of labels, linguistic and reading abilities should be evaluated over time. (Refer to Catts & Kamhi [2005c] for an in-depth discussion.)

Although it may be useful to understand the patterns and educational needs of different subgroups as Catts and Kamhi (2005c) and others suggest, can one get caught in the trap of spending too much time testing and looking for clean diagnostic categories and not enough time teaching and providing language intervention for those who need it (Christensen, 1992; Wallach, 2004; Whitmire, 2005)? In one of the most pointed and poignant statements on the issue of too much testing and labeling, and not enough appropriate teaching, Christensen (1992) wrote about the overlapping nature of learning- and reading-disabled categories and questioned the usefulness of trying to distinguish between the groups:

> Thirty years of psychometric approaches have failed to provide satisfactory answers to the learning disabled dilemma. A continuation of such a quest [for a distinct group] should not be conducted without addressing the serious social, ethical, and moral issues involved in the pursuit of this select group. (pp. 276–277)

In a similar vein, speech-language and other professionals who work with school-age students might ask a related question: How much valuable time should be spent asking whether Billy has attention-deficit disorder (ADD), attention-deficit/hyperactivity disorder (ADHD), or central auditory processing disorder (CAPD)? Might we consider more descriptive approaches that look into Billy's classroom and the curriculum—the contexts in which his problems are occurring—as well as assess his overall linguistic and metalinguistic abilities? (See the discussion of the culture and language of schools later in this chapter.) Likewise, would it be more helpful to recognize the cycle of reduced language learning that occurs for children with reading, writing, and spelling problems? Are children with "pure" reading disabilities (if they exist) at a disadvantage? Does having a reduced access to what print has to offer, including exposure to literate forms of language, new and rare vocabulary, advanced text structures, and so on, have a negative impact on spoken language (ASHA, 2001; Catts & Kamhi, 2005d; Silliman et al., 2002; Westby, 2005)?

Indeed, the reciprocity between spoken and written language systems, that is, the two-way street, comes to mind and reflects a more integrated way to consider the difficulties children may have across time. That language disorders are both a *cause* and *result* of reading disabilities (Catts & Kamhi, 2005a), as noted in Chapter 1, should say something about the way intervention is approached and the type of services children receive (Wallach & Ehren, 2004; see Chapter 3). Again, one's beliefs and knowledge about what "language" is, what "reading" is, what "learning" is, and the intersections among them influence "who does what to whom" in the real world.

Speaking specifically about dyslexia and the misperceptions that exist about what it "looks like," Wadlington and Wadlington (2005) suggest that regular educators who may be among the first professionals to see vulnerable children in their classrooms also need to understand more about the nature of reading disabilities. For example, the idea that dyslexia has something to do with letter reversals is an erroneous belief, a misconception that Hight (2005) also found among the teachers she surveyed. Thus we can all learn more about children and adolescents in academic trouble and we can work at assessing the perceptions we bring to the instructional and intervention table. Moreover, we can reevaluate the productivity of the turf wars that sometimes exist among professionals who cannot decide who does what to whom. In all fairness, defined roles and responsibilities are not always clear to professionals who share in the education of students with LLD, as noted by Silliman and colleagues (2002), a reality that was not necessarily facilitated by the separate categorization of disabilities (*language* impairment vs. *learning* disability) that were "codified in the Individuals with Disabilities Education Act (IDEA '97) for over twenty-five years" (p. 8).

Alternatives in Our Midst? Providing statistics from the U.S. Department of Education (2001), Troia (2005) indicates that "the prevalence of LD among children in school has increased by more than 200%...so that, currently, students with LD comprise about 50% of the school-age special education population" (p. 106). These are staggering statistics that have sparked a national debate. Perhaps change has been too slow in coming, but shifting policies on the federal level, coupled with the nationwide concern for the increasing numbers of students being referred for special education services, are having an effect on the ways we assess and manage students with LLD. Troia (2005) notes that the 2004 reauthorization of the Individuals with Disabilities Education Improvement Act (IDEA '04) opens the door to alternative approaches for identifying and classifying students who have learning disabilities/reading disabilities, the majority of which are language based—the perspective of this text and not necessarily Troia's. The reauthorization of IDEA, among its provisions, includes changes in the way "LD" is determined. First, it moves away from the IQ-achievement discrepancy model (i.e., cognitive referencing) to determine the gap between "expected" potential and performance; second, it shifts from a "wait-to-fail" mentality to a prevention mentality, especially for children who are not identified until their problems surface in academics (Whitmire, 2005).

The alternative provides for a three-tiered model termed *responsiveness to intervention* (RTI). Students "travel through" the tiers with varying degrees of support in an intervention/management approach that differs from the more traditional "diagnostic labeling into special education" approach. Troia (2005, p. 109) presents a model for RTI (Box 2-2). In tier I, all students receive instruction based on evidence-based practices. The classroom teacher "delivers" the curriculum with adaptations made as necessary with consultation from appropriate professionals as needed, including speech-language pathologists (SLPs). In tier II, interventions might supplement and complement the curriculum. It isn't until tier III that students receive the specialized intervention (including specifically tailored language therapy) that may have to supplant

BOX 2-2	*Tiered Model for Responsiveness to Intervention* (RTI)

The RTI model functions in a dynamic assessment mode; instruction and adaptations to the curriculum are its focus. It is supplemented with monitoring, in-class, and curricular support as needed.

Tier I

All students receive instruction based on evidence-based practices. Classroom teachers "deliver" the curriculum and adapt as necessary based on consultation with appropriate professionals, including speech-language pathologists.

Tier II

Interventions may supplement and complement the curriculum.

Tier III

Students receive specialized intervention (including specifically tailored language therapy) that may replace classroom instruction; the student may then be referred for special education placement, if necessary.

Data from Troia, G. A. (2005). Responsiveness to intervention: Roles for speech-language pathologists in the prevention and identification of learning disabilities. *Topics in Language Disorders, 25,* 106–119.

the classroom instruction (and the student may then be referred for a special education placement).

Ehren and Nelson (2005), among others (e.g., Staskowski & Rivera, 2005; Troia, 2005; Whitmire, 2005), look at RTI models with a special eye toward the ways language and literacy intersect with the curriculum, and the particular role of SLPs in the process. Figure 2-2 presents a summary of Ehren and Nelson's (2005) model. They point out that although RTI models offer opportunities to modify the way services are delivered to children and adolescents with diverse types of academic problems, the success of operationalizing this model will be influenced by many variables. The variables include understanding the role of language in learning and what it really means to have a shared responsibility in literacy learning (Wallach & Ehren, 2004; see also Chapter 3).

Ehren and Nelson (2005) echo the points made earlier in this chapter about labels changing over time. They point out that "learning-disabled" and "reading-disabled" labels often supplant "language-disabled" (SLI) labels. They write that "language-based difficulties in upper grades masquerade as school failure of varying etiologies, most of which are not attributed to language problems by those who work with [learning-disabled students] daily" (Ehren et al., 2004, as cited by Ehren & Nelson, 2005, p. 123). Consequently, if the core of many students' problems are actually language based, the roles of SLPs in RTI models should be more visible than they are now. For this expanded SLP visibility to happen, they must transition from a "caseload" to a "workload" mentality (ASHA, 2003; Ehren & Nelson, 2005). And although RTI models are far from

Tier I–Scientifically-based language-sensitive classroom instruction

Students receive language-sensitive literacy instruction in the general education classroom along with screening of language and literacy development.

SLP consults with general education teachers about instruction and screening.

Tier II–Intervention in general education

Students who struggle with language and literacy receive more intensive language-based intervention in small groups in general education.

SLP collaborates with other professionals to administer and interpret language assessments (spoken and written) and to plan and provide small-group intervention.

Tier III–LI Identification

Students who do not succeed in Tier II are considered in need of intensive therapeutic intervention from the SLP.

SLP collaborates with others to determine LI eligiblity based on lack of responsiveness to prior intervention and other evidence and provides language therapy in collaboration with others.

Figure 2-2 ■ The responsiveness to intervention (RTI) model and the speech-language pathologist (SLP). *(Redrawn from Ehren, B. J., & Nelson, N. W. [2005]. The responsiveness to intervention approach and language impairment.* Topics in Language Disorders, 25, *120–131. Copyright B. J. Ehren and N. W. Nelson.)*

perfect, they offer alternatives to some of the "traditionalism" in testing and placement. They also move professionals to a preventive mode, at least for some children. The pervasiveness of language disorders remains a reality for others.

Ehren and Nelson (2005) sum it up as follows:

RTI can circumvent problems SLPs encounter when identifying LI [language impairment] using standardized norm-referenced tests, especially as related to providing an alternative to cognitive referencing. In addition, the prevention of LI identification among students who need good language development in the classroom and more explicit intervention in general education may help SLPs identify a smaller group of students for intensive therapeutic services. (p. 129)

Although RTI models are becoming more prevalent in discussions among clinicians and educators today, we still have a steep slope to climb to create and implement fully collaborative programs for students with LLD (Wallach & Ehren, 2004). Progress is certainly being made, as reflected in RTI models as an example, but professionals' understanding of language learning and language proficiency varies greatly. Nonetheless, this area of research and its practical applications offer additional promise. As we look ahead to where we have been and where we are going in LLD, the following two themes are discussed that add to our knowledge base:

1. The continuum of language learning
2. The language-loaded nature of school

Language Proficiency, Literacy, and Schools Revisited

Language Learning on a Continuum of Change

The top part of Figure 2-1 (p. 30) represented what the continuation of early language disorders looks like. The bottom part of the image suggests a parallel track. Although children are changing, so too are the language demands they face daily. The two tracks, language disorders and language learning changes across time, give practitioners a way to conceptualize highly complex behaviors. As with all models as noted in Chapter 1, the continua model is not meant to represent a literal translation from theory to practice. What the model does do is help practitioners describe prototypes of language across time and situations (e.g., informal conversation vs. expository academic-like text). In the real world of language use, behaviors often overlap and intermingle (Kamhi, 1997; Wallach, 2004). Thus while approaching a study of the continuum with caution, clinicians may ask themselves yet another question: How can knowledge about the changing nature of language have a positive influence on the intervention goals set for their students?

Conceptual frameworks, including those discussed by Scott (1994, 2005) and Westby (1984, 1994, 2005), and introduced in Chapter 1, view language learning as having various styles and purposes; as a result, these changes can be described along a continuum that stretches from the most informal types of communication exchanges, such as *chat*, to the more formal types of communication, such as *planned written discourse/planned academic language.* Between the two extremes—combining informal and formal characteristics—are discourse events such as narratives, keeping personal journals, and writing letters to friends. Scott and Westby indicate that as children move up the grades, they have to become more proficient in using and processing language that is formal, planned, impersonal, and written. They also develop a more sophisticated understanding of ways that personal/informal and impersonal/formal dimensions cut across modalities. For example, it is appropriate to use informal writing styles *in certain situations,* such as writing e-mails to close friends. However, it is important to shift to more impersonal and formal language styles in other situations, such as presenting at a national or state convention. (See classic and recent discussions by Scott [1988, 1989, 1994, 2005] for more details.) Similar to Scott's notions, Westby (1994) uses the terms *orality* and *literacy* to describe language changes across time. She talked about how children progress from oral styles of communication to literate styles of communication across spoken and written domains. Many of these concepts relate to expanded definitions of literacy, which were outlined in Chapter 1.

Silliman and Wallach (1991; cited in Wallach & Butler, 1994a, p. 9) talk about the expectations facing children in schools and the assumptions made about

As children advance through the grades, they have to become more proficient at using and processing formal, planned, impersonal, and written language.

their oral-to-literate abilities. They noted that in addition to managing new content encased in difficult language, that is, the curriculum and instructional language, children also have to shift their *oral* presentation styles to fit the "formality" required in school settings. Children not only have to learn to read but they also learn to "*talk* (and write) more like books" (Silliman & Wallach, 1991; Wallach & Butler, 1994a). Box 2-3 outlines some of the changes that occur

---

BOX 2-3   *Three Aspects of Oral-to-Literate Transitions Made by Students from Students' Perspectives*

Talking Like Books
- This style is a great idea if you can read and write.
- Your talking starts to sound like books if you have been read to a lot and after you have learned how to read.
- Teachers might expect you to talk like books even if you do not read and write well.
- This style comes in handy in class, with the principal, on job interviews, in speeches and broadcasts, and when talking is formal.
- This is not the style of talk you have to use on the basketball court.

Writing Like Talking
- You only write the way you talk in some situations, and writing is always different from talking.
- It is important to know when to use this style because writing like talking usually does not work well on the printed page.
- This style is not allowed in school for too long.
- Writing like talking is great for the "personal stuff," when you are writing speeches for a character, when you are keeping a journal, and when you are reminding yourself about something.

Writing Like Books
- This style is a great idea if you have the books, you can read, and you know grammar.
- You will need to know how to write like books because it's the language of school, texts, and reports.
- This style gets very formal and specific and a little impersonal.
- You have to plan ahead and make specific choices and really "know" your language.
- After Grade 4, this ability is a must and stays that way for most of your life.

From Silliman, E. R., & Wallach, G. P. (1991, November). The communication process model for LLD children: Making it work. Short course presented at the American Speech-Language-Hearing Association annual conference, Atlanta. As cited in Wallach, G. P., & Butler, K. G. (1994). Creating communication, literacy, and academic success. In G. P. Wallach & K. G. Butler (Eds.), *Language learning disabilities in school-age children and adolescents: Some principles and applications* (pp. 2–26). Boston: Allyn & Bacon.

in both spoken and written language along the oral-to-literate continuum. Silliman and Wallach (1991) indicate that school-age children move from talking like books, to writing like talking, and finally to writing like books. Written from students' points of view, one gets a glimpse of a number of language abilities and stylistic changes required to succeed academically.

Understanding and studying language learning and disorders by considering the changes that occur across time is one of the dimensions that help frame language intervention goals at school-age levels. Understanding the cultural and linguistic diversity of schools is another.

School as a Unique Language and Culture

"Regular" Language versus "School" Language. When children enter a school building and become students in an academic world, they leave their homes and communities for a new, different, and usually more demanding world. The assumption that children come to school with intact (and very good) language was the norm in years past. This notion may be changing as a result of shifts in the population and the statistics mentioned earlier (p. 32) relating to the overwhelming increase in referrals to special education. For the most part, however, entering school means bringing with you preschool experiences that will help you make the transition from home-based activities and *contextualized* language (the oral side of the continuum) to academic-based activities and *decontextualized* language (the literate side of the continuum). It is assumed that children entering school (as early as kindergarten) have mastered many aspects of orality (or informal language) and some aspects of literacy.

> Because of a number of statistics, including recent population shifts, the idea that children come to school with intact and proficient language can no longer be assumed.

It is assumed, for example, that children have been read to, have books in their lives, and have had practice with sound/letter correspondences (van Kleeck, 1998). In addition, many children enter school with strong inferential processing skills that they have acquired in the shared reading experiences with parents and other adults (van Kleeck et al., 2006). With this assumed background, students are better equipped to manage the shift from informal to formal uses of language in school. Children now adopt a "talking to learn" strategy, and they shift from a "learning to read" to a "reading to learn" approach (Bashir et al., 1998; Fey et al., 1995). Indeed, when children come to school, they also move to that second layer of language learning and participate in more "metalinguistically heavy" activities (van Kleeck, 1994).

In their classic article about schools and school discourse, Berlin and colleagues (1980) wrote:

> The goals of schools are embodied in the curriculum. In teaching subject areas such as science, math, art, and physical education, the school attempts to enhance children's level of functioning. Because language is clearly one of the skills that the school wishes to foster, it too has become part of the curriculum. Thus, just as one teaches history, math, and geography, one *teaches language.* (p. 54)

Recognizing the way that language weaves its way throughout the school curriculum, Berlin and colleagues make the point that the language of schooling and the curriculum is somewhat removed from everyday discourse. They say that most classroom discourse exchanges "compartmentalize" language (teaching separate units of vocabulary, syntax, etc.) to such a point that this process actually "interferes with the child's understanding of the way in which oral and written discourse actually develops" (Berlin et al., 1980, p. 55). Expanding on their ideas, Blank (2002), writing more recently, reiterates the point that classroom discourse is filled with verbal concepts. Children must master new topic knowledge (new language content) while, at the same time, deducing implicit meanings from what they hear and read, for example, figuring out what the teacher really wants. Blank notes a twofold challenge for all children, especially for language learning disabled students. She reminds practitioners to think about school language for what it really is: (1) the language of school is informationally loaded, and (2) school discourse presumes a good deal of "already known" information, as well as inferential and integrative processing ability.

Indeed, processing and comprehending instructional language includes many skills that children bring with them into the classroom, including metalinguistic abilities (i.e., talking about language, reflecting on language, and analyzing language). Succeeding in schools also means successfully accessing textbook language and using strategies for correcting misunderstood content information (Wallach, 2004). Summarizing the challenges of classroom discourse beautifully, Bashir and colleagues (1998) say that "within instructional exchanges, including discussing, questioning, responding, and summarizing, teachers and students construct and make explicit the content of the curriculum" (Bashir et al., 1998, p. 10).

In addition to managing the language-loaded curriculum, meeting classroom expectations includes many other verbal (and sometimes nonverbal) abilities, including responding to the teacher's signals of task reorienting, knowing when to try for the teacher's attention, and knowing how to pass a turn or guess appropriately. Peer interactions such as soliciting help in acceptable ways and times, giving appropriate help to classmates, and participating in group decision making through appropriate conversational rules of turn taking are also part of the process of classroom discourse (Nelson, 1998). These pragmatic functions discussed by Nelson (1998) also touch on the culture of schools and the special rules—implicit as they sometimes are—that students must learn to be successful.

Home Culture versus School Culture. Although mastery of a school curriculum presents new challenges for many students, it presents a particular challenge for students with spoken and written language learning problems who have to master simultaneously the curriculum's content and the social-communicative rules that regulate access to the curriculum (Nelson, 1998; Wallach & Ehren, 2004). Language learning disabled students may not "come with" the language required to meet the needs of the fast-moving curriculum. In addition, these students' "styles" of language may be different from their teachers' expectations. Indeed, teachers also bring with them curricular and pedagogical knowledge, skills, experiences, and expectations. These teacher qualities interact with the strategies students bring for "studenting" and curricular expectations. Classroom materials have their own structure and format, couching subject matter and topics in language. And classroom groups take on lives of their own. The class may function as a whole group, and there may be small group activities,

The knowledge, skills, and expectations teachers and students bring to school and the structures and formats of materials and group dynamics combine to make classrooms a complex environment.

specified instructional groups (e.g., reading or math groups), and peer group activities (Blank, 2002; Weade & Green, 1985). This complex system of interconnected factors, about which volumes have been written, reminds us that "problems are not just within children—and neither are solutions" (Nelson, 1998, p. 12).

Wallach and Ehren (2004) point out that sharing information about a child's performance within the framework of a school's or classroom's culture can offer an excellent opportunity for collaboration among professionals. For example, they note that teachers and SLPs can share information about the following:

■ What are the personal frames of reference students bring to a lesson (or a therapy or resource room session) that might influence their participation?
■ What will be the social and academic expectations for participating?
■ Do students "read" both the social and academic requirements for participating?
■ How will groups be organized and how will expectations for participating vary within and across groups?
■ How will turn-taking procedures be organized?
■ When a student responds to a question inappropriately, what happens?

These are only a few of the many questions one could pose, and the opportunities appear golden for professionals who work both within and outside of classrooms to create a dialogue around these types of questions. Chapters 3 and 4 will provide additional information on the subject of collaboration.

In Summary: Language Underpinnings and the Curriculum

Developing and implementing curriculum-relevant, appropriate, and innovative language intervention for students with LLD is a masterful balance among a student's inherent abilities (what one "brings" to the task of language learning and academic learning), the demands of a specific grade's curriculum (driven by state standards), and the numerous ways a curriculum is packaged and delivered to students (the way task demands and teacher demands intersect). Wallach and Ehren (2004) asked a number of key questions about these complex relationships. Two key questions they raised were, What language abilities are necessary to become literate? and What are the *language underpinnings* of academic tasks? In other words, ask Wallach and Ehren (2004), "What does it 'take'?" That is, what language abilities are necessary to perform well on any number of academic tasks? These questions frame language intervention at school-age levels. Clearly, understanding the transitions from orality to literacy (back to the continuum) and the ways in which the demands of the curriculum intersect with instructional language and teachers' styles are part of the process of deciding "what to do" for students with LLD.

Thus clinicians in the business of facilitating language should see language as the dynamic system influenced by context and content (see Chapter 1). The linguistic and metalinguistic knowledge, skills, and strategies a student has (or "doesn't have") in his or her repertoire, in addition to other information-processing skills (e.g., Gillam et al., 2002), may "match" or "clash with" the knowledge, skill, and strategies required to succeed in social studies, history, English, science, math, or another subject (Ehren, 2003). The meshing of Nelson's (1998, 2005) "inside" and "outside" factors creates a challenge for professionals who work within and outside of classrooms. For SLPs, language intervention at school-age levels includes these two major components (what the child brings and the context and content he or she is faced with in the classroom). It follows that the answers to "what to do" reside not only within a student's inherent abilities but also in the textbooks, classroom pragmatics, and demands of the academic tasks (see Chapters 3 and 4).

Looking Ahead

In 2004, Wallach summarized the state of the art in LLD by talking about the "good news" and the "bad news." Fortunately, she saw more good news on the horizon. The good news included a wealth of research that is available in language-based learning and reading disabilities, some of which was summarized in this chapter. Research in the area of information processing has also added to our knowledge base (e.g., Caccamise & Snyder, 2005; Lahey & Bloom, 1994; Windsor et al., 2001; see also Chapters 7 and 8). This research has helped to drive intervention in new and more appropriate directions. Ehren's numerous works (e.g., Ehren, 2000, 2005b, 2006a, 2006b), along with those of her colleagues (e.g., Ehren et al., 2004), have contributed much to the meaning of strategic-based language intervention. In addition, we have learned a great deal about the culture of schools and the multifaceted and language-loaded, print-heavy nature of the curriculum. Added to the good news that surrounds us is the influence of RTI models, which show promise in terms of the ways we identify children in trouble in schools (Ehren & Nelson, 2005; Troia, 2005).

The downside to the good news includes the ever-present search for the "silver bullet" or quick fix for students with LLD that is sometimes reflected in the latest program or the promises of workshop leaders. There is also some ongoing confusion among professionals about their roles and responsibilities in shared literacy, although the era of collaboration has led to significant improvements in this arena. But there are, no doubt, school administrators and supervisors who are still asking, "Why is my 'speech' pathologist involved in reading?" Likewise, the resurgence of intervention practices that approach a child's "problem" as an isolated tree in the forest remain too removed from the "outside" pieces of the problem—the curriculum and the classroom. Kamhi's (2004) recent discussion of why some concepts remain popular in language assessment and intervention while others take longer to catch on helps us appreciate two things: (1) we have to rethink the usefulness of espousing popular practices because it's "the way it's always been done," and (2) we must take a hard look at approaches that propose overly simplified solutions for the complex problems manifested by students with language learning difficulties. (See Chapter 5, p.124–125, for a more detailed discussion of Kamhi's [2004] "meme" theory.)

As the old advertisement reminded us: "We've come a long way." We will go even further as we continue to evaluate current research and theoretically solid practices. Our knowledge and understanding of new models of identification and service delivery offer us opportunities to change the practice of placing too many children in special education too soon. Evidence-based practices that include solid partnerships between researchers and practitioners offer us additional opportunities to change the landscape of intervention. To understate the case might be to say that we have much to learn about children and adolescents with LLD, and part of the learning process includes leaving some of the old myths and legends in language intervention behind in the narratives of the past (Wallach & Madding, 2005, 2006). The chapters that follow look forward, and sometimes back, encouraging readers to enjoy the journey.

2

A Practical Framework

PART OUTLINE

3   What Language Intervention "Looks Like" at School-Age Levels

4   Creating "Curriculum-Relevant" Therapy
   Making the Tough Choices

A Practical Framework

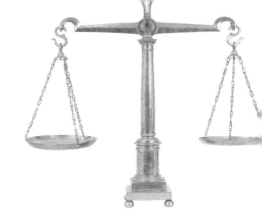

*W*hen attempting to facilitate new [language] behaviors, one wants to lighten the use of resources for other behaviors. For example, in teaching a child to write stories, clinicians might consider the conditions of low stress, familiar lexicon, mental models that are easy to construct and not too complex, and use of simple syntactic structures.

(Lahey & Bloom, 1994, p. 369)

3 What Language Intervention "Looks Like" at School-Age Levels

SUMMARY STATEMENT

Chapter 3 presents an overview of what language intervention "looks like" in the school-age period. We focus on the school-age period from Grade 1 to high school in this text. We include kindergarten in our discussions because kindergarten has become what Grade 1 "used to be." The changing demands of kindergarten create additional challenges for students who come to school with a history of language disorders. Within the context of knowing the academic demands that face children as they enter school, this chapter asks readers to reflect on the whys of their intervention choices. What drives the decision to work on a particular aspect of language? For example, narration and expository text are popular intervention targets. Are they relevant and meaningful choices? Why? The chapter also asks clinicians to consider the ways that their intervention decisions connect to classroom and academic success. Continuing with the text's format, a number of questions set the tone for evaluating the decisions clinicians make about "what to do" with students with language learning disabilities (LLD). The notion of creating relevant, strategic, and focused intervention is emphasized as a recurring theme in this text. And as we strive to attain these intervention goals for the students in our care, we ask yet another question: Have we "watered down" the curriculum for students with LLD so much that their opportunities to acquire language learning and thinking skills are more restricted than they should be (Ellis, 1997)?

KEY QUESTIONS ■■■■■■

1. What language abilities underlie many academic tasks? And what language abilities do students "bring" (or not bring) with them to these tasks?
2. How does facility with specific aspects of language influence academic success? Do we know?

3. Is the reciprocal relationship between spoken and written language reflected in language intervention decisions?
4. What is meant by strategic and curriculum-relevant language intervention?

INTRODUCTORY THOUGHTS

Snapshots of School-Age Language Disorders

SNAPSHOT 1

A clinician is working with a 14-year-old student with language learning disabilities (LLD). The student (JG) has many strengths in linguistic and nonlinguistic areas. For example, he is engaging, enthusiastic, and quite verbal. He loves to talk and interact with people, loves movies and books that he is able to read, and is a creative cartoonist. In this excerpt, JG is reviewing with the clinician some of the information that appears in a unit he and his classmates have participated in for the last few weeks, "The Roman Empire."

> Speech-language pathologist (SLP): Let's look at the title of this class unit you've covered. It says "The Beginning of the Roman Empire." As we have done before, let's look at the words to check comprehension and see how the title helps us to understand what's coming up in the chapter. What is an *empire*?
>
> JG: . . . like a princess.
>
> SLP: Is "empire" a person or a place? (*They have worked on people, places, and things in previous sessions.*)
>
> JG: I'm not sure. I think it's a place.
>
> SLP: So can "princess" be an empire?
>
> JG: No,'cause they're not towns.
>
> SLP: O.K. So an empire is a place. It has towns, cities, and countries.
>
> SLP: O.K., Now let's look at "Roman."
>
> JG: Roman is like an empire...It means men, too, because it says "Ro...man." It means people.
>
> SLP: Right. The empire is a place and the people who live there are the...

JG: Romans.

SLP: Good. Let's talk about the place and the people.

SLP: What city...this is a place...is the center if the Roman Empire?

JG: I'm not sure.

SLP: Let's look at the word "Roman." The city name is a part of Roman.

JG: Is it Rome?

SLP: Great. That's where this chapter will take place. Let's look at the people we're talking about.

JG: Romans must mean people.

SLP: Good! Where do they live?

JG: (*Points to Rome on the page after a long pause.*)

SLP: (*Goes on bit with the people and places. Then she asks:*) Where do Americans live?

JG: I think, California.

The "Roman Empire" scenario provides a very abbreviated view of some of the difficulties encountered by students whose language disorders, although changed (and as noted in the previous chapters), are still pervasive and serious. The gaps in both background and language knowledge contribute to JG's academic difficulties. His particular difficulties with the semantic and morphophonemic areas of language, reflected in his spoken language and metalinguistic awareness, interact with his overall difficulties with decoding and reading comprehension. JG's morphophonemic gaps were evidenced further as the sessions progressed. For example, he had difficulty expressing the relations between words such as *senate—senator, Italy—Italians*. JG's spoken and written language difficulties are reminiscent of Catts and Kamhi's (2005b) notions of the ways language and reading "play off" one another.

SNAPSHOT 2

A clinician is working with a group of language learning disabled students within their classroom. There are six students in the group, four boys and two girls. The students range in age from 11 to 12 years old. The clinician is working with students on the concept of how titles can help a reader prepare for what is coming in the text. (JG also worked on using titles in the previous snapshot.) She is using titles that appear in their Grade 6 social studies text and some titles that she has collected over the years. A title from a classic article by Hennings (1993) is one of her favorites. The brainstorming session goes like this:

SLP: OK, I have a tricky title that is one of my favorites. Let's see if we can figure out what it might mean and what the chapter will be about. Ready?

CP: Oh, I love these tricky ones.

SLP (*Showing the title in print and reading it for the students.*) "Christopher Columbus: How History was Invented."

AR: Oh, oh, I know. Columbus discovers America.

SLP: Yes, that's a piece of it. Columbus discovered America.

RB: We don't have off that day. It's not a holiday here.

SLP: That's true.

(The brainstorming goes on for a while. The students know who Columbus was but they do not know [or cannot express or recall] too many details and facts about his life and his voyages.)

GS: I know. The word "invented" is like...you make something new. So since Columbus discovered America, it's like he found something new.

CP: Right, we're going to read about Columbus going to America and finding the Indians and new lands.

The students in snapshot 2, who have participated in this activity numerous times, are certainly "playing with language." It is the SLP's goal to help them develop *strategies* they can take with them to other academic and communicative situations. Her next step is to take them through the chapter that follows and help them connect what they have predicted via the title and what the chapter, that is, what the print, actually says. On reading further, it was "discovered" that the students had some of the elements correct. The chapter was about Columbus and the newly found land of America. However, the core concept or message in the chapter (i.e., its "main idea"), missed by the students, was that Columbus may not have been the hero (or person) we thought he was. Although it was recognized that he took the road less traveled, he did many things to the native peoples that were not worthy of praise. The chapter was trying to say that we have to look deeper to find our "real" history. Thus the wording of the title, thought to be facilitative, would only work if the reader interpreted its figurative meaning. Nonetheless, the text would (and should) clear up any misinterpretations. Proficient readers would use their background knowledge, plus the text, to validate or invalidate first impressions to construct meaning (Caccamise & Snyder, 2005; DeKemel, 2003c; Ehren, 2005b; Lahey & Bloom, 1994; see also Raphael & Au, 2005, Chapter 8, this book, pp. 229–234). For students with LLD, constructing meaning from text may be no easy task.

SNAPSHOT 3   Written samples were elicited from a 13-year-old student with LLD about 2 months apart. LA was asked to provide a personal account of her recent vacation to the lake with her family (shown in sample 1). She described another vacation with her family and cousin, Yoko (in sample 2). LA's spoken language has improved, especially in its "micro" aspects, including syntactic and morphological proficiency. By contrast, her connected discourse still requires a great deal of work. Her decoding and reading comprehension have also improved, although she is still about 1½ to 2 years behind her Grade 8 peers in reading comprehension. Her clinician has been working on organizational techniques to improve her connected speech (in both narrative and expository genres) and her written expression.

Sample 1

In the morning, we hiked to pear lake and it took us about 3 hours to get to pear lake. While we were at Pear Lake, we walked around and around and have a little picnic.

Sample 2

My family and Yoko are going to the Grand Canyon because Yoko has not gone there before. We feel happy and Yoko feels excited. After we picked up grandma, we headed there. When we got there, we unloaded and we went on a hike. The canyon was beautiful and it looked like a big whole in the ground. We were scared that we would fall off the rim if we got to close to it. There were people on donkeys taking rides down the canyon. It was so fun.

The student in snapshot 3 has spent a great deal of time working on written expression with her SLP in collaboration with her teachers. Her ability to create and organize monologues in both spoken and written language has improved with a variety of scaffolding techniques, including questions to guide her talking and writing and visual maps such as those suggested by Singer and Bashir (2004) and Bashir and Singer (2006), among others. Her written samples show progress in the form of better "setups" (where the family is going), use of affective language (how participants "feel"), more elaboration about what is seen and done (what the canyon looks like, etc.), and some closure, albeit abrupt, to end the piece ("It was so fun"). Her intervention will continue to focus on expressing herself in connected discourse and comprehending narrative and expository text.

Language Intervention at School-Age Levels: The Basic Questions

Readers of this text probably recognize some of the students in the snapshots presented in the previous section. No doubt they could contribute additional snapshots to represent students with LLD on their caseloads. Indeed, school-age students with LLD challenge us each day we step into our respective school buildings. Creating relevant language intervention programs includes the ongoing search for "what will work" to help students survive and thrive in their classrooms. The key elements include consideration of the linguistic skills a student brings to the classroom, the requirements of the curriculum, and the classroom context itself. Assessment and intervention approaches that focus *only on the student,* omitting curricula and classroom variables, miss significant pieces of the puzzle.

A number of questions drive language intervention at school-age levels that are different from the questions that drive preschool language intervention. These questions are discussed next and summarized in Box 3-1:

1. The major question we should pose is, *What language abilities are assumed to be intact to complete academic tasks?* This question suggests that language practitioners must know something about the curriculum and the demands of the classroom to make language intervention relevant.

2. Related to the first question is the one that follows logically for SLPs and hits directly at the "what-to-do" question in language intervention: *How do language intervention choices reflect this understanding of curricula and*

| BOX 3-1 | *Questions that Drive School-Age Language Intervention* |

1. Which language abilities are assumed to be intact to complete academic tasks?
2. How do language intervention choices reflect an understanding of curricula and classroom concerns?
3. Do traditional assessment and intervention approaches account for spoken and written language reciprocity?
4. How does language intervention lead students to perform activities independently?

Summary Question
What does language intervention "look like" at school-age levels?

classroom concerns? This question suggests that working with school-age students with LLD means understanding which language abilities *underlie* academic tasks (Ehren, 2000, 2004, 2006a; Wallach & Ehren, 2004). In other words, which language patterns and behaviors are most relevant to school success and, by contrast, which might be *irrelevant?*

3. The third question involves the systemic, reciprocal nature of spoken and written systems: *Does our assessment/intervention approach account for spoken and written language reciprocity?* This question hints at the challenge facing SLPs who work on spoken language only as their focus of intervention. Is intervention that focuses solely on speaking and listening enough?

4. Last, *How does language intervention lead students to do it "on their own"?* This question raises the issue of generalization. How do we help students "take ownership" of the language skills we have facilitated when we are not "there" to be their scaffold? When do students become "strategic" (Ehren, 2000, 2003)?

In sum: *What does language intervention at school-age levels "look like"?* Its goals and objectives created and its techniques and materials used should address (and answer) the questions raised in this section.

Language Intervention and Academic Success: Which Language Abilities Are Assumed?

In this section, we return to the classroom on Monday morning. We remind ourselves that mastering the curriculum for children and adolescents with LLD is a daunting challenge. This mastery of various subjects and their content is a challenge for many of our students today, including some students without identified language disorders. In addition, the curriculum, that is, the content the student must absorb in each grade, is delivered via complex language, often in the form of expository text (Blank, 2002; Westby, 2005, 2006). As children progress through the grades, they must also demonstrate what they know in written form. One could say that to be successful in school students have to manage the "triple threat" of language proficiency: They have to comprehend and absorb new and complex information that is couched in

Triple threat of language proficiency:
1. Comprehend and absorb new and complex information...
2. ...within formal, literate styles of language...
3. ...and demonstrate that knowledge in written connected discourse.

more *formal, literate styles* of language, and demonstrate what they know in *connected discourse* that is *written*.

The school curriculum has been developed with the assumption that the children and adolescents using it have intact language (Bashir et al., 1998; see also American Speech-Language-Hearing Association, 1982, for a classic discussion). Children who are beginning their educations are assumed to have enough linguistic ability needed to perform well in classrooms as early as kindergarten. Kindergarten has become a greater challenge today than it was in the past because of its focus on more structured and academic-like endeavors. For example, in some kindergarten classrooms in California, children are involved in phonics activities that may be too complex for many 5-year-olds (e.g., blending sounds, identifying sounds, relating sounds to animal sounds and images, and completing worksheets). Including and beyond kindergarten, children must deal with the more literate and formal language of the classroom, as mentioned earlier (moving across the oral-to-literate continuum as per Chapter 2). They must also participate in various classroom activities such as shared reading groups, following directions, responding to questions, and discussing curricular topics (Bashir et al., 1998).

Much preparation for school is rooted in children's preschool experiences. Children who come to school with rich language and preliteracy experiences from their homes and preschool environments have an advantage over children who come with experiences that are not as rich and literacy intense (Boudreau, 2005; Dickinson & Tabors, 2001; van Kleeck, 1998; van Kleeck et al., 2006). Likewise, the early experiences of preschoolers with language disorders are understood today in terms of how early language disorders influence later school performance (as noted in the previous chapters). Speech-language pathologists (SLPs) and early elementary teachers should have knowledge about the communicative, linguistic, and metalinguistic abilities children bring with them to kindergarten and evaluate whether these experiences are sufficient for success. Recognizing the reciprocal relationship between spoken and written language, as well as the assumptions made about children's preschool preparation, Dickinson and Tabors (2001) wrote the following:

Children who come to school with rich language and preliteracy experiences from home and preschool have an advantage over children who have not had these experiences.

> In the past it was assumed that the primary task of children in the preschool years was exclusively language development. It was thought that children first developed language well during the years prior to schooling and then learned reading and writing when formal education began in kindergarten or first grade. With the increased availability of research on younger children..., we have come to recognize that children acquire important early literacy skills beginning at birth and that success in reading at the first grade is largely dependent on how much children have learned before they get there. (p. xv)

Thus the assumptions about what children know about language and literacy set the pace for what happens in the primary grades. As mentioned previously, children with language disorders have a particular challenge making the transition to school.

Speech and language pathologists are in the unique position by virtue of their training and expertise to complement, rather than replicate, the knowledge and expertise of their educational partners (see additional information in Chapter 4). The language intervention goals, techniques, and materials they choose for school-age students, as the questions raised earlier suggest, should start with the context that students "live in" for a good portion of their lives—school. Although not excluding the language demands at home and in life in general, in this text the focus remains on the connection between language intervention and academic demands. Thus among the questions reiterated are, What language abilities does it "take" to succeed in school? More specifically, What language abilities underlie the academic and classroom tasks students face daily? By posing these questions, SLPs can provide supportive information to teachers who may not have the background knowledge or training in language development and disorders to evaluate the language abilities, spoken and written, meta and nonmeta, that are required to complete the classroom tasks they require of their students during the school year. Likewise, SLPs may share information with their learning disability specialists and school psychologists about the "language load" of various standardized tools and programs (Wallach, 2004; see also Chapter 4).

Which language abilities are necessary to succeed in school? Which language abilities underlie academic and classroom tasks students face?

Examples of What It Takes from the Student Snapshots

The student snapshots presented at the beginning of the chapter provide examples, albeit brief, that remind us about the layers of language involved in each of these tasks. History and social studies curricula are steeped in unfamiliar and complex language content that is wrapped in sophisticated language form. And, as noted, demonstrating what one knows through the written mode is evidenced in most of the assignments and requirements of test and nontest activities (Bashir & Singer, 2006; Nelson, 2005; Scott, 2005; Singer & Bashir, 2004; Westby, 2005). We can see in all the snapshots that these students lack (or have difficulty with) some of the language skills needed to acquire the information presented in their texts and classrooms. The last student example (LA in snapshot 3) reminds us of the role of written language intervention to help her perform more effectively as a student.

But *what does "it" take* to complete assignments such as the ones sketched out in the snapshots? That is the question to which SLPs must return. Wallach and Ehren (2004) offer some answers. They point out, for example, "that a headline [in a newspaper] or title [in a textbook] can facilitate comprehension and prepare students for what might be coming up in a text *if* both language knowledge and background knowledge are available and applied to the task" (p. 46). The first title, "The Beginning of the Roman Empire," is straightforward in terms of summarizing what the chapter is about. Nonetheless, one can see how much language knowledge is "assumed" to make the title useful. By contrast, the second title, "Christopher Columbus: How History was Invented," is less direct than the first one. The students have difficulty comprehending the precise meaning of the phrase, "how history was invented." This changes the author's intent of the Christopher Columbus passage (Hennings, 1993; Wallach & Ehren, 2004). Consequently, while headlines and titles may serve as facilitative cues to the meaning in text (and may be a strategy we would like to help students acquire), practitioners must be aware of the background and linguistic savvy assumed to be intact to make them useful. Students not only have to understand the individual words (have the lexical knowledge) in the titles, but they also have to understand the figurative meanings of an author's word choices. In addition, students have to use the titles actively—asking themselves questions about the title and how it "tells" them to prepare for what might be coming up in the text; students must bring to the task their prior knowledge about the topic and, eventually, use the text to validate their hypotheses (Caccamise & Snyder, 2005; Kaderavek et al., 2004; Kintsch, 2005). The strategy of using titles to facilitate comprehension is made even more difficult when students are poor readers.

Snapshot 3, as mentioned previously, reminds clinicians and other practitioners to consider what students' written compositions say about their spoken language and metalinguistic abilities. Pointing out the different perceptions about what might be important to consider for intervention or classroom work, Wallach and Ehren (2004) wrote, "While one might be tempted to focus on the spelling, grammar, and punctuation in written language pieces, it might be more important to observe what the piece says about what a writer knows about language" (p. 47). In other words, we go back to the question of what language abilities are "assumed" to be intact in order to produce a piece of writing that is elaborated, yet concise, accurate, and interesting at the same time. LA's spoken language, while improved significantly as noted, still required work in connected discourse for both narrative and expository genres. Her abilities to plan, self-correct, and monitor her comprehension are aspects of LA's language intervention that cut across spoken and written modalities (Bashir & Singer, 2006). LA's example and the others presented in the snapshots remind SLPs and teachers that written products reflected in both narrative and expository pieces are influenced by spoken language experiences and advancing metalinguistic and metacognitive abilities (Kaderavek et al., 2004). Flipping the coin, however, we are also reminded of the two-way street concept mentioned in Chapter 1—that is, that written language proficiency also influences spoken language organization and planning.

Remember the two-way street from Chapter 1? Written language proficiency is influenced by advancing spoken language abilities, and spoken *language proficiency is, in turn, influenced by written language advancements.*

Language Abilities That Underlie School Tasks: A Key Piece of the Puzzle

Ehren (2003) asks language clinicians to think about the differences among *knowledge, skills,* and *strategies* (Box 3-2). She points out that speech and language pathologists should consider these distinctions because understanding the differences among these terms may clarify the focus we take in language intervention. Moreover, acknowledging the distinctions among knowledge, skills, and strategies may provide a clearer role definition for SLPs. *Knowledge* is the information one already has; *skills* are those actions or procedures for which you have competence; and *strategies* are approaches you use (bringing into play your knowledge and skills) in specific situations. SLPs might help students acquire the language skills needed to manage the curriculum, whereas teachers might focus more directly on the content knowledge required by the curriculum, with shades of gray in between professionals' roles, as the next chapter suggests.

BOX 3-2	*Knowledge versus Skills versus Strategies*

> **Knowledge:** Information a person already has
> **Skills:** Actions or procedures for which a person has competence
> **Strategies:** Approaches used in specific situations

Data from Ehren, B. J. (2006, October). *Curriculum-based intervention.* Workshop presented for Region 10 of the Corona-Norco Unified School System, Norco, CA.

Ehren (2003, 2006a) provides an example that brings knowledge, skills, and strategies together. She points out that paraphrasing is a popular reading comprehension strategy. Knowing that teachers might use paraphrasing activities in the classroom or that they might expect students to "have" paraphrasing as a comprehension strategy, SLPs could then ask, What language abilities are required (or are assumed to be intact) to use the paraphrasing strategy? The *knowledge* piece, writes Ehren (2003), includes having synonyms for words, and the *skills* piece includes having a repertoire of syntactic forms. Understanding the purpose of paraphrasing and knowing when to apply the strategy completes the knowledge, skills, and strategy triad.

The creation of meaningful language intervention at school-age levels starts with the question, *What language is required* to complete academic tasks? This question (and its answers) is far from the place where standardized tests live. For example, what language abilities are assumed to be intact when asking students to unravel and retain material from their core course textbooks? We saw some aspects of this question reflected in the example of the Christopher Columbus title in snapshot 2. Linguistic ability—that is, syntactic and semantic ability—and expository text knowledge are necessary to unravel the information in the Christopher Columbus chapter, not to mention skills related to fluid and automatic decoding (Blank, 2002; Butler & Venable, 2003; Troia, 2004). In addition, since connected text, like textbook language, is not just a linear sequence of strings of sentences, students must learn to appreciate what Blank (2002) calls "the hidden logic that connects the sentences so that they [understand] the text's intended meaning" (p. 156).

To understate the case would be to say that students in middle school with and without language problems are challenged by the metaphorical double-edged sword of complex content and structure as they try to absorb the information across many subjects from school textbooks (Wallach, 2004). Clinicians are also challenged by the many questions facing them as they move from school to school and class to class (Wallach & Ehren, 2004):

■ What language abilities underlie the successful completion of a math story problem?
■ What language abilities form the foundations for participating in a science project successfully?
■ What language abilities are required to edit one's work? To reorganize a composition? To debate in class?

■ What language abilities are needed to construct a writing piece that recounts events, tells an imaginary story, and lists the accomplishments of an author?

Understanding Language Expectations: What It Must Be Like to Have a Language Disorder

How can we begin to understand what it must be like to be language disordered in school and have to deal with a fast-moving and complex curriculum? We can try to imagine having a language disorder in our primary language and the language we must learn through. For example, we might think about experiences we have had trying to learn a new skill (e.g., skiing, sailing) in a "classlike" situation with a group of people and a teacher/instructor. The simulation of LLD comes home to us when we have trouble "getting it" while everyone else in the group is succeeding seemingly with ease. Now imagine taking the skiing or sailing lesson in a language (e.g., Japanese or French) with which we have limited proficiency. Clearly, the new "curriculum," plus the language through which it is delivered, presents a double-edged challenge to us. Using an example such as taking skiing lessons in Japanese reminds us of the intersection of background knowledge (how much experience have we had skiing), language abilities (how much Japanese do we bring to the lesson), and other factors (maintaining motivation, the teacher's modification of language, etc.) when faced with learning something new.

We can also understand language disorders by thinking about what it is like to comprehend, talk about, or write about a topic that is less familiar to us. For example, *what does it take* to write a piece on "the relationship between interest rates and the bond market" or "the role of free agency in baseball" if we are unfamiliar with these topics? Perhaps our linguistic knowledge (how one structures a paragraph, composition, etc.) would help us begin the task, but we would be hard pressed to write an enlightening essay without embarking on the appropriate level of research. This phase of writing an essay on an unfamiliar topic, that is, embarking on the research, encourages us to ask, yet again, *What language abilities does it take* to begin to undertake the research necessary to complete the assignment successfully? Indeed, practitioners are reminded with the examples presented in this section that there are many questions to ask about "what it takes," that is, what language is required or assumed, to underlie the tasks facing their students. Many researchers and clinicians remind us to pay close attention to both the way texts are written and what a text has to say (see also Blank, 2002; Bransford et al., 1999; Ehren, 2005; Scott & Windsor, 2000; Westby, 2005).

Blank (2002) provides another wonderful example for clinicians and teachers to consider by "creating" a language disorder. The example provided in Box 3-3 reminds teachers, SLPs, and other professionals who work with school-age students to consider not only the complexity of school texts but also the knowledge (background experiences, vocabulary, etc.) and abilities (syntactic, inferential, etc.) that are, once again, "assumed" to be intact to access, retain, and comprehend the information presented in both spoken and written texts. She presents the following excerpt from a primary school textbook. To help us understand what it might be like to "miss" the meaning, seven of the original concepts were replaced with nonsense words. In the completed

BOX 3-3 What It's Like to Have a Language Learning Disability

---

Sample Textbook Excerpt
Modified Version
Smith had made a promise. But could Turboland keep it? By 1961 some jabots had reached a few hundred kiloms up into the surrounding belt. But the glerf was almost a quarter of a million kiloms away! A trip to the glerf and back would take eight yims. By 1961 only one turbian had even been up in a jabot—and for only fifteen stashes!
(The passage continues with nonsense words substituted for key concepts.)

Original Version
Kennedy had made a promise. But could America keep it? By 1961 some rockets had flown a few hundred miles up into space. But the moon was almost a quarter of a million miles away! A trip to the moon and back would take eight days. By 1961 only one American had even been up in space—and for only fifteen minutes!

From Blank, M. (2002). Classroom discourse: A key to literacy. In K. G. Butler & E. R. Silliman (Eds.), *Speaking, reading and writing in children with language learning disabilities: New paradigms in research and practice* (p. 155). Mahwah, NJ: Lawrence Erlbaum Associates. [Original text passage from Donnelly, J. (1989). *Moonwalk: The first trip to the moon* (pp. 19–20). New York: Random House.])

---

version, a total of 17 words, or 12% of the passage, was changed, resulting in a profound effect on comprehension.

Blank's example illustrates the "language-heavy" nature of school texts. It demonstrates how even a small percentage of unknown words can influence comprehension dramatically.

The Culture of Schools Encased in Teacher Talk: More of "What It Takes"

In their classic article, Berlin and colleagues (1980) wrote that "verbally-based teaching is the medium of instruction through which all other learning is to be fostered" (p. 48). They also point out that the complexity and amount of language used in classroom settings presents students with an ongoing challenge. They go on to write what all clinicians and teachers know: "Faced with the seemingly endless flow of words, [students with language disorders] might retain only fragments of the total utterance or more likely "tune out" the auditory stream" (p. 50).

Most teachers are aware that not every student can match their expectations. Nevertheless, they bring into the classroom expectations about politeness, about how conversations are carried out, about attitudes children "should" have toward teachers and education, and about what children have experienced outside school (Creaghead, 1992; Weade & Green, 1985; Westby, 2006). These expectations influence much of what transpires in the classroom. Teachers refer to things they assume their students have experienced or about which they have knowledge. They assume students can understand classroom rules, whether spoken or not. They assume students will be able to engage in conversations within the classroom, both with the teacher and with peers. They assume students will be able to follow instructions and carry out assignments arising from these instructions. They assume that students will be able to come to class prepared with the appropriate materials and information, particularly if they have been given instruction about what constitutes "appropriate."

Beyond these basic assumptions, teachers make largely unconscious presuppositions about the type and level of language to use in teaching. Teachers make great use of rhetorical questioning in their teaching. Although there is evidence that teachers in the earlier grades modify their language according to the developmental level of their students, teachers after approximately fourth grade typically make frequent use of nonliteral language forms such as idioms, analogies, similes, sarcasm, and indirect polite forms (Blank, 2002; Nelson, 1994; Westby, 2006). Children without language disorders are able to handle some aspects of nonliteral language by age 8, but many nonliteral forms are acquired as late as 13 years old (Nippold, 1998; see Chapter 9). Students with LLD, including those represented in the snapshots at the beginning of this chapter, are especially vulnerable as language, especially classroom language, becomes more abstract.

Blank (1986) and Blank and colleagues (e.g., Blank & Marquis, 1987; Blank et al., 1994, 1995) discuss discourse in ways that may be useful to consider when evaluating the demands of classroom instruction. First, they encourage clinicians to assess the level of reasoning required by teachers' instructions. Second, they ask clinicians to evaluate teacher-student interactions.

According to Blank and colleagues (1978) and Berlin and colleagues (1980), there are four levels of discourse that can frame our interpretations of student-teacher interactions (Box 3-4). Level 1 is called *matching perception*. Matching perception demands encourage the child to focus on the immediate environment. The language is generally matched to the here and now. Demands such as "What is this?" "Point to the pencil," and "Give me the spoon" are considered Level 1 demands. Level 2 is called *selective analysis of perception*. Level 2 demands are more refined than Level 1 because the child has to focus on some more salient aspect of the environment. Questions such as "What color is the pencil?" "What's happening in the picture?" and "What shape is the bowl?" are examples of Level 2 commands. Levels 3 and 4 require thinking beyond the immediate situation. Level 3 demands are called *reordering perception*. Demands such as "Show me the ones that are not red," "Tell me what I put in the bowl before I added the eggs," and "Show me the part of the egg we don't eat" are Level 3 demands. Level 4 demands are called *reasoning about perception*. With Level 4 questions, the child must think about what could happen or what might happen. The child also has to think about cause-and-effect relations when asked Level 4 questions. Questions such as "Why is the boy wearing a raincoat?" "Why did you pick that one?" and "What will happen to the cookies when I put them in the oven?" are Level 4 examples. Discrepancies between teacher-child levels might encourage us to modify our language,

Evidence indicates that after approximately fourth grade, teachers typically make frequent use of nonliteral language forms such as idioms, analogies, similes, sarcasm, and indirect polite forms.

3

BOX 3-4	*Levels of Discourse in Teacher-Student Interactions*

Level 1: Matching Perception
These demands encourage the child to focus on his or her immediate environment.
Examples: "What is this?" "Point the pencil."

Level 2: Selective Analysis of Perception
These demands are more refined than those in Level 1; they force the child to focus on a more salient aspect of his or her environment.
Examples: "What color is the pencil?" "What shape is the bowl?"

Level 3: Reordering Perception
These demands require thinking beyond the immediate situation.
Examples: "Show me the ones that are not red." "Show me the part of the egg we don't eat."

Level 4: Reasoning about Perception
These demands require the child to think about what could or might happen and focus on cause-and-effect relations.
Examples: "Why is the boy wearing a raincoat?" "What will happen to the cookies once I put them in the oven?"

Data from Blank, M., Rose, S., & Berlin, L. (1978). *The language of learning: The preschool years.* New York: Grune & Stratton; and Berlin, L. J., Blank, M., & Rose, S. A. (1980). The language of instruction: The hidden complexities. *Topics in Language Disorders, 1,* 47–58.

Obliges: Form of classroom discussion that require a response from the student
Comments: Statements that accompany actions; no student response required

the contextual cues, or the topic so that students with LLD can succeed. We return to the concept of discourse levels in Chapters 7 and 8.

Blank and colleagues (1994, 1995), expanding on Blank (1986), discussed what they call the oblige/comment distinction in classroom discourse. The oblige/comment notion expanded on the four levels of abstraction described in the previous paragraphs. *Obliges* (such as the demands listed in the four levels of perception) require a response from the student. For example, "Why do we think history was invented when we talk about Christopher Columbus?" is a Level 4 oblige. By contrast, *comments* are statements that accompany actions (or lessons) without requiring a response from the student. "We say that history was invented when we talk about Columbus because he was not the hero we thought he was" is a Level 4 comment that might accompany a picture of Columbus coming back from the new world. The comment form exposes students to more sophisticated language, but they are not placed in an immediate failure situation because they do not have to respond. Obliges are different from comments because obliges require a response from students. Obliges that might be less complex in a Christopher Columbus lesson could include "What is Columbus doing in the picture?" (Level 2) and "What are the names of his ships?" (Level 1).

Blank (1986) suggests observing the ratio of obliges and comments that occur in a language session or a classroom lesson. She reminds us to note whether teachers are always in an oblige mode, as follows:

■ Do teachers continually ask students to respond to questions without giving them enough opportunities to initiate conversations at higher levels of discourse?

■ Do teachers' lessons include a rich variety of comment levels?

■ Is there a balance between obliges and comments, with comments being given at higher levels of discourse?

■ And, clearly, what are the assumptions made about what level of language students can manage?

Although there are many descriptions of classroom discourse and instructional language (see, e.g., Westby, 2006), Blank and colleagues have provided an interesting way for SLPs (in collaboration with teachers; see Chapter 4) to consider another piece of the curricula/classroom puzzle. Although not necessarily used widely, Table 3-1 presents a simplified version of an oblige/comment analysis that offers promise.

In more recent work, Blank (2002) reiterates a number of concepts she has refined over the years. She reminds us that the "talk of the classroom...revolves around written language; specifically the texts of the curriculum" (p. 152). In addition, she notes that students spend a great deal of time in discussions about assigned readings. The assumption, yet again, is that students come with both background knowledge and linguistic ability (both spoken and written) to engage in these activities. Presenting a number of scenarios, Blank (2002) looked at (1) the verbal concepts of text and (2) the implicit, invisible meanings in text. In the example presented earlier with the substituted words (p. 56), she writes that school language, which may occur in teacher talk or in a textbook, contains complex verbal concepts in which "words are critical to the meaning. [Moreover, words] pile on, one after another, like an avalanche of information" (p. 154). As we saw in the "moon passage," readers are able to keep up with the text's meaning because they *already know* the words that are critical to meaning (Blank, 2002). Blank (2002) adds that students

Table 3-1
Discourse Oblige and Comment Analysis Outline

Participants	Obliges	Comments
Clinician/teacher	How many obliges occur at Levels 1 to 4 during the lesson?	How many comments occur at Levels 1 to 4 during the lesson?
Child/student	How many opportunities did the child/student get to initiate Level 1 to 4 obliges?	How many Level 1 to 4 comments did the child/student make?

From Blank, M., Marquis, A. M., & Klimovitch, M. (1995). *Directing early discourse.* San Antonio, TX: Communication Skill Builders. (Based on original in Blank, M. [1986]. *Natural language exchanges and coding techniques.* Workshop presented at the Language Learning Disabilities Institute, Emerson College, Boston, MA.)

must also manage the implicit, invisible meanings in text. This means that listeners and readers must pull together what they hear or read by linking sentences together, making inferences (reading between the lines), and monitoring comprehension along the way (see also Caccamise & Snyder, 2005; Kaderavek et al., 2004).

Blank (2002) provides another classic example of classroom language. It is from a junior high school social studies class. With the excerpt that follows, she provides a glimpse of teacher talk that includes both complex concepts and implicit meaning. She notes that the teacher's language is less direct (in terms of what she wants) than it could be. Nonetheless, students have to negotiate the sometime "implicitness" of classroom discourse to succeed.

Teacher: OK, current events. Glenn?
Student: Pablo Casals, the well-known cellist died at the age of 96.
Teacher: OK, shush, Jim?
Student: The war in the Middle East is still going on.
Teacher: Is it going on in the same way? Frank?
Student: Egypt asked the Syrians to intervene. They want a security meeting or a quick meeting of the U.N. Security Council.
Teacher: OK. For what reason? Do you know? Anyone know why Egypt has called a meeting of the Security Council of the U.N.? What has the Security Council just initiated?
Student: A cease fire.
Teacher: A cease fire. So what is Egypt claiming?
Student: Israel violated...
Teacher: Israel violated the cease fire. And what is Israel claiming?
(Blank, 2002; original from Peshkin, 1978, p. 102)

Blank (2002) points out that the topic for discussion (the Middle East situation) is not explicitly stated. It becomes clear as the teacher's feedback evolves. It is "assumed" that Glenn has figured out that his response about Pablo Casals was incorrect at this time for this discussion. This awareness may or may not be in Glenn's repertoire. A more explicit way to let students know what is wanted might be to say something like the following: "Our next activity is current events. We are going to discuss the latest developments in the Middle East." But, clearly, both the verbal concepts that fill classroom discussions and the implicit nature of classroom discourse and texts provide two great challenges for students with language disorders. Think back to the challenges facing JG (snapshot 1, p. 46) in his Grade 7 classroom.

There are many factors within the classroom context that influence the creation and delivery of language intervention programs at school-age levels. Teachers' expectations about what children know and the language they use to teach new concepts also have a tremendous effect on students' performances. Many subtle communicative rules, both social and academic, underlie classroom exchanges. Weade and Green (1985) formulated several questions as additional guidelines for classroom observations; these are outlined in Box 3-5.

Thus language intervention at school-age levels requires that SLPs take into consideration both the language of the curriculum in particular and the

BOX 3-5   *Weade and Green's Guidelines for Classroom Observations*

1. What are the personal frames of reference students might bring to the lesson that might influence their participation (books they have read or been exposed to, television shows they might know, cultural experiences, etc.)?
2. What will be the social and academic expectations for participation (formal lesson format, game, more casual conversational format)?
3. How will the group be organized (whole group doing one lesson, one group doing math, another doing reading, different group levels)?
4. How will turn-taking procedures be organized (bid for turns by raising hands, respond in unison)?
5. What forms of response are required (name the word, say the number, complete the sentence, produce a monologue)?
6. What frames of reference for completing the lesson will be shared by teacher and students (the same way we did the lesson the last time)? Which students did not get it the last time?

From Weade, R., & Green, J. L. (1985). Talking to learn: Social and academic requirements of classroom participation. *Peabody Journal of Education, 62,* 16.

language and culture of school in general. Westby (2006) provides a reminder of the expectations that change at each grade level. Box 3-6 summarizes some of the challenges facing children as they move through the grades.

In a number of the chapters that follow, student, teacher, and curricula interactions will be explored further. In the next section of this chapter, we ask the following question: How does knowing what we know about the language skills and abilities that underlie school performance influence the intervention choices we make about "what to do"?

Helping Students Access the Curriculum and Instructional Language: Thinking about "What To Do"

Ehren's (2003, 2006a), Blank's (2002), and Wallach and Ehren's (2004) examples, among others from the literature, remind practitioners that meaningful language intervention connects the linguistic skills and abilities students "bring with them" to the realities and expectations of school. When students lack or have difficulty with language, we must recognize how these difficulties "play out" in the classroom. Those of us, such as SLPs, who work (or have worked) traditionally "outside" classrooms now recognize that we must understand the expectations that set the tone for academic learning. In addition to absorbing the information set by each grade's curriculum and state standards, students must learn to manage the sometimes fast-moving language of teachers and the social nuances attached to learning within a dynamic and ever-changing group situation.

In part, we have begun to answer the "what-to-do" question. Developing meaningful language intervention programs (i.e., what school-age intervention should look like) includes asking the relevant questions about the language

<table>
<tr><td>**BOX 3-6**</td><td>*Expectations at Three Different Grade Levels*</td></tr>
</table>

Preschool
- Language is related to arriving and going home
- Participates in "show and tell"
- Sits while being read to and answers story questions
- Has many of Berlin and colleagues' (1980) discourse skills (at least Levels 1 and 2; see also Box 3-4)
- Has conversational and some school language (early "meta") ready for school

Primary Grade (Grade 1 focus)
- Tells/retells stories and events in logical order
- Expresses ideas in a variety of complete sentences
- Completes homework
- Creates rhyming words
- Sounds out words when reading
- Stays on topic and takes turns in conversation

Secondary Grade
- Completes oral reports
- Completes written reports
- Follows teacher lectures
- Takes notes
- Works with peers
- Participates in class discussions
- Manages spoken-written expository text

Modified from Westby, C. E. (2006). There's more to passing than knowing the answers: Learning to do school. In T. A. Ukrainetz (Ed.), *Contextualized language intervention* (pp. 319–387). Eau Claire, WI: Thinking Publications; and Creaghead, N. A. (2002). Healthcare and school service: More coalitions and collaborations. *The ASHA Leader, 7*(4), 35; see also ASHA, 2005.

abilities that underlie school requirements. As Wallach and Miller (1988) noted, the questions are formulated and modified by a continuous evaluation of how our language intervention goals fit in with the student's real world. As asked in Chapter 1, "How does this syntax lesson, metaphor unit, auditory discrimination activity, or word-naming exercise relate to Monday morning in the classroom?" To move on from the initial question, school-based practitioners may "go" to several sources of information to find some of the answers to the complex questions that drive school-age language intervention.

Intervention as a Complex Balance of Many Variables: Chewing Gum and Walking at the Same Time

The quote by Lahey and Bloom (1994) that opens this chapter hints at a way to begin to evaluate the variables one must consider (or control) when attempting to help students acquire new linguistic skills. As discussed throughout this text, we know that students with LLD are overwhelmed when content, form, and language use come together to create a tidal wave of complexity. Intervention choices include decisions about which piece of language (or context) to "control" so that our students can "experiment" with new and more difficult language demands (Lahey & Bloom, 1994). As the Lahey and Bloom (1994) quote suggests, if our goal is to have students write longer and more coherent texts, we might *start* with topics with which they have significant background knowledge and experience. If we want to help students become more "meta" about stories—for example, by identifying and organizing stories into their various components (setting, theme, plot)—we should use familiar narratives initially. Likewise, if we are asking students to comprehend an expository passage, we might present that passage with a great deal of contextual support (e.g., pictures, prereading discussion, visual map). Indeed, language intervention, unlike school, should provide students with the intense and specialized help they need (Ehren, 2000). Making choices that provide students with ways to "get" the language they need includes understanding which variables to manipulate across time.

Lahey and Bloom (1994) talk about language processing as a limited capacity system (see also Caccamise & Snyder, 2005; DeKemel, 2003c; and Snyder et al., 2002, for more detailed discussions). They say that when the system is strained, for example, when students are faced with complex content (e.g., the Roman Empire, Christopher Columbus's true character) embedded in complex language forms (unfamiliar vocabulary, expository text), something has to "give." Faced with complexity or difficulty on all sides, trade-offs in performance will occur.

Using a wonderful example of learning to drive a manual shift car, Lahey and Bloom (1994) clarify limited capacity/competing resources concepts. This example also helps us to think about the difference between doing something automatically (without much effort) and doing something requiring a lot of effort. For example, many people learning to drive a stick shift car (something we often have to do in Europe) have trouble steering, using the pedals and clutch, and shifting at the same time. Indeed, few beginners (we hope) would even think about talking on a cell phone during the learning period. However, after drivers become more proficient at shifting gears so that all the movements involved in shifting and steering are automatic, resources are "freed" from all the focus and concentration needed for the driving itself. At this point, cell phones are likely to reappear (especially in California, where people seem to drive and talk on their phones all the time). Many of our students with LLD are faced with too many demands competing for resources and not enough "freed space." Since language is already an issue requiring more effort, that is, more resources and energy, one can see why it may be difficult to do all the things required in the classroom.

What is also fascinating about Lahey and Bloom's take on the limited capacity/competing resources concept is that it helps clinicians to consider some of the variability (sometimes called "inconsistency") in students' performances. Lahey and Bloom (1994) ask clinicians to think about the

When students with LLD are faced with complex content embedded in complex language forms, something has to "give" because their resources are strained.

"synergistic interaction of several processes with each other, with context, and with the material to be processed rather than emphasizing a specific ability" (p. 355). Thus looking at the changes in contextual support, the specific nature of the tasks at hand, and the language required for participation and success come into play in both assessment and intervention. Language intervention includes making choices about which aspect of language to teach, as well as how to balance the resources that may be competing for a student's focus (see also Snyder et al., 2002).

In addition to the concept of a limited capacity mechanism in language, Lahey and Bloom (1994) discuss the related concept of mental models and language performance. They point out that we construct and hold in mind mental representations (mental models) that underlie the expression and comprehension of language. The more we hold in memory, that is, the stronger our mental models are, the less support we need from external sources to "trigger" thoughts or ideas. For example, a 5-year-old with language disorders may be able to tell a simple story such as the *Three Bears* as long as the pages of the book are in front of him. In other words, his mental model (or story frame) may not be as stable as it will be as he develops and has more experience and familiarity with the story. As his mental model strengthens for the *Three Bears* story (and for story structure in general), the same child should be able to tell the story without the picture book. In other words, he can generate a mental model of the story from memory, rather than from external sources. Lahey and Bloom (1994) point out that the concept of mental models relates to children's move from "here and now" talk to "there and then" communication. They summarize the implications for intervention and remind clinicians to be cautious about their goals and recommendations, as follows:

> The important point is that both familiarity of content and the strength of contextual cues influence the ease of constructing a mental model. Strength or usefulness of contextual cues could vary with the child (e.g., pictures may help one child but constrain or hinder another...). Intuition might suggest that retelling a story would be easier for a child than making up a new story [but the results] will depend upon how easy it was for a child to develop a mental model from the original presentation of the story...For a familiar story, this may be easy, but for an unfamiliar story, it may be a very difficult task. (Lahey & Bloom, 1994, p. 360)

Lahey and Bloom's chapter is an excellent resource for speech and language pathologists. It brings to life and makes accessible many complex concepts from information processing theory and language disorders. We will return to these concepts throughout this text.

Viewing Language on a Continuum: Revisiting a Framework

Westby (2000b) provides a framework for assessment that works well for intervention (Figure 3-1). The framework also helps to operationalize some of Lahey and Bloom's (1994) concepts. Although Westby (2000b) relates the concepts in her framework to culturally and linguistically different students, the framework is very useful for students with LLD. She says that clinicians should be aware of the language activities they choose in terms of how they vary in task demands and the contextual support present.

Westby's Four Quadrants

Cognitively Undemanding

Exchanges greetings
Uses language to request and
   command
Carries on conversation
Follows spoken directions with
   contextual supports
Describes classroom objects and
   persons
Gives directions to peers

Relates personal experiences
Talks about familiar topics
   without contextual support
Reads notes, signs, directions
Writes from direction
Answers questions about stories/text,
   with familiar content

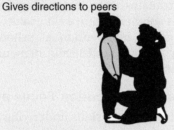

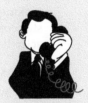

Context-Embedded	**Context-Reduced**

Follows directions for academic
   tasks
Understands contextualized
   academic content
Talks about less familiar topics with
   contextual support

Understands lectures on academic
   content
Uses language to predict, reason,
   analyze, synthesize, evaluate
Tells/writes imaginary stories
Tells/writes explanations, persuasions
Engages in deductive thought
   experiments

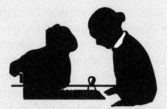

Cognitively Demanding

Figure 3-1 ■ A framework for language assessment and intervention. *(Redrawn from Westby, C. E. [2000]. Multicultural issues in speech and language assessment. In J. B. Tomblin, H. L. Morris, & D. C. Spriestersbach [Eds.], Diagnosis in speech-language pathology [2nd ed., pp. 35–62]. San Diego, CA: Singular Publishing Group.)*

For example, Westby (2000b) says that very familiar and undemanding tasks or activities (those that Lahey and Bloom [1994] would say have strong mental models and are at more automatic levels) require little or less active thinking. These are tasks the child/student has mastered. By contrast, unfamiliar and demanding tasks, such as many academic tasks, require more active involvement. If one goes *across* the Westby quadrants, one sees that the tasks at the top are considered less demanding whereas the tasks at the bottom are considered more demanding. Adding the contextual variable to the mix, we go *from top to bottom*, noting that the left side of the quadrant contains tasks that are contextually embedded or supported whereas the right side of the quadrant contains tasks that are contextually reduced. Westby's four-quadrant model is another resource clinicians can consult in the decision-making process. Language intervention at school-age levels should help students handle many of the linguistically demanding and context-reduced activities of quadrant four.

Choosing a Language Intervention Focus and Sequence

Once we understand the language skills underlying academic tasks along with the linguistic demands of curricula and instructional language, the challenge facing us is making a decision about which aspects and sequences will form a student's language intervention program. In this age of evidence-based practice (EBP), we are still learning about "what to do" and how to do it effectively. We certainly know much more than we knew as recently as a decade ago. Nonetheless, decisions about what to do may vary from clinician to clinician, as noted in Chapter 1. For example, one speech-language clinician might decide that because a student such as JG (our student from snapshot 1) has word-naming and word-retrieval problems, she will focus on spoken language production for the next few weeks. JG's teacher might decide that his bigger problem is poor word recognition/decoding for reading. She will focus on JG's phonics program. Ideally, clinician and teacher should question themselves about the priorities involved in their choices, as well as communicate with one another about the connection or reciprocity between JG's "two" problems (see Chapter 4). They should also be thinking about naming/retrieval difficulties that interfere with JG's ability to "get" the content of the curriculum. JG's teacher and SLP should also consider which metacognitive and metalinguistic strategies will facilitate language and learning (e.g., Bashir & Singer, 2006). As will be seen in JG's language intervention goals later on in the chapter (see Box 3-7), his current SLP combined text and word-finding and analysis strategies with decoding and meta activities. Spoken and written language activities were also combined in his language intervention goals and objectives.

Decisions about which aspects of language to facilitate are never easy to make. The first step is to view the curriculum and the classroom as a backdrop for intervention. As we look to the language abilities students bring (or do not bring) to school, we must remember to get beneath that proverbial tip of the iceberg mentioned in Chapter 1. Indeed, we must try to keep the horizon in mind while, at the same time, we evaluate the relevance of our goals and

Creating meaningful language intervention involves both *inside* (individual language skills) and *outside* (task demands, materials, techniques, contexts) endeavors.

objectives for communicative competence and classroom learning. And, as Nelson (1998) points out, we must also consider what students *can* do, as well as what we think they *cannot* do. Lahey and Bloom's (1994) work, among others, including Nelson's (2005) recent works, remind us that creating meaningful language intervention is an *inside* (student's language skills)–*outside* (task demands, materials, techniques, contexts) endeavor.

As we know, research from many different fields may provide guidelines about the significant language and meta acquisitions that influence school success. Information about task complexity provides another knowledge source for developing intervention techniques and sequences. In addition, the role of background knowledge and how to help students acquire and *use* background knowledge cannot be minimized (Alan Kamhi, personal communication, 2006). As practitioners we must use each of these pieces of information with caution, considering available data about evidence-based practices as they become available (Hegde & Maul, 2006). We cannot "give" our students with LLD everything they need to know, but we are able to help them acquire knowledge by helping them acquire the linguistic skills and strategies that may override the specifics of any classroom lesson or intervention session (Ehren, 2000, 2003, 2006a). But, to state what may be an obvious point, we must also remember to keep in mind the heterogeneity that exists in children and adolescents with and without LLD, the very long and gradual nature of language acquisition, and the complexity involved in learning new things.

Can the Language Development Literature (and Other Research-Based Literature) Provide Guidelines for Intervention?

We have talked a great deal about understanding expectations in this chapter. The curriculum at each grade level and the expectations therein provide information about some of the challenges facing our students. Likewise, the other suggestions presented in this chapter, such as Westby's four-quadrant model, also help us to develop frameworks for language intervention. The example presented next is more specific because it focuses on sentence comprehension. Originally presented by Wallach and Miller (1988), the example that follows is used here for three reasons:

1. It demonstrates how a clinician's knowledge of language learning (or cognitive) sequences can be another way to evaluate and develop language intervention choices.
2. Practicing clinicians often include sentence-level work in their therapy sessions.
3. Sentence processing as an area of study—and processing in general—is widely misunderstood among school-based clinicians.

Although the study of sentence comprehension became a bit obscured as the focus of research shifted to connected text, syntactic proficiency and sentence processing remain important aspects of language proficiency (Eisenberg, 2006; see Chapter 8 for additional information). In terms of one misunderstanding that exists, the processing of complex sentences involves more than "counting clauses."

As noted in Chapter 1, the notion of creating an intervention sequence that progresses from "one-step," to "two-step," to "three step" commands, and so on, simplifies processing into a linear event (like beads on a string), ignores the influence of content and context on processing, and omits consideration of the dynamics of the capacity/resource notions discussed earlier (Wallach, 2003; Wallach & Madding, 2005).

Sentence Comprehension

Some General Points. In the preschool period, children are highly dependent on extralinguistic cues, such as facial expression and context, to understand what they hear. When language occurs in a context-heavy environment, it is generally easier to understand. Thus, if a mother is cooking and says "Mommy is cooking" (a Level 1 comment according to Blank et al., 1994), the child has the benefit of context to comprehend what Mom is saying. When the language and the context are different, comprehension tends to be more difficult. Thus, if, while cooking, the mom says "The Lakers won last night," the language and the context are unmatched. One has to attend to "the language itself" to get the message. Clearly, younger children and some children with LLD are more comfortable in contextualized language situations. They use the context to figure out what people are saying. Younger children are also oriented toward "probable events." They are "semantically oriented." That is, preschoolers use their knowledge of the world and logic to figure out what things mean (Owens, 2005; van Kleeck, 1994). Adults visiting foreign countries where they cannot speak the language also use contextually based and semantically oriented strategies. They look at other cues such as facial and gestural cues, as well as what's going on in the situation, and make "educated guesses" about what people are saying. (See Chapter 5 for a detailed discussion of language comprehension and auditory processing.)

As children age and advance toward kindergarten, they get better at listening to key words, piecing the words together, and making some accurate guesses about connections. These are good *strategies.* Young children pay little attention to the actual word order or structure of sentences unless there is a specific reason to do so (e.g., there is a communication breakdown). As children approach school age and move into the early elementary grades, they develop a more heightened awareness of word order and sentence structure. In addition, as they begin to read, they become more "meta" about their language. Older children, not as dependent on semantically oriented strategies, pay attention to word order, sentence structures, and smaller linguistic units (e.g., conjunctions, prepositions) to make sense out of what they are hearing. School-age children are more structurally oriented than preschool children and they are more proficient at handling language that is decontextualized. Students with LLD must also make these language transitions from semantically oriented strategies to structurally based strategies and from contextualized to decontextualized language.

Some Classics from the Psycholinguistic Literature. Consider the passive sentence, "The pictures are being painted by the artist." A passive sentence is generally more difficult structurally/syntactically than an active sentence, for example, "The artist is painting the pictures." If both sentences are closely matched to the context in which they are spoken, however, they might be processed equally well. For example, suppose the passive sentence was used by a speaker to a child while walking through an art show (as the child and the speaker watch an artist). In this case, the spoken sentence is matched to the situation. The sentence's somewhat confusing word order (pictures-painted-artist) is less important than the context and the extralinguistic cues that accompany it (such as gesture). When sentences (and other aspects of language) are taken out of context or have less contextual support, comprehension "correctness" may change. For example, asking children to manipulate objects or point to pictures to demonstrate comprehension takes the language out of context and is, consequently, a more decontextualized task.

Classic studies such as those by Bever and others from the 1970s and 1980s (e.g., Bever, 1970; Daneman & Carpenter, 1983) have provided information about sentence comprehension and the strategies that children use, especially when sentences are less bound by context. More recent works have added to the database (e.g., Gorrell, 1998; Montgomery, 1995, 2000, 2002). Bever (1970) (and discussed by Owens, 2005) talked about some of the predominant strategies that appear in child studies. One predominant comprehension strategy is what Bever (1970) and others called a *word-order strategy*. Thus a passive sentence such as "The dog is chased by the cat" could be interpreted as "The dog chases the cat," if a word order strategy (dog-chase-cat) were employed. A word order strategy involves interpreting the noun-verb-noun as if it were the actor-action-recipient of the sentence. Unlike the passive sentence presented earlier, "The pictures are being painted by the artist," which has a semantic constraint (artists can paint pictures but pictures cannot paint artists), the dog/cat sentence cannot be "second-guessed" on a semantic basis alone. Dogs and cats can both be "doers" of the chase action in the sentence. To reiterate: Research tells us that in the earlier phases of development, children are more comfortable with "second-guessing" what they hear, using semantically based strategies that are rooted in context or world knowledge (Owens, 2005; van Kleeck, 1994). As they move through the early school years, children's syntactic strategies are refined, partially due to metalinguistic advances, as well as advances in reading and writing (van Kleeck, 1994). Eventually, of course, children must become aware of the smaller linguistic units such as *by, or, if,* and so on that change meaning (Wallach & Ehren, 2004).

Studies of complex (two-clause) sentences provide clinicians with additional information and shed light on the "one-step," "two-step," "three-step" command dilemma. Sentences such as "Brush your teeth before you go to bed" and "Pick up the plane before you pick up the block" represent word order and meaning matches. The order in which one says the sentences follows the order of events. An *order-of-mention strategy* means the order one hears in the clauses is the order one follows in interpreting the sentence. Sentences such as "Before you go to bed, brush your teeth" and "Before you pick up the block, pick up the plane" represent word order and meaning mismatches. The order in which one says the sentences violates the order of events. Reversing the word order in the brush/teeth sentence, for example, "Before you go to bed brush your teeth," should not make

An *order-of-mention strategy* means that the order in which the clauses of the sentence appear is the order in which those events happen.

the sentence tremendously difficult because of its *real-world relevance* and *routine* that usually accompanies the utterance. The block/plane sentence becomes quite difficult when word and clause order are reversed because there is no real-world relevance attached to the sentence. In addition, the spoken or written word order is the opposite of the order of events. Other issues such as clause order also influence comprehension (see Chapter 8).

Many of the intervention choices for school-age students with language disorders focus on students' processing difficulties. Although individual sentence processing is only one of the aspects to consider, the examples remind us to look at some of the approaches children use when attempting to comprehend spoken and written sentences. Rather than counting clauses as a measure of success or as an intervention goal, consider the principles gleaned from the research. One principle informs us that children use semantically oriented strategies when they are younger. They are also more dependent on context to disambiguate messages. The second principle informs us that children progress from almost exclusive use of semantically oriented strategies to use of more structurally and syntactically oriented strategies. As children advance linguistically, they learn that one speaks to one's teacher differently from the way one speaks to peers. They learn to take others' perspectives, and they learn how to handle language away from context. Among the sentence processing strategies used are the following:

1. Use contextual cues to get the message.
2. Try word-order and order-of-mention strategies to get the meaning.
3. Use probable events strategies to "second-guess" word order.

Although these strategies may be helpful in certain situations, students also must learn when to reject or modify strategies.

From Theory to Practice: An Example. How can we begin to translate the information from the comprehension literature into a language intervention plan? Wallach and Miller (1988) originally presented a template in the form of a cover sheet that would serve as a guideline for clinicians. It would develop into a more detailed intervention session or sessions. The cover sheet presented in Figure 3-2 (which might ultimately be in the clinician's head) represents an understanding of what we are doing and why we are doing it. In other words, each clinician might ask the following questions that underpin language intervention decisions:

■ Is there a theoretical base for my decision to focus on an aspect of language and to present it in a particular sequence?
■ What type of language/cognitive strategy is involved in the choice?
■ What am I trying to help the student accomplish? Am I working on contextualized or decontextualized language?
■ Does this language skill have anything to do with the curriculum or the classroom?
■ Is there evidence for the practice employed?

The next step would be to convert this information into an actual language intervention session (or sessions). The clinician might choose to use complex sentences (such as *before/after* sentences, among others) as her stimuli. She might find the sentences in the student's history or social studies texts (using the curriculum as a backdrop). But she has made a decision that this work at the

COVER SHEET FOR SEMANTIC-SYNTACTIC COMPREHENSION UNIT: SENTENCE PROCESSING LEVEL

Theoretical Principle(s):

A. Children move from semantically oriented strategies to syntactically oriented strategies.

B. Children move from word order and order-of-mention strategies to an understanding that word order/clause order does not always lead directly to meaning.

Type of Strategy:

Focus on word order and order of mention. Student uses strategy across subject areas; shows knowledge of modifying strategy.

"Level" of Language:

Decontextualized and metalinguistic (language is taken out of context; e.g., student is manipulating objects, pointing to pictures, discussing strategy, etc.)

Clinician Questions:

1) Why has this aspect of language been chosen?
2) Is it appropriate for student's language and metacognitive/metalinguistic level?
3) How do I modify or change the plan (the level of scaffolding) as needed?
4) Have I accounted for competing resources?
5) How is the language session related to (and integrated with) classroom activities and the curriculum?

Figure 3-2 ■ Cover sheet used to guide clinicians to ask questions about what they have chosen to focus on in language intervention and why.

"micro" or sentence level is relevant. It has to be "brought back" to the context of the classroom and the curriculum. This focus might be taken to introduce the student to more literate forms of language. It might help the student develop more grammatically proficient written language (at the sentence level). It is always important to recognize that this kind of activity may be completely irrelevant and inappropriate for some students. The cover sheet for the lesson helps the clinician to begin to specify more precisely the goals for each student. The cover sheet also helps us to evaluate our intervention decisions.

A Phonemic Segmentation Cover Sheet. Most speech and language professionals, other specialists, and teachers are aware of the role that phonological awareness plays in early literacy experiences and reading acquisition (see Troia, 2004). We will return to this topic later in the text (see Chapters 5, 8, and 9). A sample cover sheet for this aspect of language and metalinguistic ability reminds clinicians to continue to be analytical, research oriented, and evidence based about their choices (Figure 3-3). Although phonological awareness

---

COVER SHEET FOR A PHONEMIC SEGMENTATION UNIT: INDIVIDUAL SOUND LEVEL

Theoretical Principle:
Children appreciate larger units of speech before they are able to break up speech into its component parts. Children move from phrase, to word, to syllable, to sound segmentation abilities.

Type of Strategy:
Analytical; phonemic (break words into sounds)

"Level" of Language:
Metalinguistic (focus on manipulating sounds of the language)

Clinician/Educator Questions:
1) Why have segmentation activities been chosen?
2) Is the student ready for this <u>phonemic</u> level of speech segmentation?
3) Am I prepared to back up and do word/syllable activities if the student has difficulty with sound segmentation?
4) Are the segmentation activities related to the student's reading/writing program?
5) Can the segmentation activities be integrated into word knowledge, narrative, and other meaningful language/classroom activities?
6) Am I keeping the focus on comprehension and the purpose of reading clear to the student?
7) Are the words chosen for the segmentation activities with the student's naming repertoire? Is the vocabulary related to curricula/content areas?

Figure 3-3 ■ Cover sheet used to guide clinicians involved in language intervention for phonemic segmentation.

activities of all types have become a very popular route, we must evaluate the when, how, and why of our choices.

The Questions Continue: Keeping Language Intervention at School-Age Levels Systemic, Strategic, and Relevant

This chapter has provided a brief overview of various ways to think about language intervention at school-age levels. The themes introduced in this chapter will be weaved throughout this text. In the next chapter, we will explore some of the shared responsibilities of team members and highlight some of the differences between teaching curricula content and providing therapeutic language intervention (Ehren, 2000) and creating a balance between these two prongs of language learning and academic success. In chapters that follow we will also review some of the classic mistakes we sometimes make in intervention. For now, the following questions continue to be raised:

For language...
■ Why have I chosen to work on a particular aspect of language?
■ How does my choice relate to classroom discourse? To academic performance?

- Which sequence will I follow?
- How will I combine spoken and written aspects of language?
- Am I trying to facilitate the first layer (spontaneous) or the second layer (metalinguistic) of language?
- What are the verbal (and nonverbal) demands of the lesson?
- Are my instructions making the demands explicit for the student?
- Am I moving the student from the oral side to the literate side of the continuum?

For tasks and techniques...

- Are the tasks chosen appropriate?
- Am I trying to do too many things at once, overloading the student with too many demanding tasks couched in unfamiliar and new content?
- Have I given the student too little information or the appropriate information (or scaffolding)?
- Are the materials making the task easier or more difficult for the student to perform well?
- How much inferencing does the task/lesson require?
- Am I balancing the linguistic and the nonlinguistic demands of the task so that the student's learning strengths are utilized most efficiently?

Pulling the Pieces Together

Another Example from the Literature. Table 3-2 and Box 3-7 relate to our student, JG. He is the 14-year-old adolescent presented in snapshot 1 at the

Text cont'd on p. 77

Table 3-2
Ellis' Revised Thinking About "Watering-Up" Curricula for Students with Language Learning Disabilities

Goals of "Watered-Up" Curriculum	Ideas from Ellis (1997)	JG's Intervention*
1. More emphasis on *constructing* knowledge. (*JG fails to use knowledge he has or revise thoughts based on incoming knowledge.*)	Knowledge and understanding of facts is relative, not static. Students need to learn how to revise and delete information using background information plus text.	Activities work toward activating prior knowledge. Prepare JG for what's coming up in text; use K-W-L technique.†
2. Think *depth of comprehension,* less superficial coverage.	Facilitation of quality of deep knowledge structures ("core ideas") rather than	Keep the "bigger picture" of text in mind. Link activities across macro-micro components.

*This summary is only a partial look at JG's language intervention program. It is used to demonstrate how we may apply concepts from the literature to help students with LLD thrive in their classrooms. Ellis's (1997) idea of "watering up" the curriculum is a powerful one.
†The K-W-L technique refers to Ogle's (1986) three column graphic organizer that encourages students to monitor their comprehension along three dimensions: (1) what I *know* (K), (2) what I *want* to know (W), and (3) what I *learned* (L). (See Box 3-7, p. 77, for additional information.)

Continued

Table 3-2
Ellis' Revised Thinking About "Watering-Up" Curricula for Students with Language Learning Disabilities—cont'd

Goals of "Watered-Up" Curriculum	Ideas from Ellis (1997)	JG's Intervention*
(JG tends to focus on irrelevant facts instead of main ideas.)	quantity of content is stressed. Factual details should be taught if essential to understanding core concepts.	JG is led with questions and other scaffolds to see how new information connects to his real-life experiences.
3. Focus on *archetype* (broad) *concepts, patterns, and strategies,* such as problem-solution intent and connections and cause-effect relations. *(JG has difficulty recognizing the use of "larger" concepts or underlying structure to comprehend text and create solutions to problems.)*	Graphic organizers and other visual and mapping supports can help facilitate understanding of "larger" patterns of text and the ability to conceptualize relationships and to solve problems.	Practice with expository text structures before reading helps JG recognize the author's facilitate comprehension of content. Archetype concepts in text structure relate to real-world situations in JG's life.
4. Consider ways to encourage student *elaboration of ideas.* *(JG requires scaffolding and help with elaborated language to understand core concepts.)*	Starting with one's own words to explore topics is recommended; work toward helping students acquire paraphrasing and summarization strategies for comprehension.	Client and clinician role-play with elaborated language, meta work, and cloze procedures for lexical development and proficient decoding. JG has to acquire the underlying language skills that "lead to" paraphrasing and summarization abilities.
5. Keep the horizon of *developing more effective habits of mind,* higher-order thinking and information processing, and learning strategies in mind. *(JG has underdeveloped meta skills; he has difficulty making semantic connections.)*	Thinking skills should be thought of as having equal importance as content being taught in the curriculum.	JG uses several graphic organizers to monitor thinking and approaches he will take to complete tasks. Focus on when and why certain organizers (and other strategies) are used. Color-coding is used to identify main ideas, facts, and details while reading and for prewriting.

Modified from Ellis, E. (1997). Watering up the curriculum for students with disabilities: Goals of the knowledge dimension. *Remedial and Special Education, 18,* 326–347; and Christie, J. (2006, November). Report prepared for CD 669C, *Child Language Clinic.* Long Beach, CA: Department of Communicative Disorders, California State University at Long Beach.

BOX 3-7

Sample of Selected Language Intervention Goals and Objectives for JG

Goal 1*

JG will apply the K-W-L Plus (Carr & Ogle, 1987) model (what I *know*, what I *want* to know, what I *learned*) to expository text to facilitate his ability to comprehend and organize the text, as follows:

  Objective 1: JG will outline at least three "what I know" ideas about a familiar topic presented in an expository text format.

  Objective 2: JG will generate at least three "what I want to know" questions about a familiar topic presented in an expository text format.

  Objective 3: JG will indicate three "what I learned" concepts about a familiar topic (from selected materials) presented in an expository text format.

  Objective 4: JG will use a graphic organizer to outline the key elements of a familiar topic (the title, the main idea, the supporting details) to prepare for writing a report on the topic and to integrate the K-W-L pieces of known and new information.

Curricular materials are used as the goals are modified to move to less familiar and more difficult topics. Subtypes of expository text are fleshed out as well. Compare-contrast, problem-solution, and cause-effect texts are among the subgenres used in intervention (see Goal 5).

Goal 2

JG will apply self-monitoring strategies (including self-questioning and word awareness strategies) to facilitate his ability to check comprehension and integrate word knowledge and discourse structure in narrative text, as follows:

  Objective 1: JG will use lexical analysis techniques to comprehend the way titles relate to corresponding text in personal and imaginative narrative text.

  Objective 2: JG will apply "K" knowledge (K-W-L above) to narrative text themes using clues about the narrative with the clinician (exploiting background knowledge).

  Objective 3: JG will identify story grammar elements from familiar passages in a narrative text. The main elements of focus will be identifying the main characters, their problems, and the resolution.

  Objective 4: JG will select key vocabulary words and phrases that relate to the elements of a narrative.

  Objective 5: JG will practice self-questioning strategies to promote understanding of the key content words of a passage.

  Objective 6: JG will monitor himself as he reads a narrative passage (by evaluating whether he understands what he is reading using practiced strategies).

Intervention moves from more familiar to less familiar content; see Goal 3.

*Goals and objectives are presented to highlight some of the main areas covered with JG. Some of the specific techniques and materials used are covered in later chapters of the text. It should be noted that successful outcomes are not viewed from a criterion-referenced perspective that puts a percentage correct on each objective within the clinic (e.g., "JG will perform at 80% level correct"). Rather, success is evaluated across intervention sessions and within classroom and curricular contexts. Outcomes are also measured in terms of "events" (e.g., JG's discourse structures demonstrate the addition of various elements such as the story elements within a narrative or the number and type of arguments within a persuasive piece). The SLP and JG's teachers work within a strong collaborative framework (see the summary section within this box).

Continued

BOX 3-7

Sample of Selected Language Intervention Goals and Objectives for JG—cont'd

Goal 3
JG will demonstrate comprehension of unfamiliar text at the paragraph level. He will use contextual (guess from surrounding words) and word-specific strategies (e.g., decode and look up meaning) to find the meanings of unknown words for comprehension of narrative and expository text, as follows:

  Objective 1: JG will read *sentences* from an unfamiliar *narrative text* and will answer wh- questions with verbal prompting and utilization of a dictionary to facilitate his comprehension of the text.

  Objective 2: JG will read *paragraphs* from an unfamiliar *narrative text* and will answer wh- questions with verbal prompting and utilization of a dictionary to facilitate his comprehension of the text.

  Objective 3: JG will read *sentences* from an unfamiliar *expository text* and will answer wh- questions with verbal prompting and utilization of a dictionary to facilitate his comprehension of the text.

  Objective 4: JG will read *paragraphs* from an unfamiliar expository text and will answer wh- questions with verbal prompting and utilization of a dictionary to facilitate his comprehension of the text.

Goal 4
JG will demonstrate morphophonemic awareness, building from the base words to new, related words to increase his word knowledge abilities in spoken and written language (e.g., electric—electricity—electrons; Rome—Roman; senate—senator), as follows:

  Objective 1: JG will pick the base word from a group of related words with different morphological endings.

  Objective 2: JG will produce the meanings for different morphological units (e.g., "-ed" means past tense).

  Objective 3: JG will construct new words given a base word and a morphological ending.

  Objective 4: JG will decode multisyllabic words with derivational endings, open syllables, and closed syllables in a decontextualized context.[†]

Goal 5
JG will compose a paragraph summarizing a passage of expository text including a topic sentence, supporting facts and details, and a closing sentence, as follows:

  Objective 1: JG will identify all parts of an expository paragraph including topic sentence, supporting facts, details, and closing sentence using highlighters of different colors to indicate the distinctions among these features of text.

  Objective 2: JG will outline an expository passage of three paragraphs showing the relevant features (see Objective 1) of the paragraph using the color-coded highlighters to represent the features.

  Objective 3: JG will compose a paragraph summarizing a passage of expository text including a topic sentence, supporting facts, details, and a closing sentence.

[†]Word knowledge/decoding practice with semantic component; words practiced and unfamiliar are embedded in connected discourse as part of previously mentioned goals and objectives.

BOX 3-7

Sample of Selected Language Intervention Goals and Objectives for JG—cont'd

(Appropriate scaffolding from the clinician occurs as needed with spoken and written prompts; see also "stoplight organization" in Chapter 8.)

JG Summary

JG is personable and motivated to learn. He has good conversational skills and is a creative artist. He has deficits in background knowledge that limit his reading and verbal comprehension of curricular content. His poor reading skills, in a reciprocal relationship with spoken language, contribute to his background knowledge gaps. JG needs a considerable amount of time to process linguistic information. Frequently, while reading he substitutes words that are phonemically similar (not monitoring the "logic" of the word choice). The long latency period for processing, combined with his word-by-word reading and his limited knowledge of text structure, contributes to his reading comprehension problems. He also has difficulty recognizing (or identifying) and monitoring his comprehension gaps. Intervention should continue to help him take "ownership" of practiced strategies in the clinic.

Contextual support and the use of familiar topics set the tone for intervention. Less familiar topics (curricular content) are added to the mix as he becomes more familiar with the various structures across genres. The roles of decoding, word knowledge, and background knowledge are considered in the intervention efforts geared toward helping JG comprehend and produce connected text. Intervention goals for the next semester should continue to focus on building effective strategies for decoding within a semantic framework, that is, developing comprehension of word meanings, to facilitate more fluent reading. JG should work on increasing his knowledge of the morphophonemic aspects of words (e.g., working on morphological endings, building words from a base word). He should continue to use specifically tailored graphic organizers across narrative and expository text to help develop his (internal) mental models of text. A "macro" goal that weaves its way through all the intervention goals is to help JG develop and refine his self-monitoring skills while reading. The macro goal is related to increasing his semantic knowledge and association skills so that summarization and paraphrase strategies may be added to his reading comprehension repertoire.

NOTE: These intervention goals are across two semesters and approximately 25 weeks. Additional but related goals were included in the complete program and modified according to JG's needs over time.

beginning of this chapter. Table 3-2 represents an adaptation of Ellis's (1997) conceptualization of "watering up" the curriculum for students with LLD. Ellis (1997) points out that, very often, the curriculum is too "watered down" for our students. That is, it frequently contains language that is disjointed and it emphasizes memorization of insignificant facts. In a similar vein, poor readers often spend less time reading and are exposed to reading materials that are "less language rich" than good readers (a phenomenon that is sometimes called the "Matthew effect"; see Catts & Kamhi, 2005d, p. 97). "Watering down" the curriculum, according to Ellis (1997), has a negative influence on students' abilities to develop mental models that represent interrelationships among different concepts and information. As summarized by Christie (2006) and modified for this text, Table 3-2 presents five examples of Ellis's goals for "watering up" the curriculum and also demonstrates how these concepts relate to JG's intervention plan.

An Example of JG's Language Intervention Goals. Box 3-7 summarizes the goals and objects for JG, the student in snapshot 1. They represent a combination of goals set for a 25-week period (approximately across two university semesters) with "in" and "out of" class intervention and collaboration with JG's classroom teacher. JG's language intervention goals and objectives provide another window into the original question: What does language intervention "look like" at school-age levels? It is an example from one student and is not intended to represent all students with LLD. Some of the SLP's goals are aimed at improving JG's life in his Grade 7-8 classroom. Her focus includes helping JG acquire some of the linguistic skills and strategies necessary to manage the curriculum. Intervention includes work on comprehension monitoring skills, semantics (word knowledge plus decoding), and comprehension, expression, and meta-analysis of narrative and expository text.

In Closing

Students bring various abilities and disabilities with them to school. They may have or they may lack the knowledge, skills, or strategies (or a combination of all three) to be successful academically. Students with LLD may not have the strategies needed, or the resources available, to perform school tasks well and to keep up with a fast-moving curriculum that gets tougher every year. In some cases, students have strategies for learning available to them but they are unsure of when and how to use these strategies (e.g., paraphrasing). In other cases, students with LLD may not have the background knowledge and language skills required to acquire a strategy and use it effectively. Some students with LLD apply what they have learned in more concrete and rigid ways to a task. In other words, they do the same thing the same way for every task. They may not know how to modify strategies or use their linguistic skills to meet the needs of a particular situation. For example, memorization will often fail to facilitate retention and comprehension. Sequencing may be a more important element to pay attention to in a recipe or when giving directions to someone's home than it is for a descriptive piece. As practitioners involved in the business of helping children and adolescents develop the language knowledge, skills, and strategies needed to succeed in school, our first task is to understand the numerous possibilities that influence both language and learning success, including some of the critical variables that influence our language intervention decisions.

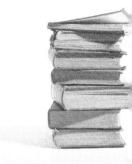

T o understand the task facing a child or adolescent sitting in a real-life classroom, researchers and speech-language pathologists (SLPs) must consider the integrated workings of multiple systems and the challenges of allocating attention, sorting external and internal sources of information, making sense of details and the broader picture in parallel, acquiring basic skills, and learning higher language and thinking skills—in short, becoming educated.
(Nelson, 2005, p. 232)

4 Creating "Curriculum-Relevant" Therapy

Making the Tough Choices

SUMMARY STATEMENT ▰▰▰▰

Chapter 4 builds on a number of the issues raised in the previous chapter. The chapter continues to explore what language intervention should look like at school-age levels. Examples from math and history bring the concept of curriculum-based intervention into focus. The chapter provides a brief look at some of the language skills and abilities required to master content area subjects. This is an ongoing theme of the text. Chapter 4 also presents a more detailed discussion of the roles and responsibilities of different professionals involved in the education of students with language learning disabilities. It also provides information from our colleagues in education and curriculum development. What are they asking about curricular demands? Some of the similarities and differences between classroom "instruction" and language "intervention" are explored with recognition that the lines between the two may blur occasionally. A major theme of the chapter, that is, what "shared responsibility" in language and literacy really means, is highlighted. The responsiveness to intervention (RTI) model, which was introduced in Chapter 2, among others presented, is revisited. We take another look at delineating professionals' roles in school-based settings with a particular focus on the evolving responsibilities of speech-language pathologists.

KEY QUESTIONS ■■■■

1. What are some of the challenges attached to the creation and delivery of "curriculum-relevant" language intervention?
2. What is meant by "shared responsibility" in language and literacy-based education approaches?
3. What are some of the "do's" and "don'ts" of language intervention?
4. How do professionals develop language-based programs that complement, rather than replicate, each other's expertise and training?

INTRODUCTORY THOUGHTS

Curriculum-Based Intervention: Some Beginnings

Examples That Challenge Students and the Professionals Who Serve Them

Box 4-1 contains several examples of mathematics problems within curricula in Grades 2 and 6. The examples are referenced in the discussion that follows, so readers are encouraged to fully review this box before moving on.

BOX 4-1

Mathematics Samples from Grades 2 and 6

Grade 2

Grade 2 students are asked to "solve each problem" (problems 1 and 2), as follows:

1. Lee has 2 quarters, 2 dimes, and 1 penny. How much more money does he need to buy a toy for 79 cents?
2. Maria has 67 cents. Her aunt gives her 3 dimes. She buys a ruler for 22 cents. How much does she have now?

Students then are asked to "write about it" in problem 3. The textbook shows the following:

■ Pictures of five coins:
  ■ A fifty cent piece
  ■ A quarter
  ■ Two dimes
  ■ A nickel
■ The correct total is **$1.00.**

Problem 3 is stated as follows:

3. Mai makes a mistake counting her coins. She counts them this way.

The values are shown under each coin as they are added together by Mai: 50, **60,** 70, 80, 85. The total shown is 85 cents, which is incorrect. The bold shows the "mistake," which is *not* shown in the problem for the second graders. They are asked to solve the problem by "writing about it."

Mathematics Samples from Grades 2 and 6—cont'd

EXPLAIN what Mai does wrong.
(The response is required in written form in a complete sentence or more.)

Grade 6

The following examples provide additional insights into the complexity of language in curricula content. Grade 6 students are asked to "solve" the following (problems 4 and 5):

4. Rosa is making piñatas out of newspaper, glue, and colored tissue paper. The supplies she needs to make one piñata cost $1.79. If Rosa has $7.00, does she have enough money to make five piñatas? EXPLAIN.

5. In Gabriel's history class, the students took notes for 15 minutes, watched a video for 8 minutes, and discussed homework for 10 minutes. The time remaining was spent working on research projects. If the class was an hour long, how much time did the students spend on their projects?

Then in problem 6, Grade 6 students are asked to "write about it" as follows:

6. Solve each problem. Use correct math vocabulary to explain your thinking.
    Mike is going on a bike ride with five of his friends. Each of the boys will drink 2 pints of water during the ride. Mike's mom asks how many quarts of water they will need in total for the ride. Mike quickly calculates 6×2 and says they will need 12 quarts of water.
    a. Explain what he did wrong.
    b. Show how to find the correct answer.

Curriculum examples from *Mathematics* (2002). (California ed., Grade 2 [p. 184], Grade 6 [pp. 53, 199]). Boston: Houghton Mifflin.

One has only to glance at these math story problems to appreciate that Carlson and colleagues (1980) were quite accurate when, more than 25 years ago, they wrote: "Math encompasses more than the factual operations of addition, subtraction, multiplication, and division. More than any other subject, it requires a basic language and conceptual repertoire as prerequisites for the development of abstractions necessary for problem solving" (p. 60). Carlson and colleagues (1980) provided some provocative suggestions that are still current. They reminded speech-language pathologists (SLPs) to evaluate a number of critical aspects of language that both underlie and interfere with success in math. They noted that children with language learning disabilities (LLD) (and perhaps others) may not understand some of the vocabulary that surrounds the math problem. Words and phrases such as *some, and, altogether, how many,* and so on can be confusing in certain problems. For example, *Some of the children were ice skating. Three were girls and nine were boys. How many children were skating altogether?* In addition, the idea that "girls" plus "boys" equals "children," a form of linguistic cohesion, may also complicate the math problem.

One could make similar observations to those made by Carlson and colleagues (1980) and Gruenewald and Pollak (1990) about the problems presented earlier from Grades 2 and 6. For example, we could also consider the impact of specific words and phrases such as *how much, more, enough, needs, time remaining, how long,* and so on. In addition to the specific lexical items that might be more "math specific," such as the meaning of *quarter*, *nickel*, and *dime*, we could take into account the difficulty a student may have processing and comprehending the connected text of the math problem (as per Chapter 3):

■ Does the student understand, for example, that "Maria/her/she" (see Box 4-1, problem 2) are linked cohesively, that is, the pronouns all refer to "Maria"?
■ Likewise, does the student understand the linguistic cohesion reflected in "Mai" and "she" and "coins" and "them" (see Box 4-1, problem 3)?
■ Can the student handle the complex *if* structures reflected in Box 4-1, problems 4 and 5?
■ Can the student hold in memory the three events (taking notes, watching a video, and discussing homework) in Box 4-1, problem 5?
■ Does the student understand what *how long* (see Box 4-1, problem 5) and *calculate* (see Box 4-1, problem 6) mean?

Carlson and colleagues (1980) and Gruenewald and Pollak (1990) raise another interesting point that relates to the vocabulary of math but also cuts across curricula areas. They say that students may use math and other curricula words correctly in specific situations but fail to use those words in different situations. For example, the word *first* may have different meanings, including spatial, quantitative, or temporal meanings; however, the student may have "mastered" only one meaning of the word. We might consider this notion of restricted word knowledge in relation to words such as *same* and *different*, *before* and *after* (see also Chapter 3, p. 70). It follows, then, that students should be exposed to different uses of words in different contexts (and across subject areas) (Gruenewald & Pollak, 1990; see also Chapter 9).

Beyond our analysis of the math problems themselves from lexical, semantic, syntactic, and textual variables, we can consider the additional demands of the "math" tasks. For example, what language skills are required to "write about it," "explain," or "use correct math vocabulary?" *What does it take* to explain what "isn't right" about an answer in problems 3 and 6? As noted in these examples, children are being asked to *write* their responses, as well as identify a mistake, as early as Grade 2. These demands assume a reasonable degree of linguistic ability, including the syntactic and semantic ability necessary for expressing oneself in writing. The problems also remind us to consider what Blank (2002) and her colleagues (see Chapter 3, p. 58) would say is the ability to "reorder" one's perception. Level 3 demands require moving from thinking about what *is* to thinking about what *is not* (correct). The response from one Grade 2 student without language problems for problem 3 (see Box 4-1) was, "She conted the second corter wrong." (The spelling represents the child's rendition, perhaps a "trade-off" of resources as per Lahey & Bloom, 1994; see Chapter 3, p. 63. The math concepts, the expression of reasons, plus writing may have competed for the child's attentions.)

As students progress through the grades, one might not be surprised to observe the level of problem solving required and the degree of linguistic abilities assumed to be intact by sixth grade. By observing the progression from Grade 2 to 6 (see Box 4-1), one may note that tasks build on those taught and, hopefully, learned in the earlier grades. By the time students arrive in Grade 6,

Lexical, semantic, syntactic, and textual variables add to the demands a student is faced with when asked to solve a mathematics problem.

they have practiced *writing about* and *thinking about* what's "wrong" in the problems. But one can also see how difficult the Grade 6 problems would be for students with LLD. Problem 6 (see Box 4-1) brings home to us the possibly overwhelming demands placed on our students. Not only do they have to comprehend and absorb the connected, expository text, but they also have to know the difference between a "pint" and a "quart," for example, and be able to express that difference in writing.

The "language-heavy" curriculum, although challenging, presents SLPs with golden opportunities to use what they know (language disorders and language development) to shed light on the interaction among what language abilities a student brings to school (or not), task requirements, and the instructional demands he or she faces daily. In an excerpt from a Grade 6 mathematics textbook, students are reminded of the following: "Understanding math language helps you become a successful problem solver" (*Mathematics*, 2002, p. 205). Using boxes that are brightly colored in the original textbooks, a black-and-white rendition is shown in Figure 4-1. We can see from Figure 4-1 that students are also encouraged to exploit the reciprocity between spoken and written language. This is good advice for our students with LLD who need specific and intense intervention to help them acquire the "math" language required to succeed.

To say the least, Figure 4-1 shows that the language skills required or "assumed" to be available to students by Grade 6 are rather complex. It includes writing definitions, comparing and contrasting concepts, and comprehending and expressing the "why" of relationships. Getting students with LLD to the point where they can participate—to *"write* about it" and *"talk* about it"— becomes the linchpin of language intervention at school-age levels. Language intervention is not teaching the curricula content but facilitating the language skills required to partake in it (Ehren, 2000; Norris, 1997; Wallach & Ehren, 2004). And although we recognize that "content" (semantics) is also language, SLPs and teachers need to find ways to balance the language learning load so that they, too, exploit their strengths and the unique training and knowledge they bring to the education of students.

Language intervention is *not* teaching the curriculum but instead involves facilitating the language skills required to partake in it.

Write about it!   Talk about it!

Use what you have learned to answer these questions.

8. Write your own definitions of translation, rotation, and reflection.

9. How is a rotation different from a translation?

10. How is a reflection different from both a translation and a rotation?

11. Why is it important to identify the point about which a figure is being rotated?

Figure 4-1 ■ Assignments from a sixth-grade mathematics book encouraging students to use written and spoken language. *(Redrawn from* Mathematics *[2002]. [California ed., Grade 6, p. 429]. Boston: Houghton Mifflin.)*

Roles and Responsibilities: The Long Road to Clarification

As implied in the final sentence of the previous section, there are some key issues (and misinterpretations) that come to mind when discussing curriculum-based intervention (and the role of SLPs in the process). We could use many examples across subject areas including and beyond math to demonstrate the power and influence of language on learning. A history example will be presented at the end of this chapter. We saw, for example, the difficulty attached to the "moon landing" passage in Chapter 3 (p. 56). These examples help us to appreciate what it might be like to be a student with LLD who has to keep up with a math or social studies lesson. We could also return to the Christopher Columbus lesson and analyze the chapter's language for additional clues to students' difficulties. We could also study the language of science, a topic we will cover in forthcoming chapters. Understanding the demands of the curriculum (and the classroom, as noted throughout this text) provides a direction for creating relevant language intervention. As Cirrin (2000) noted: "Effective assessment of the language of curriculum materials requires that [SLPs] *read the books and worksheets that the student is expected to read*" (p. 304).

But here's where confusion sometimes reigns. We know that for any subject area there is a set of explicit vocabulary words and concepts that students must master (Cirrin, 2000). An issue that often clouds the lines between teacher and SLP is, Who "teaches" that vocabulary? Isn't it the role of the science teacher to teach the vocabulary of science? The social studies teacher to teach the language of social studies, and so on? The simple answer is "yes." But shouldn't the SLP help students with LLD master the curriculum by "reinforcing" it (reviewing/reinforcing the vocabulary words of the subject area)? Shouldn't the SLP "review" student worksheets with them and help them complete the worksheets? The simple answer is "no," as suggested by the earlier statement that we help our students *access* the curriculum. While recognizing that there are no "simple" answers to complex questions, we believe that trying to keep up with the curriculum (plugging in "missed" pieces) and "teaching" subjects (e.g., algebra or geometry) for which an SLP might have little or no background is not the best use of his or her expertise and training. By contrast, using the curriculum as a context for language intervention and finding ways to help students *use* the background knowledge they bring to tasks, as well as learn how to acquire knowledge, are goals we should consider as we move through the maze of evolving roles of the professionals who share in the education of students with LLD. But, again, we must stress that there are differences of opinion regarding the road one might take. And there are always "shades of grey" that influence the perspectives taken about what SLPs can and should do, that is, should they teach or reinforce subject area content or should they teach the strategies needed to access that content (Kamhi, 2006, personal communication).

Ehren (2000) addresses the role of SLPs in curriculum-based assessment directly. She reminds SLPs to "maintain a therapeutic focus." In an earlier work, Norris (1997) also cautioned SLPs about falling into the "tutor trap." Both Ehren and Norris encouraged SLPs to use their expertise appropriately by making distinctions between "classroom instruction" and "language intervention." In a wonderful and important piece of work, Ehren (2000) provides examples of activities that are "recommended and not recommended for in-classroom services in order to maintain a therapeutic focus and share responsibility for student success" (p. 227). For example, she recommends working on the language in the math problems presented. According to Ehren (2000), a student's math worksheet or textbook becomes the context for intervention.

Relating Ehren's concepts to the math problems presented, language therapy goals might include improving comprehension of complex sentences such as *if/then* and *before/after* sentences (depending on the student's needs and the math problem). Language intervention might also include work on core vocabulary (e.g., *more/less*) that is needed to solve the problem. In addition, language intervention might include work on managing connected text in the form of an objective to improve a student's understanding and use of cohesive devices. An activity that is *not* recommended, as noted by Ehren (2000), would be to "take the math worksheet and help the student on the caseload complete the problems [because] completing the worksheet with the student does not address therapy goals specifically" (p. 227). Working on the nonrecommended activity, according to both Ehren (2000) and Norris (1997), is tutoring.

Ehren (2000), Wallach and Ehren (2004), and Wallach (2004) talk about the ways SLPs can provide complementary and appropriate intervention for students with LLD. They say that some vocabulary words might be thought of as being the "linguistic glue" that holds concepts together. Ehren (2000, 2003) adds that these words are "assumed to be known" by students who then can use their resources as discussed by Lahey and Bloom (1994) (and Chapter 3, p. 63) to focus on the "new" content words of the curriculum. For example, smaller linguistic units and phrases such as *if, or, because, was caused by, as a result of*, and so on may be difficult for some students with LLD and may interfere with their ability to manage the additional, unfamiliar content of the social studies, math, science, and other subjects. Meltzer and colleagues (1996) also talk about "tricky" words such as *always, but, only, not/never*, and *except* (using the mnemonic ABONE) that may interfere with students' comprehension of curricula material, including the ability to interpret test/instructional questions correctly. Other key words such as *prewar, postwar, cause*, and *effect*, among others, remind us that history also has its smaller, sometimes problematic words that surround the key content words of the curriculum (Hennings, 1993).

Complementary programming (and services) are delivered when teachers teach the specific curricula content (e.g., the names of the generals and battles of the Revolutionary War) and SLPs help students with LLD comprehend and use what Wallach and Butler (1994a) called the "linguistic glue" words and phrases (such as those mentioned previously) and other key words that are assumed to be intact. Ehren (2006a) points outs, for example, that words such as "conflict," "democracy," and "freedom" might be ones to consider working on with our students with LLD since it is assumed that students without LLD "have" these core words in their repertoires. This may be a false assumption, but, nonetheless, Ehren's ideas speak to the need for SLPs to make intervention choices that might have a greater impact on students' knowledge and that move beyond "reinforcing" or "reviewing" what teachers are doing.

Complementary services can be delivered when teachers focus on the specific curriculum content and SLPs help students comprehend and use key words and phrases within that content.

BOX 4-2   *Cirrin's Five Basic Curricula Demand Concepts*

---

1. *Classification:* Organizing and grouping (e.g., words such as *same as, different from,* and those expressing size, shape, and texture)
2. *Conservation:* Understanding the constant attributes of an object (e.g., words such as *more, less, all, half, taller than*)
3. *Time:* Expressing sequential order and relations among events (e.g., words such as *first, before, during*)
4. *Seriation:* Understanding relations between objects and their order (e.g., words comparing sizes, lengths, height, space/time, amount)
5. *Space:* Locating objects in relation to others (e.g., words such as *over, under, above, top, bottom*)

Data from Cirrin, F. (2000). Assessing language in the classroom and curriculum. In J. B. Tomblin, H. L. Morris, & D. C. Spriestersbach (Eds.), *Diagnosis in speech-language pathology* (2nd ed., pp. 283–314). San Diego, CA: Singular Publishing Group.

Cirrin (2000) also encourages SLPs to think in broader terms when they create language intervention goals and objectives. He points out that several key concepts relate to different subjects at different points in time. Some of this vocabulary knowledge is assumed to be intact when students face the specific content of the curriculum. He outlined five basic concepts that relate to curricula demands: classification, conservation, time, seriation, and space (Box 4-2).

Classification involves organizing and grouping things. For example, in science, students might have to group (and understand similarities and differences) between classes of plants and animals. Words and phrases that might be needed to express classification are *same as, different from,* and others that specify *shape, size, texture,* and so on. *Conservation,* in the Piagetian sense, includes understanding that "certain attributes of an object are constant, even though the object may change in appearance" (Cirrin, 2000, p. 305). According to Cirrin (2000), "the ability to conserve is basic to the understanding of number, measurement, and space" (p. 305). Depending on the nature of the task in a math or science lesson, the vocabulary associated with conservation includes words such as *more, less, all, half, whole, taller than,* and *shorter than,* among others. *Time* encompasses the expression of sequential order and relations between events. Time concepts cut across many academic areas. In social studies, one might have to understand dates and time lines. In English literature, one must understand the ways events connect in a story. There are many vocabulary words to express sequence, including *first, second, before, after, during, next,* and so on. Words that can express event relations in time include *morning, afternoon, today, yesterday, long time,* and others. *Seriation* includes understanding relations between objects and their order. Some of the vocabulary connected to seriation concepts include number concepts (*first, second, third*), size concepts (*big, bigger, biggest*), length (*long, longer, longest*), height (*tall, taller, tallest*), space/time (*in front of, behind,* etc.), and amount (*least, most,* etc.). Finally, *spatial concepts* locate objects in relation to others. Words from this category include *over, under, above, top,* and *bottom.* Both seriation and spatial concepts cut across many subject areas.

Cirrin (2000) provides a checklist that may prove to be a useful tool for SLPs and teachers as they sort through the intersection of language underpinnings and curricula requirements. Figure 4-2, Cirrin's adaptation of work by Gruenewald and Pollack (1990) and Prelock and colleagues (1993), outlines the areas that might be covered in a dialogue (spoken or written) between SLPs and teachers.

Modifications can be made based on the grade level and needs of individual students. But, again, the importance of knowing something about each grade's expectations is a critical step in the creation and implementation of relevant language intervention at school-age levels. The first section of the checklist (see Figure 4-2, section A) may provide the SLP with a *context* or *backdrop* for intervention. It tells the SLP about the expectations a teacher has (based on state/curricula guidelines) for a particular unit. Section A, as noted in our discussions in this text, is *not* meant to be a directive for the SLP to "review" or "reinforce" the particular vocabulary of the science or social studies lesson. An SLP might ask the teacher what she or he is covering in the coming weeks and which concepts the teacher expects the students to "have." Section B in Figure 4-2 provides insights into the focus of particular lessons or units. It is helpful to know how teachers view these concepts in relation to what they are teaching. This information can be expanded on when the SLP assesses a student's comprehension and use of the vocabulary (covered in the previous section) that might be used in textbooks and other curricula materials. Section C in Figure 4-2 provides a number of interesting suggestions for obtaining information about the way students are required to "show what they know" in a particular classroom or unit of study. The examples that follow under each of the categories can be modified based on grade levels, although the ones listed offer a broad spectrum of possibilities.

Figure 4-2 presents one example of a tool that can be used to obtain information about selected classroom/curricula expectations. But it can also be used to obtain information about a student's performance from the teacher's perspective. Each category could include a "student performance" section along with an "expectations" section. And although the checklist offers some guidelines about behaviors to observe, the list can be expanded (or shortened), as mentioned earlier. For example, in section 2 of Part C (see Figure 4-2), we could ask specifically about inferential versus literal questions. We could also include questions that relate to paraphrasing activities (see Chapter 3, p. 54). The checklist is useful because it can provide direction for further evaluation by SLPs.

After gleaning information from teachers, classroom observations, state standards, and other sources, SLPs can then make judgments about which language goals and objectives will be the most appropriate and relevant for the student from contextually based information. Clearly, collecting information directly from students' teachers may be most useful, but this is not always possible for school-based practitioners to orchestrate. Nonetheless, finding ways to understand the curriculum and the expectations that students face daily is key to successful intervention. For example, using abbreviated, written checklists that are

A. Vocabulary Review of Curriculum

1. Identify prerequisite vocabulary necessary for achieving lesson objectives:

2. List new vocabulary to be introduced:

B. Concepts Necessary for Achieving Lesson Objectives

Check appropriate line for underlying concepts required in the instructional task:

- ❏ Conservation (number, size, length, amount)
- ❏ Time (temporal order, duration)
- ❏ Spatial
- ❏ Causality (cause/effect)
- ❏ Classification (sorting, inclusion/exclusion, regrouping)
- ❏ Order/seriation (number, length, height, space/time, amount)

C. Language Requirements Review

1. Comprehension: Student must demonstrate comprehension by (check all that apply):

- ❏ pointing/showing
- ❏ sequencing pictures/words/sentences/numbers
- ❏ role playing
- ❏ following oral directions
- ❏ demonstrating or restarting directions
- ❏ other (please specify):
- ❏ circling, drawing
- ❏ manipulating objects
- ❏ answering questions
- ❏ following written directions

2. Oral Expression: Student must express self verbally by (check all that apply):

- ❏ defining vocabulary
- ❏ talking in complete sentences
- ❏ answering and asking questions
- ❏ explaining answers
- ❏ other (please specify):
- ❏ storytelling or retelling
- ❏ reciting known information
- ❏ oral reading
- ❏ clarifying responses

3. Written Expression: Student must express self in writing by (check all that apply):

- ❏ writing numbers/letters
- ❏ spelling words
- ❏ making outlines
- ❏ writing stories
- ❏ writing explanations
- ❏ writing equations/formulas
- ❏ other (please specify):
- ❏ copying numbers/letters/words
- ❏ filling in sentences
- ❏ writing complete sentences
- ❏ writing book reports
- ❏ creating word problems

Figure 4-2 ■ Selected vocabulary concepts and language requirements of the curriculum. (*Redrawn from Cirrin, F. [2000]. Assessing language in the classroom and curriculum. In J. B. Tomblin, H. L. Morris, & D. C. Spriestersbach (Eds.),* Diagnosis in speech-language pathology *(2nd ed., p. 307). San Diego, CA: Singular Publishing Group. Data from Gruenewald, L. J. & Pollak, S. [1990]. Language intervention in the curriculum and instruction [2nd ed.]. Austin, TX: Pro-Ed; & Prelock, P., Miller, B., Reed, N. [1993].* Working with the classroom curriculum: a guide for analysis and use in speech therapy. *San Antonio, TX: Communication Skill Builders.*)

shared between SLPs and teachers may be more practical than meeting face to face. Surveying selected textbooks and worksheets to find clues to the linguistic demands of a task will provide SLPs with additional information about students' difficulties managing the curriculum. Finally, reviewing state standards (see Chapter 9) is another strategy, among many, that SLPs may find useful to connect language intervention with academic learning and success.

Shared Responsibility in Language and Literacy Learning: A Closer Look

The suggestions made in the previous sections and in chapters that will follow remind practitioners that there are ways to create and implement programs for students with LLD that reflect a shared responsibility among professionals. Wallach and Ehren (2004) point out, as do others who write about collaboration, that the road to working together begins by understanding that professionals bring different perspectives to the table. These differences, reflected in diverse backgrounds and training, represent the proverbial double-edged sword. Speech-language pathologists, reading specialists, and special and regular educators may share similar ideals and goals, for example, to help children and adolescents succeed academically and socially, but their goals and objectives are often packaged in diverse philosophical slants gleaned from different bodies of research (Wallach & Ehren, 2004). Nonetheless, one reality remains constant, that is, "creating opportunities to explore each other's unique contributions might represent a small first step toward developing truly collaborative language-based literacy programs" (Wallach & Ehren, 2004, pp. 41–42). Professionals' roles, when complementary and collaborative, guide students through the culturally different, discourse-dense, and informationally loaded world of school. (See Wallach & Ehren, 2004, for a more detailed discussion of collaborative models.)

Viewing Language Teaching on a Continuum: One Way to Explore Professionals' Roles and Choices

Ehren (2000) described the shared, yet unique, roles of professionals working with students with LLD as existing on a "language teaching continuum." She pointed out that curriculum-relevant intervention grows out of an understanding and implementation of the following four basic concepts:

1. Professionals' roles match their expertise and maximize what they can do, especially when team members (e.g., teacher and SLP) share students.
2. Professionals understand the differences between "instruction" and "intervention" (or therapy), and this understanding is reflected in their language/literacy/learning goals.
3. Professionals can articulate ways in which teaching the content of the curriculum versus teaching its language underpinnings reflect different levels of training and expertise.
4. Professionals understand the populations for whom each professional is responsible.

Figure 4-3 represents Ehren's "language teaching continuum."

Using Figure 4-3 as a visual aid, Ehren (2000) (and as summarized in Wallach and Ehren, 2004) asks professionals to consider four aspects along the continuum: (1) the *what*, (2) *how delivered*, (3) *by whom*, and (4) *for whom*. The model helps professionals appreciate their uniqueness while, at the same time, recognizing

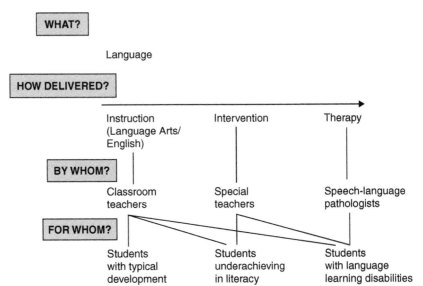

Figure 4-3 ■ The language teaching continuum of service delivery. *(Redrawn from Ehren, B. J. [2000]. Maintaining a therapeutic focus and shared responsibility for student success: Keys to classroom speech-language services. Language, Speech, and Hearing Services in Schools, 31, 219–229. Copyright 2000 by B. J. Ehren.)*

that there are shades of gray and modifications that may be necessary in the "real world" of schools. Indeed, some adaptations may occur as responsiveness to intervention (RTI) models (see Chapter 2, p. 34, and the next section) grow in visibility in educational settings. As noted by Wallach and Ehren (2004), there are always times when professionals may cross boundaries to find creative ways to meet the needs of students in their care.

The What. Language arts is the content area discussed by Ehren (2000). We could also talk about any other subject (history, science, math, social studies, etc.). But regardless of the subject matter, all students must use language, as we have discussed throughout this text. In a framework of shared responsibility, all professionals might "deliver" language to their students, but the delivery will occur in different ways and for different purposes. The "what" aspect in the model provides an example of how "language" as a subject area has a different focus and purpose when it is packaged as "language arts" or "language therapy." Similarly, the math examples presented in Box 4-1 remind us that SLPs would "handle" math requirements of the classroom (the *what* in the model) with a different focus from teachers. Although teachers and SLPs might both use the same math materials, they would be doing so in different ways and for different purposes. In the best of worlds, the collaborative nature of math's delivery occurs when SLPs and teachers communicate, making "instruction" and "therapy" effective complements of one another.

How Delivered. Teachers are involved in "delivering" the curriculum and its content to students. According to Ehren (2000), this is *instruction*. Language arts

Curriculum-relevant therapy involves helping students master language foundations that will enable them to access the curricular content.

is one of the subjects that students are exposed to as part of their curriculum. When instruction is insufficient to produce the mastery required in the curriculum, schools respond by offering a variety of *intervention* services (e.g., reading recovery, English as a second language [ESL] programs, speech-language therapy). In this continuum, *therapy* is a very specific, more intense type of intervention (see Ehren, 2000). As outlined in Figure 4-1, students with LLD may require therapy, which is different from a more "typical" language arts curriculum. Our theme is reiterated here in that curriculum-relevant therapy includes helping students master the language foundations or underpinnings that will enable them to access the curricular content (Ehren, 2000, 2002). For example, therapy might include learning how to process and use expository text structure for handling social studies pieces such as the "moon landing" piece presented in Chapter 3 (p. 56).

By Whom and for Whom. As we consider new models and changes in federal legislation (see Mastropieri & Scruggs, 2005; Whitmire, 2005), the roles played by teachers and specialists will continue to evolve. Ehren's model represents one way to consider professionals' "core roles." In other words, what is their *primary* responsibility? We might ask, for example, for which population is the SLP *primarily* responsible? As we look to RTI models as alternatives to more traditional testing and placement, professionals (including SLPs) may have expanded or modified roles in the collaborative process, which is a critical component in RTI models. Speech-language pathologists who are involved primarily with students with *identified* LLD and who are providing language intervention/therapy for these students (tier III in RTI models) may also play important consultative roles as "vulnerable" students move through tiers I and II as depicted in Box 2-2 (see Chapter 2, p. 33). The perspective underlying Ehren's model is that the SLP, reading specialist, and other specialists are not *primarily responsible* for typical learners, as Figure 4-3 suggests. Similarly, students who are underachieving in literacy may be involved in the intervention arena serviced by special education teachers and other specialists who are generally not SLPs. But, again, the model does not suggest that professionals never cross disciplinary lines. The model merely helps professionals find a centered understanding of a "best fit" for their expertise and training. It encourages professionals to continue to ask themselves "where" their choices originate from— choices that relate to the *what*, the *how*, the *by whom*, and the *for whom* (Wallach & Ehren, 2004).

Responsiveness to Intervention Approaches Revisited

A New Set of Questions. In Chapter 2 (pp. 32–35), we presented a description of the responsiveness to intervention (RTI) model. The model outlines three tiers of service that are available to students as they move through the system. Several examples for SLPs' involvement in each of the tiers were summarized by Ehren and Nelson (2005) (see Box 2-2, Chapter 2, p. 33). In an expanded discussion of RTI approaches and curriculum-relevant practices, Staskowski and Rivera (2005) make a number of points. They indicate the following:

■ RTI initiatives have the potential to prevent some literacy and learning difficulties and school failure.

- Many SLPs are already involved in curriculum-relevant service delivery that cuts across the three tiers.
- RTI initiatives may introduce new roles for SLPs, especially for those who have been practicing (by choice or otherwise) within more traditional frameworks.

Staskowski and Rivera (2005) suggest that as school districts plan RTI initiatives, "new opportunities [will arise] for SLPs to extend curriculum-relevant practices to students with and without communication disorders" (p. 136). Although school-based SLPs may read this statement with alarm, given current time constraints and caseload realities, the shift in thinking with RTI models may offer promise for the creation of more reasonable "workloads" (see Chapter 2, p. 33) in the future. For example, students who may have been placed on caseloads in the past may be better served in tier II. RTI's prevention and intervention-early and in-class focus may result in fewer students remaining on caseloads (and working "outside of" their classrooms) for their entire school careers (DeKemel, 2003b). Staskowski and Rivera (2005) present an excellent summary of SLPs' changing roles through the "three-tiered model" across three evolving service delivery approaches: the traditional medical model, the curriculum-relevant model, and the RTI model.

As seen in Table 4-1, Staskowski and Rivera's (2005) descriptions provide an overview of the different roles and responsibilities that reflect, in a sense, the evolution of language intervention in schools. Many articles, books, workshops, and other materials have covered the questionable effectiveness of medical model orientations (diagnose-treat-cure) and traditional service delivery models in schools (e.g., Merritt & Culatta, 1998; Miller, 1989; Simon, 1987; Wallach, 2004; Wallach & Butler, 1994a). Table 4-1 shows the particularly limited role that SLPs play within a traditional model framework. For example, tier III activities with their focus on standardized tools provide little connection to the classroom and the curriculum. Traditional models tend to focus on "inside the student's head" problems only. By contrast, curriculum-relevant models (the middle column in Table 4-1) move SLPs out of their broom closets (as per Simon, 1987) and "speech" rooms into classrooms. Curriculum-relevant models have also helped to bring SLPs face-to-face with the contexts and materials that their students struggle with daily. RTI models may move us further. And while the primary work of SLPs may still have a tier III focus, as Ehren (2000) suggests, there may be more opportunities to collaborate with colleagues in different ways. As noted in Chapter 2, the curriculum is language. Thus SLPs can play important roles, as also expressed by Troia (2005), in the creation of "high-quality services" within the general education classrooms and beyond (tiers I and II) while still maintaining their "therapeutic" focus as noted by Ehren (2000) (among other tier III activities) in the process.

SLPs might ask themselves a number of questions to evaluate "where" they are in their own evolution as school-based professionals. Inspired by Staskowski and Rivera (2005), the questions posed in Box 4-3 may provide some useful insights.

The questions in Box 4-3 serve as guidelines for self-reflection. They may also provide a helpful way to share perceptions and opinions with colleagues in speech and language. The questions focus mainly on the curriculum-relevant model.

Table 4-1
Comparison of the Roles of Speech-Language Pathologists Across Three Models of Service Delivery

Tier	MODEL		
	Traditional Medical Model	Curriculum-Relevant Model	Responsiveness to Intervention Model
Tier I: All students	No role	Participate on school improvement and curriculum teams. While working in classrooms that include "caseload" students, collaborate with teachers to provide group instruction for all, targeting, for example, phonemic awareness, vocabulary, participation in class discussions, strategies for following directions, social skills for interacting with peers, oral comprehension, reading comprehension, and writing processes.	Work at the school building or district level to plan professional development and group instruction for all, focused on language and literacy, whether or not the classroom includes students "on the caseload," targeting, for example, phonemic awareness, word-decoding skills, self-talk to assist in self-regulation, social skills for interacting with peers, strategies for following directions, reading comprehension, and note-taking strategies.
Tier II: At-risk students	Provide in-service activities to help teachers recognize the symptoms of speech-language impairments and know how to refer them for assessment. Screen for the presence of speech-language impairments in selected grades or classes.	Provide information about relationships of language development and learning or social interaction difficulties. Consult with child study teams and teachers when they are concerned about particular students about when to refer. Observe students in the classroom. Problem-solve ways to assist students in the classroom before initiating formal diagnostic activities.	Work with other school support team members to monitor progress of "at-risk" students. Help others design and implement specialized instruction for those who are not responding adequately to general classroom instruction. For example, might involve small-group instruction for students having difficulty learning phonics and other word-decoding skills or with reading comprehension.

Continued

Table 4-1

Comparison of the Roles of Speech-Language Pathologists Across Three Models of Service Delivery—cont'd

	MODEL		
Tier	**Traditional Medical Model**	**Curriculum-Relevant Model**	**Responsiveness to Intervention Model**
Tier III: Students with disabilities*	Use diagnostic procedures (primarily formal tests) to diagnose impairment and identify students eligible for special education services. Use test results to develop IEP goals and plan intervention. Provide treatment and monitor progress toward goals. Reassess periodically to decide whether child remains eligible for SLP services.	Use curriculum-relevant diagnostic procedures (e.g., interviews, curriculum-based language assessment, dynamic assessment, and relevant standardized tests) to identify students who are eligible for and need speech-language assessment intervention services. Use assessment results to plan collaboratively with teacher, student, and parents what curricular areas and related language-literacy abilities to target in intervention. Provide services in classroom or therapy room that are relevant to goals to progress in the general education curriculum. Monitor progress using curriculum-relevant assessment procedures and decide whether the student continues to need special services.	Before any special education services are recommended, it should be determined that the student has difficulty benefiting from high-quality services within the general education classroom (tier I), within gradually more intensive small-group instruction (tier II), or from even more intensive individualized instruction (tier III).

From Staskowski, M., & Rivera, E. A. (2005). Speech-language pathologists' involvement in responsiveness to intervention activities: A complement to curriculum-relevant practice. *Topics in Language Disorders, 25,* 137.

*RTI models differ. Three-tier models are common, but even they differ in whether or not students in tier III are identified as having disabilities and being in special education.

IEP, Individualized education plan.

More positive responses indicate the use of curriculum-based approaches to speech-language services in schools. Parts I and III are reversed from the sequence presented in Table 4-1. Part I questions focus on tier III activities. These questions are presented first because the activities reflected in tier III should be familiar to many SLPs. The questions here help SLPs determine the

BOX 4-3

Self-Evaluation Questions for Speech-Language Pathologists

Part I

1. Do you know what the curricula requirements are for the students on your caseload with LLD? (Specify and reflect on your choices. For example, why do you know more about the language arts curriculum than the math curriculum?)
2. Do you use curricula materials when you assess your students? When you create language intervention goals and objectives? (Discuss which ones and why they were chosen.)
3. If you have answered "no" to question 2, how do you determine a student's language intervention goals and objectives? (For example, do you use standardized tests? Do you "teach to" the tests?)
4. Do you consult with students' teachers or observe within the classroom to determine or develop language intervention goals?
5. Do you conduct your therapy within the classroom or in a separate room? (Percentage of time in each setting?)
6. How do you decide when a student continues (or not) to need language therapy?
7. Do you include written language intervention goals for your students with LLD? (Percentage of oral-to-written work?)
8. Do you participate in any activities related to general education or special education curriculum development?

Part II

1. Do you work with "at-risk" students? (Percentage of time?)
2. Do you consult with child study teams and teachers when they are concerned with particular students?
3. Do you observe in classrooms and offer suggestions to teachers for students who may need help but have not been referred for formal testing at this point?
4. Do you run in-service activities or find other ways to provide colleagues with information about language and its relationship to school success?
5. What is the purpose of your work in question 4? In other words, is it focused toward developing "high-quality" instruction and intervention? Is it focused on improving the referral process?

Part III

1. Do you participate on any curriculum development/improvement teams in your school?
2. Are you involved in any prevention-related programs? (Explain your role.)
3. Do you provide instruction for your "caseload" students only when you go into the classroom?
4. Do you run "all class" demonstration lessons for teachers in specific language areas such as phonemic awareness, story comprehension, and so on?
5. Do you participate in district-wide activities for the creation and implementation of more effective educational programs for all students?
6. Do your principals know how speech-language pathology has evolved?

Data from Staskowski, M., & Rivera, E. A. (2005). Speech-language pathologists' involvement in responsiveness to intervention activities: A complement to curriculum-relevant practice. *Topics in Language Disorders, 25*, 13–147.

nature of service delivery that is predominant in their settings. Ideally, fewer speech-language professionals are locked into medical model formats, although these models of service delivery are alive and well. The questions in part I are focused toward the assessment and management of identified students with LLD. The last question (question 8 in part I) relates to the RTI model. Part III questions relate to tier I, and part II questions are matched to tier II. School-based SLPs who are participating in curriculum-relevant service delivery may have an easier time building on services if and when schools initiate RTI models. The more involvement SLPs have in prevention, consultation, and intervention with students who are not yet in special education, the more experience they are obtaining that relates to RTI initiatives. As put by Staskowski and Rivera (2005):

> Many SLPs already have moved from the traditional model of service to a more curriculum-relevant approach to provide increased support to teachers and students in their quest to achieve state standards and adequate yearly progress. The RTI initiative builds on these efforts by providing a structure to identify students with language and literacy risks, shape early literacy programs, and utilize dynamic assessment techniques to prevent school failure and ensure greater success for students at risk as well as for those with disabilities. (pp. 145–146)

They go on to say that as SLPs take on leadership as well as participatory roles in RTI initiatives, they will not only have an impact on the future achievement of students, but they will also increase their perceived value to schools (Staskowski & Rivera, 2005).

Questions from the Education Side of the Fence. Speech-language pathologists and other specialists are among the school-based professionals who are asking questions about how their roles and responsibilities may change in RTI models. We have explored a number of possibilities for SLPs in this chapter and in Chapter 2. Ehren and Nelson (2005), Straskowski and Rivera (2005), and Troia (2005), whose work has been discussed, have articulated their views about the shifting roles that SLPs may play in the RTI era. Similarly, educators are also studying the changing roles of classroom teachers in the general education stream. Echoing a number of concepts discussed in this text, Gerber (2005) says that students' "responsiveness" to instruction and intervention includes an understanding of schools' and teachers' roles in the process. He writes:

> Individual differences in responsiveness to instruction are not in any sense *inside* students. Responsiveness to instruction is embedded in but not separate from a complex educational context that includes institutional as well as teacher variables. (Gerber, 2005, p. 516)

Gerber goes on to say that teachers' perceptions of students' responsiveness are variable and must be considered carefully when RTI initiatives are implemented in school systems.

Mastropieri and Scruggs (2005) continue Gerber's discussion by asking a number of questions that speak to the feasibility and the challenges related to the implementation of RTI models in schools. They ask professionals to think about teacher training and experience, the types of monitoring that will be required to ensure that RTI procedures are implemented fully and appropriately, who will be "in charge" of the monitoring and follow-up, the differential needs of elementary versus high school levels in RTI formats, and funding processes (between general and special education). They ask professionals to think about the following:

■ Who prepares all general education teachers to deliver instruction using scientifically based approaches?

■ What does seventh grade science instruction at tier 1, tier 2, and tier 3 look like? How long will students remain in a tier?

■ How is a determination of "nonresponsiveness" to intervention made? In other words, will all teachers use a standard cutoff score on classroom tests?

■ Who has the ultimate decision-making power to move students up and down the tier system?

■ What exactly are diagnosticians and school psychologists doing and when?

Although SLPs are not mentioned specifically in the article, Troia (2005), Ehren and Nelson (2005), and Staskowski and Rivera (2005) offer some suggestions that relate to some of the possibilities that appear on the horizon. Although SLPs would fall under Mastropieri and Scruggs' "diagnosticians," the omission of mention is interesting given the predominance of language learning in the academic equation.

Mastropieri and Scruggs (2005) raise a number of critical questions that will no doubt be on the table for the next decade and beyond. Remaining optimistic, they see what they call "RTI-type" services as having promise. They think that change should occur in general education, first at tier I and II levels. In other words, in their view all students should be assured of an evidence-based, quality instruction early on. But they also believe that RTI-type services are "greatly needed to provide appropriate services to the many students caught in the middle—those not 'disabled'…and yet struggling to keep up in school" (Mastropieri & Scruggs, 2005, p. 529). Exercising caution, they remind educators to avoid getting on new bandwagons too quickly and add that professionals "would be wise to consider questions regarding the efficacy, reliability, validity, and utility of RTI prior to wide-scale adoption" (p. 530). Indeed, both opportunities and challenges face educators and specialists as they search for relevant and appropriate ways to reach students with and without LLD. It is clear that SLPs, reading specialists, and regular and special educations will face future challenges together.

Curriculum-Relevant Therapy: An Historical Example and Some Final Thoughts

We have been asking a number of questions in this text. One basic question—What does language intervention "look like" at school-age levels?—has led us to a study of the curriculum and the contexts in which students must learn. Another question—What language knowledge and skills underlie school tasks?—underpins our language intervention goals and objectives. Looking through history, science, geography, and other textbooks at different grade levels is a daunting experience. The language savvy required, plus problem-solving skills needed, place students with LLD in a most difficult situation. And students without language learning problems are often challenged as well by curricula materials, not because they have disabilities but because the materials and teaching techniques are less effective than they might be. It is interesting to learn something about what our education colleagues are saying and doing about the current state of the art in curriculum development and change.

This endeavor provides SLPs with an excellent perspective from the other side of the desk.

History presents a challenge for many students. In addition to the complexity of history and the way it is transmitted to students, middle and high school levels of instruction include many of the following components of instruction, some of which have been mentioned earlier in the text: lectures are delivered by the teacher to the whole class; there is usually a rapid pace set by teachers with large amounts of new content; textbook information is also covered quickly; there is minimal class review or additional practice; and as the content level becomes more difficult, so too are the requirements for more conceptually oriented and abstract thinking (Mastropieri & Scruggs, 2005). These obstacles are summarized in Box 4-4.

According to VanSledright (2002a), students in history classes are frequently asked to study and memorize many facts, dates, and other information from hard-to-read textbooks. After various units, the students are often asked to take tests that rely on memory. High-stakes testing has failed to improve the situation because "such tests generally measure what history knowledge children can recall, not what they can do with what they recall" (VanSledright, 2002a, p. 133). Mirroring what we often say about various language intervention techniques, VanSledright (2002a) agrees that more empirical evidence is needed on the educational efficacy of various techniques for teaching history. Along with VanSledright, other educators and researchers are also questioning the methods, techniques, and content of the history and other subjects, including math and science (e.g., Baker et al., 2002; Kinder et al., 1992; Scruggs & Mastropieri, 2003, 2004). But the changing winds of curricula, though encouraging, may also present even greater challenges for students with LLD.

In a series of classroom teaching experiments, VanSledright (2002a) demonstrated that regular class fifth-grade students without learning disabilities were able to engage in more "strategic thinking" about history. His use of the word "strategic" should sound familiar to many SLPs. In VanSledright's study,

---

BOX 4-4   *Special Challenges to Students Studying History*

- Complexity of material
- Manner in which it is transmitted to students
    - Lectures delivered by teacher to entire class
    - Rapid pace
    - Large amounts of new content
    - Minimal class review or additional practice
- Increasingly difficult content that requires increasingly more conceptual and abstract thought

Data from Mastropieri, M. A., & Scruggs, T. E. (2005). Feasibility and consequences of responsiveness to intervention: Examining the issues and scientific evidence as a model of identification of individuals with learning disabilities. *Journal of Learning Disabilities, 38,* 525–531.

the students learned about events not by memorizing facts and dates as the main approach, but by comparing and contrasting various written and pictorial materials, analyzing what they were seeing and reading, and making judgments about events, among other activities. These activities led to gains in memory and retention for many of the fifth graders. The significant finding overall was that students as early as fifth grade were able to adopt a "strategic approach" to the history content (the American Revolution) being covered. Talking to teachers (although there are implications for SLPs), VanSledright (2002a, p. 134) reminds his colleagues that learning to think historically includes a number of skills, including the following abilities:

■ To make sense of many different sources of information from the past
■ To check evidence by comparing and contrasting information
■ To use evidence-based information when interpreting events
■ To evaluate an author's point of view in relation to events being studied

These abilities form the components of "strategic teaching" in history.

Figure 4-4 presents a summary of the history-specific strategies discussed by VanSledright (2002a) and inspired, in part, by the work of Pressley and Afflerbach (1995). He points out that students move along a *continuum* in their abilities to think historically, but we can see the value of acquiring these strategies for other subjects.

Referring to Figure 4-4, VanSledright (2002a) suggests that the ability to "use judgments to refine interpretations" (level four) by going across several sources (called *intertext* evaluations) is an end result of experience and practice with the previous levels' skills (levels one through three). For example, practice with *intratext* analysis, that is, comprehending and interpreting one document at a time, includes a number of "meta" abilities that form a base for the ones that follow. But as with other continua presented in this text, VanSledright's (2002a) hierarchy should not be viewed as representing a *rigid* step-by-step process. Rather, it should be seen as including several, sometimes overlapping processes that are influenced by students' existing background knowledge on a topic, their reading abilities, and their metalinguistic and metacognitive abilities.

Although it is not the responsibility of SLPs to teach, reinforce, or review the *core content* of fifth-grade history, they can help students with LLD acquire some of the language knowledge and skills needed to learn history. Acquiring strategies, particularly the linguistic and metalinguistic strategies, that underpin better performance in history (among other subjects) is also a critical piece of the intervention process. For example, "Using Comprehension Monitoring Strategies" (see Figure 4-4, level one) includes many "assumed" language abilities such as comprehension of a number of words (part of the content knowledge assumed), for example, "massacre" "prior to," and "incident" in an excerpt on "The Boston Massacre." These are some key words that SLPs might include in semantic units that may have a broader influence on students' comprehension of other historical events that are covered in later units (Ehren, 2006a). In addition, being able to make predictions and inferences about written documents and summarizing information, all level one strategies in VanSledright's framework for fifth graders, beg the question: What language abilities underlie these tasks? Literal comprehension of spoken and written text,

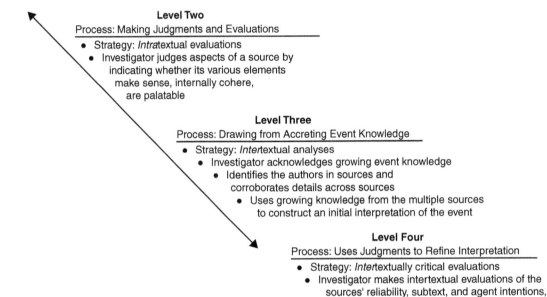

GENERAL READING PRACTICE   **HISTORY-SPECIFIC STRATEGIES**

Level One

Process: Using Comprehension-Monitoring Strategies

- Strategy: *Intra*textual analyses
  - Checks details, re-reads, summarizes,
    and/or predicts developments in the source
    - Enables investigator to make initial sense of source

Level Two

Process: Making Judgments and Evaluations

- Strategy: *Intra*textual evaluations
- Investigator judges aspects of a source by
  indicating whether its various elements
  make sense, internally cohere,
  are palatable

Level Three

Process: Drawing from Accreting Event Knowledge

- Strategy: *Inter*textual analyses
  - Investigator acknowledges growing event knowledge
    - Identifies the authors in sources and
      corroborates details across sources
      - Uses growing knowledge from the multiple sources
        to construct an initial interpretation of the event

Level Four

Process: Uses Judgments to Refine Interpretation

- Strategy: *Inter*textually critical evaluations
  - Investigator makes intertextual evaluations of the
    sources' reliability, subtext, and agent intentions,
    as a means of constructing a refined,
    evidence-based interpretation of the event

Figure **4-4** ■ History-specific strategies from the work of VanSledright. *(Redrawn from VanSledright, B. A. [2002]. Fifth graders investigating history in the classroom: Results from a researcher-practitioner design experiment.* The Elementary School Journal, 103, *131–160.)*

bringing background knowledge into play, and learning how to use and analyze words and sentences in connected text are aspects of the knowledge, skills, and strategies required to "attack" Grade 5 history.

In Closing

Acquiring knowledge about curricula expectations and understanding teaching styles and expectations contribute to setting language intervention goals and objectives that are relevant to school success. Chapters 3 and 4 have provided some answers to the question, What does language intervention "look like" at school-age levels? Chapters that follow will continue to explore principles and possibilities that underpin language and literacy goals and objectives. The position taken in this text is that language intervention at school-age levels starts by considering the context in which children spend much of their time.

The current literature in speech-language pathology, education, and related fields, while coming from different places in the galaxy, converge with the mantra that we can do better to help students "in trouble." Indeed, from the words of Vince Lombardi, legendary football coach: "Practice does not make perfect. Only perfect practice makes perfect." We may not have to go as far as Lombardi suggests, but we can certainly explore alternatives to traditional approaches, as the next chapter will demonstrate.

4

A Marriage of Conceptual and Practical Frameworks

PART OUTLINE

5 Successful Language Literacy Intervention
A Look Back to Look Ahead

6 Integrating Spoken and Written Language
An Eye Toward Becoming Literate

7 Seeing the World Through Connected Text
Bringing Structure and Content, Macro and Micro Pieces Together (Part 1)

8 Seeing the World Through Connected Text
Bringing Structure and Content, Macro and Micro Pieces Together (Part 2)

New fad diets, ineffective treatment approaches, or dangerous medical cures may spread because they are easy to implement.
(Kamhi, 2004, p. 106)

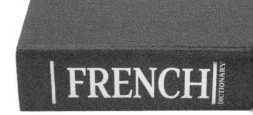

5 Successful Language Literacy Intervention

A Look Back to Look Ahead

SUMMARY STATEMENT
Chapter 5 continues to explore the challenges facing school-based speech-language clinicians and their colleagues. This chapter begins with an example from a second language learning experience as a continuation of our exploration of language learning disabilities (LLD). Second language learning experiences are used to make the case that "central auditory processing disorders" are part of a bigger picture, that is, they are symptoms of broader-based language disorders. The chapter moves in a slightly different direction from previous chapters by presenting scenarios that speak more directly to some of the "don'ts" of language intervention. While maintaining a positive view on the "what not to do" issue, we offer alternatives about what is possible when we look in authentic and functional directions. Concepts in information processing and metalinguistic development are revisited to put into perspective some current and popular practices that persist in language intervention circles. Among the questions asked are the following: Is central auditory processing a valid construct in LLD? How do we get beyond simplistic notions of processing? Is "sequencing" a foundational skill or a result of other discourse abilities? What is the role of metalinguistic awareness in language learning and language intervention? The chapter focuses on the construction of goals and objectives that are based on functional and authentic outcomes as a guide to the future.

KEY QUESTIONS
1. How can second language learning experiences shed light on what it might be like to have a language disorder?
2. What are some classic "missteps" in language intervention practices that warrant a

closer look and why do these "missteps" persist over time?

3. Which information processing concepts might professionals revisit and why?

4. How does knowledge of metalinguistic awareness help clinicians evaluate intervention choices?

INTRODUCTORY THOUGHTS

Second Language Learning Experiences: Do They Help Us Understand Language Disorders and Related Symptoms?

Consider the scenarios presented below. How do the different situations help us to understand the following?

1. Changes in language proficiency across the language continuum from oral to literate and from contextualized to decontextualized language
2. Lahey and Bloom's (1994) concept of a "limited capacity mechanism" (i.e., the trade-offs that occur when resources compete for attention)
3. Ways in which symptoms described as "central auditory processing" in origin, among others, relate to linguistic ability
4. What it might be like to have a language disorder

PROCESSING AND COMPREHENSION CHALLENGES IN FRENCH

The Language Participants

The participants are a visiting professor/clinician in communication disorders (you) and your 10 French-speaking colleagues from the University of Montreal. They speak very little English (or they are more comfortable speaking French) and you speak very little French. You are learning French, but your proficiency would be considered limited at this point.

Scenario 1

Your first stop is a restaurant. Everyone at the table is talking and laughing in a friendly and animated atmosphere. The conversation is not about food at the moment (and you are not always sure which topic is being discussed). Your companions appear to be speaking very quickly. (How can they speak so fast?) You are trying to keep up with what they are saying, with little success. You keep falling behind; you are stuck on "word three" and they seem to be on "word twenty." Anxiety is building and you feel a bit isolated. The speech stream is rushing by in a seemingly connected auditory barrage. Sometimes you are unsure where one word begins and another ends. (Is il y a one word? Where are the boundaries between n'est-ce pas?) Coming from New York, you think that it is impossible for anyone to speak more quickly than you do. Nonetheless, you are working very hard to "extract" a few words from the speech stream while watching the speakers' faces and gestures and listening to their intonation. (You laugh and smile, shake your head "yes," and engage in other nonverbal behavior when your friends do the same.) Soon, everyone shifts to the menu. You know you will be ordering the meal. Jacques asks you what you'd like to eat, and you understand him with little difficulty. Anxiety is decreasing. The topic shifts to food and drink and the restaurant. Your processing and comprehension are improving rapidly. You have to attend with less "energy" now that the topic has shifted to the immediate situation.

Scenario 2

Your colleagues take you to one of their homes after dinner for more socializing. Some of them decide to play Scrabble and others decide to talk politics. You decide to talk with the speech-language pathologist (SLP) in the group. You have less difficulty understanding her. (Is she speaking at a slower rate than the others in the group?) After a while, a Monopoly game appears (the French version, of course). You love the game so you join in. Your language comprehension is much improved while playing Monopoly. You think you will become proficient in French after all.

Scenario 3

You join Isabella, one of your colleagues from dinner, in her marketing class. You are eager to observe at the university. As you sit in class, you have a sinking feeling that your comprehension problem has gotten worse. You cannot understand what the professor is saying, but you try to maintain an attentive stance. The professor talks for quite some time; his explanations are long and involved (or so it seems). There is finally a period of time when students contribute to the discussion. Next, the professor gives the students a series of instructions. (He's talking and distributing papers at the same time.) You're not sure what is happening but the students break into small groups immediately. (You just follow Isabella, but you know you've missed the instructions entirely.) Next, the professor writes words on the board, but these "visual images" fail to facilitate comprehension for you. You still cannot get the content of the lesson or understand what's going on. As far as you can tell, however, the words appear to be related to key terminology. The whole thing is quite confusing, but Isabella will brief you (in English) after the class. She apologizes for not having the time to "prepare you" before class.

5

What the Scenarios Say to Clinicians: Factors to Consider When Creating Language Intervention Goals

The French-language scenarios remind clinicians to consider some of the ways in which language proficiency interacts with socialization and learning. The three scenarios bring to mind the continuum of language learning from contextualized to decontextualized situations. We are reminded of the work of Blank and colleagues (p. 57, this text) and Lahey and Bloom (p. 62, this text), among others, who say that when language "matches" a situation, it tends to be easier to process and comprehend. We see this phenomenon when the menus mesh with a discussion of food and ordering the meal. Put another way: Listeners *use context* to figure out what people are saying, especially when the language exceeds their ability. Familiarity with a routine also "frees up" resources to attend more closely to language. The Monopoly game provides an example of how a routine/game and language occur in a noncompeting situation. The English-speaking clinician (you) "knows" the rules and moves involved in the Monopoly game, so the language load is lessened. She can predict what might happen and can also, when necessary, attend more closely to the language without having to worry about how the game is played. (She knows, for example, that the blue and green properties are the really "good" ones.) By contrast, Scrabble requires both linguistic and metalinguistic abilities she (or you) has not yet acquired (in French).

Context and familiarity with routine both help individuals comprehend language.

From the restaurant to the classroom, one observes different degrees of *contextualized* to *decontextualized* language. Although the restaurant is a less formal (more contextualized) situation than the classroom, the visiting clinician has a difficult time processing and comprehending language when the topic and the situation are "unmatched." Indeed, at the beginning of the dinner scenario, the conversation may be about many things, including politics, recent sports events, children and grandchildren, who's been tenured or not, and so on. Topics can also shift quickly. It becomes more difficult to predict what's happening (and keep up with the speakers) from the "language alone," that is, the words and sentences coming out of the mouths of the speakers. Clearly, using facial expression, intonation, gesture, and other cues that accompany the language can be helpful to a listener. Moreover, the more you *already know* about a topic, the more successful you will be in participating in the conversation even if it is mainly as a listener. For example, if you and your French-speaking Canadian friends are devout hockey fans, you might be able to follow the conversation (and participate as a speaker) if you have sufficient vocabulary in your repertoire. By contrast, if the topic exceeds your knowledge (e.g., Canadian politics), you might be at a triple loss—the language structure, its content, and its decontextualized placement intersect to present you, an individual with language disorders, with a tough road to travel.

The triple influences of structure, content, and context are seen once again in the classroom scenario. Sorting through formal language (see Westby, 2006, and others), which carries with it more informationally loaded content than casual conversation, in the decontextualized milieu of the classroom adds to the challenges facing students with language learning disabilities (LLD). Although you "nod and look attentive" as our last scenario indicates, we may see different behavioral patterns from students with LLD. Perhaps we see what appear to be attention-deficit disorders (ADDs) or central auditory processing disorders (CAPDs) when these symptoms reflect primary difficulties with language. We might also see the "nodding and attending" when comprehension is really limited (as per the French marketing class). Suffice it to say that the classroom becomes the context where language assessment and intervention must meet to be relevant. As noted by Westby (2006), "Although [some] students may have the semantic, morphologic, syntactic, and pragmatic skills measured on many language assessments, there is no guarantee that they will be able to employ these skills in comprehending and producing conversational and textual discourse in lessons" (p. 359).

> The classroom becomes the context where language assessment and intervention must meet in order to be relevant.

As reflected in the last scenario, things happen very quickly in the classroom and students are expected to anticipate what they have to do and when they have to do it. And although some teachers, especially those in the early elementary grades, provide all kinds of contextual supports for children (through colorful pictures, actual field experiences, and show-and-tell activities that include "real" objects and other artifacts), Nelson (1994, 2005) reminds us that school learning never mirrors casual conversation even when it has contextual support. In school learning, children must recognize eventually that the important piece of the teacher's message is in "the language itself"—be it spoken or written. What the teacher is saying is more important than what the teacher is doing.

Children must learn to separate language from its context as they progress in school. They need to reduce their dependency on context as the major way to understand language and manage information.

Children have to become more proficient at "separating" the language from its context as they move through the grades. In other words, they have to become less dependent on context as the major avenue for understanding language and for managing the information in the curriculum. Although the last scenario takes place in a college-level classroom, it reminds us to consider the language-heavy and metalinguistic-focused experience facing students. It also speaks to the predominance of written instructions and materials and the dynamics of keeping up with, and feeling part of, a group. When a student is "over-whelmed" by too many difficult things at once, for example, a new and unfamiliar topic (marketing) *and* a less developed and stable language (French), resources compete for attention (the topic and language collide) so that efficient and effective performance or learning is unlikely to occur (Lahey & Bloom, 1994; Montgomery, 2002).

The scenarios help us appreciate the scope of the language continuum as contexts and the purposes of communication change. They also help us consider some of the symptoms that we see in children and adolescents with LLD (Box 5-1). For example, are our French-Canadian friends speaking faster than Americans (even New Yorkers) in the first scenario? Or is our visiting clinician predicting and comprehending "too slowly"? Slow processing is suggested since she is "stuck on word three," at least figuratively. Is the French-Canadian SLP speaking slowly in the second scenario? Or does the shared understanding of a topic (child and adolescent language disorders) influence the visiting clinician's ability to comprehend what she is saying?

Why do we "forget" what our colleagues are saying only seconds after they have said it? Does our English-speaking clinician have an "auditory memory problem"? Or is that a symptom of her underlying language difficulty? She can pick out a few key words here and there, but does she know where one word begins and others end as she tries to keep up with the quick-moving speech stream? Is this inability to "pull out" words from the speech stream, among the other examples provided in this section, indicative of a CAPD? Or are all these common symptoms representative of a tip-of-the-iceberg phenomenon (see Chapter 1, pp. 11–12)? The examples that follow in the next section ("Cases in Point") also address these questions.

The French scenarios represent another way to gain some understanding of what it might be like to have a language disorder. They also shed practical and logical light on "auditory memory problems" and "central auditory processing problems."

BOX 5-1	*Characteristics of Children and Adolescents with Language Learning Disabilities*

- Slow processing
- "Forgetting" what was said seconds after it was said
- Inability to "pull out" words from the speech stream

The readers of this text who are proficient language users would likely have "auditory memory" and "auditory perception" problems in languages they do not know or cannot speak with any level of success. The French examples and others that follow should help clinicians and teachers to think about the ways in which language knowledge influences perceptual processing. This understanding of linguistic and perceptual connections should, in turn, clarify the direction of one's language intervention goals and objectives.

In a stunningly provocative article, Nittrouer (2002) reminds her readers that children (and our visiting clinician in Montreal) must learn to *organize* incoming stimuli. She points out that children get better at speech perception when other aspects of their language develop. Using an example from her daughter's early years in a preschool setting, Nittrouer (2002) says that when her 3-year-old first started using hearing aids, the staff were disappointed because her language was not improving at the expected rate. In other words, the preschool teachers expected the hearing aids to "create" a difference in comprehension. But as Nittrouer (2002) explains, although "the signal was reaching her [daughter], she could not make sense of it" (p. 237). Fast forward to one year later and now the author's daughter, who was unable to wear her aids for a week, was perceived by the providers as having "improved hearing." In reality, her thresholds had not changed but her *language* abilities had improved to make the difference. The little girl could now make sense of the messages being conveyed even with limited hearing. According to Nittrouer (2002), her daughter's experience and other examples she provides, including foreign language examples, demonstrate "how strongly language underlies other communicative and perceptual processes affecting even the very reception of the acoustic signal" (p. 237). By contrast, limited language ability leads to less efficient processing, as the French scenarios demonstrate.

The key point made by Nittrouer (2002), among others, is that language and background knowledge influence what we *think we hear*. Gillam and colleagues (2002) make a similar point. They also reflect on Lahey and Bloom's (1994) ideas. They indicate that listeners create expectancies for what they are likely to hear. Their expectancies influence what is *attended to, perceived*, and *remembered* (Gillam et al., 2002, p. 41). As many researchers have said, a number of factors contribute to effective and efficient processing and comprehension (Box 5-2). The familiarity with information to be processed, the strength of contextual cues, the linguistic complexity, a task's automaticity, and the degree of communicative pressure come together to make things "easier" or more "difficult" (Lahey & Bloom, 1994; Weismer Ellis & Evans, 2002).

> Listeners often create expectancies for what they are likely to hear, and these expectancies influence what they attend to, perceive, and remember (Gillam et al., 2002).

Additional Examples That Help Clinicians Put Symptoms into Perspective

The resurgence of CAPD diagnoses and intervention, among other related therapies for students with LLD, is difficult to understand given the decades of research that have provided us with alternatives, some of which have been discussed in this text and in other writings (e.g., Kamhi, 2004; Nittrouer, 1999, 2002; Wallach, 2004). One aspect of both assessment and intervention that has had been a source of confusion for clinicians and teachers is the role of the phoneme (individual sounds) in spoken and written language. Decades of research have helped us understand

BOX 5-2	*Factors Contributing to Effective and Efficient Processing and Comprehension*

- Familiarity with information to be processed
- Strength of contextual cues
- Linguistic complexity
- Task automaticity
- Degree of communicative pressure

that children's abilities to "deal with" phonemes—whether discriminating them, sequencing them, or segmenting them from words (e.g., identifying first and last sounds), among other tasks—is the result of a long developmental process (van Kleeck, 1994). Understanding that words are made up of individual sounds is an abstract, metalinguistic ability (Troia, 2004; Ukrainetz, 2006a; van Kleeck, 1994). Succeeding on auditory discrimination tests requires more than "listening" and "perceiving" sound differences (Wallach, 2005).

Kamhi (2004) reminds clinicians to be mindful of the abstract nature of auditory discrimination–type activities and other activities that relate specifically to the perception, identification, and sequencing of individual phonemes in the speech stream. Although speech sounds are marked more explicitly in written language because letters represent individual sounds, phonemes are not represented as individual units in connected, fast-moving speech. (Think back to the phenomena experienced by the visiting clinician trying to process spoken French.) Discussing the complexity of speech perception and implying that clinicians should think about the tasks they use in assessment and intervention sessions, Kamhi (2004) wrote the following:

> For the last 40 years, researchers in speech perception have attempted to find the acoustic (auditory) correlates of phonetic segments (sounds). What they have found instead is that "the acoustic signal of speech shows no distinctive boundaries that might mark *where one segment ends and another begins,* and the acoustic properties that can be associated with any particular segment are spread over fairly broad temporal regions" (Kamhi, 2004, p. 107; quoting Nittrouer, 2002, p. 238; *italics added*). He continues: "In other words…individual sounds do not exist as neatly packaged and sequenced units. (Kamhi, 2004, p. 107, as per Nittrouer, 2002)

Cases in Point: Perceptual and Language Knowledge Revisited

AUDITORY DISCRIMINATION AND NEW VOCABULARY

An American clinician moves north of the border to English-speaking Canada. She shares the same language with her colleagues, but there are some differences in language, particularly surrounding the acquisition of new vocabulary. For example, some brand names in Canada do not exist in the United States. And some commercials that are unfamiliar to the clinician often have accompanying, and sometimes annoying, jingles that are used to sell the product. One jingle that the clinician hears many times in the background, but that she has not paid much attention to, suggests that "OB (or Obie) is a must-have product." The happy song tells potential buyers to "just say O B for the taste that is great...O B, O B, O B." The clinician sometimes hears herself singing the jingle but she has no idea what "OB" really means. Finally, instead of leaving the room, she decides to watch the entire commercial to solve the "OB" mystery. By doing this, she discovers two things: (1) she has misperceived one of the sounds (it isn't "OB" but "OV"); and (2) the commercial is for a Canadian beer called "Old Vienna." This is a brand unknown to her. Miraculously, however, once she learns the name, she never "hears" the jingle with an "O" and "B" but gets the "OV" quite clearly. She wonders how she ever thought it was "O" and "B" or the combined, "Obie."

What might this scenario say? First, on the surface, it may look like our clinician has an "auditory discrimination problem." The *symptom* she manifests is indeed a /b/ for /v/ substitution. Consequently, would we want to help her by creating activities that would improve her auditory discrimination ability? What intervention is recommended for our clinician? If we take a *teach-to-symptoms* approach, we might create lists of /b/ words and lists of /v/ words. We might also work on having her "feel" the vibration in her throat for these voiced sounds, look at the shape of our mouths, or have her raise her hand to identify whether a word has a /b/ or a /v/ sound in it. ("Gerry, raise your hand when you hear the /b/ sound at the beginning of a word. Now raise your hand when you hear the /v/ sound.")

But we could take a different approach. We could ask ourselves, What is the core of the clinician's problem? Is the auditory discrimination error indicative of something else; that is, is it part of a bigger picture? In this case, we would take a *language approach* to "get at" the discrimination issue. It might be more productive to help the clinician make a connection between what she knows and the new vocabulary. Does she know the names of beers that are popular in the United States? Creating a theme-based unit on "Beers of the United States and Canada" might be one way to proceed. It might be that role-playing a shopping expedition in an international food and beverage store and "talking around" the appropriate vocabulary that accompanies buying beer from different countries could be part of the intervention process. But, clearly, *knowledge of the words (Old Vienna)* and familiarity with the specific name of the Canadian beer had an influence on the clinician's perception of the "abbreviation," that is, her perception of the individual sounds in the jingle.

As Gillam and colleagues (2002) might say, it is helpful, at times, to work from a "top-down" approach (start with the *bigger* piece and work down to the smaller pieces) rather than a "bottom-up" approach (start with the *smaller* pieces and build up to the bigger piece). Although the "Beers of the World" unit serves as a humorous metaphor, it reminds practitioners to think about the direction language intervention might take. In this example, we are reminded of Kamhi's (2004) quote—that the perception and manipulation of individual phonemes is an abstract and difficult task, especially for younger children and children with language disorders. Moreover, as noted several times, it demonstrates that CAPD, and other similar symptoms, may be a *result*, not a cause, of language and metalinguistic difficulties (Wallach, 2003).

AUDITORY FIGURE GROUND AND LANGUAGE PROFICIENCY

Our American clinician is still living and working in Canada. In an effort to improve her French, she sometimes watches Canadian television's French-language stations. To maintain her attention and motivation, she tends to choose programs that she thinks are "easier" to comprehend (such as a familiar American sitcom that is dubbed in French, sports events she likes, etc.). By contrast, she avoids (or cannot stick with) programs that seem "language heavy," such as dramas with unfamiliar plots and characters, and political discussion shows that cover the Canadian economy and similar topics.

On one occasion, her self-inflicted French language lesson takes place while watching a hockey game. An important playoff is in progress and one of the Canadian-based teams wins. As with many sports' celebrations, the jubilant players are followed into the locker room for victory champagne and partying. Everyone, including the sportscasters who are trying to interview players, is getting soaked with champagne. The noise, screams, and cheers are coming through loudly and clearly in the background as the French-speaking sportscaster interviews the captain of the victorious team about the series. At this point, our clinician, who has been following the game and doing fairly well with her French (or so she thinks), cannot separate the background noise (the partying) from the foreground speech (the interview).

In frustration, she clicks to the English station that is covering the same event. Within a few minutes, the English announcer has the captain at his microphone. The hockey star is now speaking English, and he and the sportscaster are also discussing the series. The clinician notes that her auditory figure ground problem has suddenly disappeared. She has no difficulty separating the interview from the background noise, which has remained constant. She is surprised by the significant difference in her attention and comprehension. She is following the interview with ease. It makes her think about the simplicity of solutions such as "provide preferential seating for students in the classroom" because comprehension is not bound by how close one sits to the speaker (or, in this case, how close our clinician sits to the television set). One's language intervention goals would have to be more layered and strategy driven when working with students with processing and comprehension difficulties. Although there might be some advantages to placing children closer to the teacher, other factors have a more significant, long-term impact on comprehension and other aspects of language learning.

The scenarios documenting the struggles of our visiting clinician to Canada remind us to look beyond the tip-of-the-iceberg phenomena of students' symptomatology to find answers as noted in the introductory chapter of this text and elsewhere in this chapter (see pp. 114–123). They also show us that the persistence of intervention approaches that are based on outdated or limited models of language require reevaluation in this postmillennium era (Wallach, 2004). Approaches that focus on central auditory processing, auditory sequencing and other discrete skills, and oral-motor proficiency are among the intervention trends that beg for closer scrutiny (Bishop et al., 1999; Kamhi, 2004; Lof, 2003; Wallach & Madding, 2005). Moving from second language learning experiences, the scenarios that follow take readers into clinics and classrooms.

Some Classic Missteps

CASE 1

A clinician is working with a 7-year-old second grader who is suspected of having "auditory processing problems." Sean is described as a "poor listener" in the classroom. He also has difficulty following directions and learning to read. Sean is given a number of tests in the auditory processing area, and he performs poorly on tasks that involve "auditory discrimination" (e.g., judging whether two words sound the same or different) and "sound sequencing" (e.g., listening to individual phonemes and forming a word), even though he has excellent articulation and normal hearing.

As described previously, Sean's difficulties include problems dealing with the sound system of language. One of the conclusions reached about him is that he is a child with a central auditory processing disorder (CAPD). Viewed as the cause of some of his comprehension and reading/writing difficulties, it is recommended by his school team that he participate in a program that emphasizes "auditory training." Some of the team members are concerned about this recommendation because they see Sean as a "visual learner" and want to move in that direction.

What is inaccurate about this interpretation? The issues are summarized in Box 5-3.

The conclusions and recommendations made for Sean are not uncommon. They represent some of the interpretations heard at individualized education plan (IEP) meetings every day. But there are some alternative interpretations to consider. First, we need to return to the concept (see Chapter 1, p. 8–10) that language has two layers: a basic, spontaneous, *linguistic layer* and a second, reflective, *metalinguistic layer*. As noted in Chapter 1, all formal language testing involves the testing of metalinguistic awareness and ability. In formal testing, we take language out of its natural context and ask children to demonstrate what they know about language in a conscious, and sometimes unnatural, way. When we ask Sean to manipulate phonemes, we are tapping his "meta knowledge," not his spontaneous use of language. Referring back to the Kamhi (2004) quote presented earlier, we know that in the normal flow of speech, phonemes are not neatly sequenced like beads on a string. Consequently, phonemic segmentation tasks, including sequencing sounds, identifying individual sounds in words, and judging words' sameness and differences, are more difficult than they appear to be on the surface. They are later acquisitions on the continuum of

---

BOX 5-3   *Case 1: Inaccuracies in Interpretation*

- Level of language involved (metalinguistic) needs clarification.
- Simplistic analysis of symptomatology and its relationship to academics interferes with seeing the core of the child's problem.
- The focus of intervention needs rethinking. (It's more complex than identifying modality preferences.)

language learning (Troia, 2004; Ukrainetz, 2006a). Children improve on these sound-based tasks after many years of preliteracy practice (including participating in sound games and rhyming) and when they learn how to read as letters make the sound segments more explicit (Blachman, 1994; Ukrainetz, 2006a). When word pairs are presented to a child who must decide whether they sound the same or different, we are asking the child to make a *judgment* about language.

In one of the first in-depth discussions of metalinguistic ability and clinical practice, van Kleeck (1984) pointed out that making evaluation judgments about language can be very difficult for young children and children with LLD. In the case of auditory discrimination tasks, the judgment involves a phonemic one, which, again, adds to the level of difficulty. Phonemes are abstract entities. As a consequence, Sean's ability to deal with the phonemes of his language on a more conscious (metalinguistic) level may take additional time to develop. Research suggests that children appreciate larger segments of language such as words and syllables before they appreciate the smallest unit, phonemes (Blachman, 1994; Troia, 2004). Troia (2004) adds that rhyming precedes blending and blending precedes segmentation activities. Troia (2004) says that when using blending and segmentation tasks in assessment and intervention, one should "begin instruction with larger linguistic units (words and syllables) and advance to smaller units (…phonemes)" (p. 107). Viewing Sean's difficulties within the context of the phonological and phonemic awareness literature may move his intervention recommendations in a more appropriate, language-based direction.

Second, and as noted throughout this text, auditory perceptual problems should be interpreted by keeping the broader perspective in mind, that is, the way they relate to functional, meaningful language. (Think back to the Old Vienna commercial.) One could say that *we do not process auditory, we process language* (Wallach, 2003). Again, the *teach-to-symptom* approach fails to see the bigger picture. In addition to getting to the core of Sean's difficulties, it may be helpful to observe what he "does" when he is faced with tasks that are above his level. van Kleeck (1994) points out that children who are less advanced metalinguistically often respond to meta-tasks, including auditory discrimination tasks, by using a "semantic strategy." That is, a child may assume that the examiner is asking for a comparison of the word referents rather than asking for a comparison of the phonemic segments of the words. Sean may think that "lake-lake" ("Are they the same or different?") requires a "different" response because all the lakes he has seen are different. He may think that "king-ring" are "the same" because they are "almost the same" or because they rhyme. In the absence of phonological difficulties (Sean has "normal" articulation), the conclusion that Sean has an auditory discrimination problem is inaccurate. Clearly, if he speaks the language using the appropriate sounds, he has made a "discrimination" on some level. What Sean appears to be having difficulty with is demonstrating that knowledge consciously (Wallach & Miller, 1988).

Sean's case reminds practitioners that CAPD-like symptoms may be saying more than they appear to be saying on the surface. We might conclude that

Research suggests that children appreciate larger segments of language (e.g., words, syllables) before they can appreciate the smallest unit—the phoneme.

Sean's metalinguistic difficulties (should they be documented beyond what the case says at this point), or the format of the tasks used, are connected to his reading and spelling difficulties. His "listening" and comprehension difficulties must be assessed further within the contexts in which they are occurring, that is, within the classroom/curriculum, as per one of the major themes of this text. We are reminded of Nittrouer's (2002) conclusion about her preschooler's perceived and improved "listening" and "comprehension" in the absence of hearing aids: Language knowledge and ability cannot be underestimated when talking about auditory perceptual processing. Again, our clinician's experience with the Old Vienna commercial suggests that the direction of Sean's language intervention would take a different path from one that recommends a focus on improving "central auditory processing." Finally, the notion that he is more "visual" than "auditory" helps little because the strategies we use must change based on the demands of the task at hand (Whitaker et al., 2004). The categorization of children based on auditory and visual preferences requires a closer look, especially if "modality groups" relate to reading development and reading disabilities, since reading is primarily a language-based, auditory-verbal task (Catts & Kamhi, 2005b; Wallach, 2004).

CASE 2

A clinician is working with a 3-year-old child who is described as having a "language delay." Jane tends to ask questions in statement form using inflection to mark a question. She might say, "We playing now?" "We eating snack now?" and so on. As can be seen, Jane omits the auxiliary verb, which also results in a missing inversion rule for question formation in English. The lesson goes something like the following (modified from Wallach & Butler, 1994, p. 14; Wallach & Miller, 1988, p. 80):

> *Clinician:* "Now Jane, I want you to look at the blocks on the table. We have five blocks on the table. We are going to point to the blocks and say the words for the sentence. Ready?" (Clinician points to the blocks as she says each word in the sentence.) "We are eating snacks now." (Clinician instructs the child to do the same thing.)

> The child begins to do the task, continuing to omit the auxiliary verb. The clinician and the child touch the blocks together and the child begins to repeat the auxiliary. The child needs help touching the blocks to match the words. The clinician guides the child's hand as they say the sentence together. This goes on for several trials. Then the clinician moves to another use of the blocks. She says:

> *Clinician:* "Now, Jane, watch carefully. I am going to move the blocks around. We're going to make a question out of the blocks." (Clinician proceeds to move the second block to the first position of the block sentence.) "Now, let's say the question sentence together. Are we eating snacks now?"

> Jane seems confused and continues to say the sentence in statement form. The clinician shows the child the *are* block. She demonstrates the statement sentence again ("We *are* eating snacks now") and then moves the second block (the *are* block) to the beginning of the sentence to demonstrate the question form.

BOX 5-4   *Case 2: Conclusions about Language Intervention*

- The aspect of language chosen for intervention requires further consideration.
- The level of decontextualization is making the task more abstract and less functional.
- The task is too complex (too meta) for the child.

What should we conclude about this language intervention session for a pre-schooler with language disorders? Issues are summarized in Box 5-4.

The first question we might ask is, "Why is the focus for this child on improving syntactic form at this time?" This choice requires additional study, as well as knowing more about other aspects of this child's language. Are there broader goals the clinician could set for Jane (Fey et al., 1995)? We have to ask whether "correct grammar" is the most important thing we can do for her at this time. It may be an appropriate choice, but the clinician needs to question its overall communicative value for this 3-year-old. Does Jane make her needs known? Can she engage in conversations? Does she comprehend questions being asked of her during book reading routines? What are some of her preliteracy skills like? Can she participate in early monologue activities? There are many questions we could ask to evaluate ways in which the clinician's choices could be put into a broader, more functional context.

The second observation relates to the point just made. It triggers another series of questions. Is the language being facilitated in this intervention session functional? Should communication be functional for a 3-year-old child with a language delay? What is the clinician's purpose or intention? Is the clinician trying to help the child develop better contextualized language, that is, help Jane communicate with her peers, use her new forms in her life and her community—in natural settings? The clinician might use different techniques to help Jane acquire these forms if, indeed, the intention is to help Jane improve her use of language forms for the *first layer of language*. The clinician might involve Jane in theme-based, pragmatically driven activities that include modeling and other techniques that keep the sentence forms in high-context situations.

As noted in the case summary, the clinician's task is structured and decontextualized. Moreover, the statement and question sentences, represented by blocks that replicate *individual word segments*, are closer to the written word than the spoken word. (Words are separated in writing conventions but, as noted in the previous sections, they are unsegmented in the auditory stream.) The blocks fail to make the task "more concrete" for the child. The blocks and the techniques used by the clinician make the task more abstract and metalinguistic. The format of the task might be appropriate for school-age students with language disorders to facilitate segmentation abilities related to reading and writing. They require closer scrutiny for Jane. In this case, the clinician's intent and her choice of techniques and tasks are mismatched.

The task used, as with those described for Sean in the previous case, taps metalinguistic ability. It is unlikely that average developing 3-year-olds would make the word-to-block connection. The understanding that speech has segmented units (words, syllables, sounds), as mentioned throughout this chapter, involves a long, developmental period (Troia, 2004; Ukrainetz, 2006a; van Kleeck, 1994). Our second language experiences also speak to the difficulty of segmenting speech in languages that are unfamiliar to us. The choice of activities for Jane, even if we agree that the focusing on form is appropriate, should be modified.

CASE 3

Brad is an 8-year-old third grader with LLD. The clinician is working on narratives. The goal is to improve Brad's knowledge of story structure in spoken and written language. The focus is on spoken language at this time with an eye toward applying concepts learned to written language. The clinician is using a series of five picture cards to represent a story and to provide a scaffold for Brad. She asks him to "look at the pictures and tell a complete story about them." The student begins to tell a story, but it does not "hang together." There are fragments of ideas, but the story is hard to follow.

The clinician notes that Brad's stories for the sequence cards sound like a series of separate sentences. In addition, his stories omit any mention of cause-and-event relations. The clinician reminds Brad that the cards represent "one story." She reminds him to "tell one story for all the pictures." These reminders are not very effective. The clinician decides to work on sequence activities to help Brad understand that events follow from one another. For example, she works on having him tell her "what he did before he came to language therapy." She and Brad also talk about the "steps" to making a peanut butter sandwich (which he loves to eat) as part of her "improving sequencing" goals. Finally, they work on the semantic mapping of words to help him "get the main idea" of stories.

What might we need to consider in Case 3? Box 5-5 summarizes these issues.

We might say initially that working on narratives, a very popular aspect of language intervention today, may be an appropriate goal for Brad. As with the other cases, we would look at the entire picture before we reached a conclusion. For the moment, we will assume that this choice is a reasonable one. Clearly, working on connected discourse for spoken and written language represents an area of language learning that is widely studied and supported by research

BOX 5-5   *Case 3: Considerations*

- The problem may be in the cards.
- The intervention techniques that follow from the student's performance on the sequence cards should be reevaluated.
- The structural aspects of different genres (e.g., narrative vs. expository text) should be evaluated.

(e.g., Dymock, 2005; Gillam & Ukrainetz, 2006; Hadley, 1998; Scott & Windsor, 2000; Westby, 2005). Then where might we go to evaluate some of the missteps in Brad's case?

We might ask ourselves about the materials used in this therapy session. Is the use of five separate sequence cards placed in front of the student the most effective way to evaluate or facilitate narrative ability? Is there a level of inferencing ability required to "get" the concept that the pictures represent one character or related characters (or events) across time? A closer assessment of the pictures is warranted to discover whether they represent temporal or causal events clearly. For example, some cards have a temporal caste to them. Cards that represent a "story" across morning, afternoon, and evening events may not have a cause-and-effect relationship expressed in the cards. By contrast, cards that show a specific cause-and-effect event—such as two cars in an accident, which, in turn, leads to an ambulance at the scene helping injured passengers— may (but may not) present a clearer scenario for the student. Thus we would need to determine whether the materials used facilitate or interfere with Brad's performance. But, again, the use of separate cards (as compared with, perhaps, one picture with many details) may not be the most effective way to facilitate the production of a coherent narrative. This is especially true for younger children and children with LLD who may have difficulty integrating the concepts represented by individual pictures.

Other variables such as the familiarity with the content of the cards and the "preparation" and practice that preceded this activity should be considered. Likewise, the pragmatics that drives this task might also require a closer look. Consider this possibility: The therapist and her student are both looking at the same pictures. This creates a situation where the need to "talk elaborately" is weakened by the shared context. If I see it and you see it, less has to be said— or coded in language. The presupposition from the student's perspective may be that if you (the clinician) see the pictures, I (the student) need not say everything. Clearly, therapy sessions such as this one often have a "pseudo storytelling" pragmatics attached to them. This means that, at some level, the student has to catch on to the idea of "therapy talk." The "therapy talk game" has its own rules and expectations. Use of what we call a naïve listener, that is, telling the story to someone who has not heard it, adds a bit of pragmatic logic to the story-telling scenario (Hadley, 1998). As a somewhat "older" child with LLD, Brad may know how to play the "speech-language game." He may understand what the clinician wants—a clear, elaborated, detailed story, even though the clinician doesn't "need it" to follow along with the pictures. Younger children may not fare as well. Thus keeping the pragmatics of the situation in mind, something we could say for all the cases, should remain in the forefront of language intervention decisions.

The tasks that follow from Brad's difficulties with the five sequence cards also lend themselves to further analysis. The first point to address is the issue of "sequence" and "improving one's sequencing abilities" as an intervention objective. Sequence is not a "thing" we fix to other aspects of language. As mentioned throughout this text, complex behaviors cannot be categorized in simple terms. The French and Canadian language examples presented earlier remind us of the many variables that come together when a speaker and listener are involved in conversation and other language and learning activities. The clinician's notion that sequencing activities may help Brad acquire narrative-related skills makes it sound as if she thinks that this entity called "sequence" is a unified, foundational ability that will connect to narrative (and possibly other) abilities in a direct way. In some situations, sequence (like perceptual processing) is a result of other kinds of knowledge, experience, and ability. For example, Brad's exposure to and practice with story structure may be the important piece of the puzzle and may provide the *result* of improved "sequencing" ability.

In addition to the aforementioned issues surrounding sequencing, one has to ask about the types of materials being "sequenced" and for what purposes. Following directions to a friend's house may have different sequential requirements (they may be "tighter") than providing an overall description of the newest ski trails in California (a speaker can start and end where he or she wants to). The clinician's sequencing activities chosen for Brad show missteps related to these considerations. Reporting on the events one participates in before coming to "speech" does not have the same, complex structure as a narrative. While it represents a personal recount, recounts tend to have a temporal focus that is not told from the point of view of several characters involved in a theme (a conflict) and a plot (what the main character does to solve a problem). Recounts may be useful if the clinician asks Brad to structure his recounts in a particular way. For example, he could be asked to recount a morning challenge for him. He could be asked to recount the morning's or day's events as if it were a story and he was a main character. Clearly, connecting the recount more directly to narrative goals might be more useful. The second choice mentioned, the steps to making a peanut butter sandwich, is well off the mark. This is an expository text activity, not a narrative, whose content (making a sandwich) may not take Brad very far. Again, looking at "sequence" as an underlying and foundational skill creates a narrow and inaccurate direction for intervention.

Last, the choice of a semantic map also requires more careful investigation. Semantic mapping, though well intentioned, has become another popular tool for clinicians to use for any number of purposes. In many cases, the maps chosen need to be evaluated in terms of clinicians' goals and objectives. While visual maps have been shown to help students organize their spoken and written language, Singer and Bashir (2004) remind Brad's clinician that "some graphic-organizing strategies better represent text structures…than others" (p. 253) (see Chapters 7 and 8 and also Bashir & Singer, 2006; DiCecco & Gleason, 2002). Chapters 7 and 8 will provide additional information on the topic of semantic maps and language intervention goals. Suffice it to say that the maps chosen by the clinician will be a useful tool for Brad if they make story structure more explicit and if story structure explicitness is the clinician's goal.

CASE 4   Betty is asked to read the following paragraph silently:

The procedure is quite simple. First you arrange the items in two different groups. Of course, one pile may be sufficient depending on how much there is to do. If you have to go somewhere else due to lack of facilities, that is the next step;

otherwise, you are pretty well set. It is important not to overdo things. That is, it is better to do a few things at once than too many. In the short run this may not seem important but complications can easily arise. A mistake can be expensive as well. (The piece continues in the original from Bransford & Johnson, 1973, p. 400.)

Betty understands the individual vocabulary words in the paragraph. The sentences are also within her syntactic repertoire. Nevertheless, she has difficulty when asked to restate or rewrite this expository piece from memory. She fails to retain or recall very much from the paragraph, and her reproductions are missequenced and disorganized. Her teacher decides to work on "getting the main idea" in the classroom with Betty. She asks her SLP to collaborate with her. She asks if the SLP can help Betty with her memory problems. Betty's teacher informs the SLP that she will shorten the amount of information given to Betty because there are too many sentences in this paragraph and this is part of the problem. Betty can only handle small bits of information at a time.

Are there any leaps of logic in Case 4? Box 5-6 summarizes these mistakes.

Readers may recognize the paragraph presented from the classic chapter by Bransford and Johnson (1973). Their example helped us to see, yet again, that processing and comprehension are a tricky business. As with all the cases presented in this chapter, some of the interpretations that persist about why students "can" or "cannot" do things come from places that defy logic and research. We can say initially that in Betty's case, the answer may be in the text. Betty may have processing and comprehension problems, but we must look beyond the conclusions reached in this case to understand the nature of those problems. Part of this understanding comes from an evaluation of ways in which the materials are contributing to Betty's weak performance. Readers who are unfamiliar with the Bransford and Johnson (1973) paragraph may also have difficulty comprehending and remembering its details. One may be able to read the paragraph and "get" many of its "micro" pieces (individual words and sentences) without getting or holding on to the "main idea." One of the problems with the paragraph is its lack of an explicit theme or frame of reference. If a listener or reader "creates" a context (e.g., making up a title, thinking of an event that relates to the one described, etc.), memory and comprehension should be facilitated (Lahey & Bloom, 1994). To make their point about the influence of background knowledge and theme-based knowledge on comprehension, Bransford and Johnson (1973) asked readers to reread the paragraph

BOX 5-6	*Case 4: Leaps of Logic*

- ■ The problem is in the text and not necessarily in the student's head.
- ■ Less does not always produce more.
- ■ Comprehension and memory factors may interact rather than function separately.

(as noted, the original is much longer) with the following title: "Washing Clothes." Readers of this text who have never seen or heard this paragraph are asked to do the same and reflect on the effect the title has on their comprehension.

Titles, serving as linguistic frames of reference or contexts for the information that follows, have the potential to facilitate comprehension and memory. The "Washing Clothes" reference can "trigger off" background knowledge (Lahey and Bloom's [1994] mental models) that helps listeners and readers process the passage with less effort than if the experience or knowledge of washing clothes is lacking. We must ask ourselves if this additional support would help Betty. Will Betty perform better when the background knowledge she may have and other contextual supports are provided for her? Titles may help Betty anticipate what's coming up in the text if she *uses* the information, that is, if it is a *strategy* she applies to the task appropriately (Gillam et al., 2002; Wallach & Ehren, 2004; Weismer Ellis & Evans, 2002; Whitaker et al., 2004). (Recall the examples provided in Chapter 3, p. 46–48, which described the use of titles with students with LLD.) Whitaker et al. (2004) notes that the strategies we use vary based on the task. She says that we might use imagery for vivid prose or rereading a text when it is difficult, among other strategies. We change our approaches based on the demands facing us. It is clear from Betty's case that we must look at the strategies she uses to complete this task, as well as consider her performance across a number of genres (e.g., narrative vs. expository text). We must use a variety of materials and techniques to explore fully her comprehension and memory of connected discourse and text (DeKemel, 2003c; Hadley, 1998; Kintsch, 2005; Ukrainetz & Ross, 2006; Westby, 2005; Whitaker et al., 2004).

The conclusions reached about Betty, and what to do to help her, mirror many of the comments made previously. Some of the conclusions drawn about students' abilities and disabilities may be premature. As pointed out, the absence of a frame of reference in Betty's case with this particular text may have a more detrimental effect on processing (including both comprehension and memory), especially since she understands the individual words and sentences. We should always look to the text and its organization for a deeper understanding of a student's strengths and weaknesses. We should also keep in mind the notion that the processing of connected discourse, as with other aspects of processing discussed in this chapter, is far from a rigid, step-by-step, linear sequence of individual sentences. Both *bottom-up* processes (smaller units of text such as sounds and words) and *top-down* processes (larger units such as narrative structures and titles) contribute to comprehension results. Lower- and higher-level processes influence one another, forming a complex and interactive relationship; things often happen simultaneously and automatically unless problems arise (Johnston, 1999; Montgomery, 2002).

The "Washing Clothes" passage presented with and without a title gives us a taste of what can happen when information is missing. Listeners and readers do any number of things to try to *construct meaning* (DeKemel, 2003c). Providing less information is not very useful, especially if having a shorter or simplified version of a passage or story requires more inferencing, that is, filling in the blanks or missing information, on the part of the listener or reader

> The processing of connected discourse is not a rigid, step-by-step, linear sequence of individual sentences. Both bottom-up and top-down processes contribute to individual comprehension.

(Best et al., 2002; DeKemel, 2003c). Likewise, working *separately* on "memory" (one might ask, "The memory for what?") may be less effective than concentrating on strategies for activating background, structural knowledge, and other discourse activities (see Chapters 7 and 8). And although the collaboration between Betty's teacher and SLP is applauded, the "division of powers" that views "memory," "sequencing," and "comprehension" as discrete and isolated entities that can be taught separately misses the critical interactions among them.

DeKemel (2003c) tackles the complex interactions among memory, inferencing ability, and comprehension. She reminds clinicians to look carefully at the many reasons why students with LLD, such as Betty, may have difficulty managing connected text. In her discussion of narratives, she points out that, for example, some students with LLD may lack appropriate background knowledge to make the inferences necessary to understand a story, they may overuse background knowledge by not using enough textual information, and they may lack practice answering interpretation and inference questions because teachers' or clinicians' preferences may have been focused on factual questions. She reminds us, as do many other researcher-clinicians, that many factors come together to create a less than expected performance on any number of tasks. (See DeKemel, 2003c, for a detailed discussion on this topic.)

Summarizing what might be considered helpful for understanding Betty's comprehension difficulties, Ukrainetz and Ross (2006) remind us to evaluate the materials we use in both assessment and intervention contexts. They wrote the following:

> Text features have a major effect on comprehension. The meaning representation that a reader [or listener] constructs from text will be affected by the wording of the text, the idea units representing the meaning, and the text structure. Texts can be easy or difficult depending on these features and how they interact with the [listener and] reader and the activity in which they are embedded. (Ukrainetz & Ross, 2006, p. 507; also quoting Snow, 2002)

Beware of Quick and Easy Answers

Where Do the Cases Take Us?

The cases presented in the previous sections have been used to help us take a "meta-look"—a reflective, analytical view—at some of the concepts, techniques, and goals that should be familiar to many SLPs, and other professionals working in school-based and clinical settings. We have all struggled with changing theoretical and clinical orientations and trying to find a "best fit" for our students (Apel, 1999; Kamhi, 2004). Students with LLD continue to challenge us to find answers. This challenge may be exacerbated further by the heterogeneity within the population so that, as Weismer Ellis and Evans (2002) point out, "It is unlikely that a single deficit can explain the diverse pattern of language impairments observed" (p. 15). The chronic and pervasive nature of language disorders, discussed earlier in this text, adds to making any "quick fix" improbable in spite of the promises made by authors of the newest test, intervention kit, or program. Nonetheless, we keep searching for the silver bullet in LLD and other disorders, a tendency that is only human, especially in MTV-like cultures that stress "doing things faster and better." Behind this need for answers yesterday, however, is a well-meaning desire to help our children and adolescents in trouble and to meet the requirements of new high-stakes testing in schools (Silliman & Wilkinson, 2004b). But beyond the missteps seen in every school and clinic is still much good news because "our clinical practices are constantly evolving in response to changing perspectives and new information" (Wallach, 2004; Weismer Ellis & Evans, 2002, p. 15).

If we are indeed evolving clinically and educationally, why do some older and outdated practices persist? Part of the question was answered in the previous paragraph. Language disorders are difficult to "handle" from many perspectives. In a wonderful discussion of this *persistence-in-practice phenomenon*, Kamhi (2004) takes a hard look at the state of the art in speech-language pathology as reflected in his quote used at the beginning of this chapter. He presents the concept of "meme" for consideration. Kamhi (2004) says that *memes* (similar to *genes* in concept and pronunciation) are elements of a culture that are passed on, sometimes from generation to generation, person to person, or supervisor to student clinician. Examples of memes are certain catch-on phrases, ceremonies, songs, customs, fashions, scientific ideas, and technologies. Kamhi (2004) says that some memes stick better than others because "selection favors memes that are easy to understand, remember, and communicate to others" (p. 106). Other factors that favor the success of memes, in addition to ease of understanding, include who propagates a concept (e.g., a neurologist's opinion about dyslexia may have a stronger influence) and the competition related to a meme. (For example, Asperger's is a meme that has caught on quickly because it is a syndrome for which there was no specific label previously.)

The auditory processing disorder (APD) meme, evidenced in the second language learning and missteps sections, is one addressed by Kamhi in his article. Sensory integration disorders (SID) theory and practice is another. Both APD and SID memes are based on assumptions that provide a more simplistic and understandable answer to children's problems. Kamhi (2004) says that they also have a kind of "all-encompassing" and "causal" explanation for complex behaviors. They have silver bullet potential. The visually based focus in dyslexia, including the popular belief that confusing letters and reading backward is the core of the condition, is yet another meme. It has had staying power across time and in the face of decades of conflicting research demonstrating the linguistic-based reasons for so-called "reversals" (e.g., Catts & Kamhi, 2005d; Vellutino, 2003; Vellutino et al., 1994). Oral-motor training is another popular meme that has caught on in spite of what we know about functional communication and its disconnect with these procedures.

According to Kamhi (2004), language and language-based disorders are not very successful memes because they are difficult to understand and explain to others. As Apel (1999) noted earlier (see Chapter 1, p. 5) and as Kamhi (2004) reiterates in his article, *language* is defined differently by different people. Professionals have different theoretical biases about what language is and which aspects of language to facilitate (or teach) as the cases suggest. According to Kamhi (2004), *phonological disorders* is another term that is difficult to understand. What challenges the phonological meme from sticking, in addition to the

Memes are elements of a culture that are passed down—from generation to generation, person to person, or supervisor to student clinician, for example (Kamhi, 2004).

difficulty understanding what it means, is the added lack of agreement among professionals about the nature of phonological disorders. Oral-motor problem, articulation difficulty, and speech delay are memes that remain easier to communicate to others and are concepts that many clinicians cling to when working with children.

Meme theory is one way to look at why some practices maintain popularity while others, based on available research and evolving knowledge, have a more difficult time capturing clinicians' (and teachers' and parents') attention. Some of my own graduate students who are now working in school-based settings point out that ideas about "what to do" with the students on their caseloads are frequently "just passed along from clinician to clinician" without many or any changes or modifications. Although this example does not apply to every school district, or even most school districts, we can see how meme theory might work in the real world of too many children with LLD and not enough time. Although his discussion is a bit discouraging, Kamhi (2004) certainly leaves us thinking. He forces us to face reality when he says that "the playing field is one in which the truth value and logic of an idea may not be the primary determinant of its appeal and acceptance" (p. 110). But, adding a note of encouragement, Kamhi (2004) ends his article by saying that "it remains up to us to spread our language-based memes to all who will listen" (p. 111).

Creating New Memes That Will Stick

Insights from Information Processing Theory. The concepts discussed by Lahey and Bloom (1994) and others, some of which were reflected in the cases and highlighted elsewhere in this text, may offer insights into the strengths and weaknesses of students with LLD, as well as helping clinicians pay closer attention to task demands, contextual influences, and materials used. Some information processing theories, such as those that propose an underlying deficiency in temporal processing skill in children with LLD (an APD meme), have had, as noted, greater staying power.

Others that take a systemic and dynamic processing approach, offering fewer clear-cut explanations for why children with and without learning disabilities do what they do, are harder to explain (and understand). As a result, as noted by Kamhi (2004), some of the concepts from some of the current information processing theories take longer to reach day-to-day practice. But regardless of the models studied, caution in applying them to clinical practice must rule the day. Montgomery (2002) mirrors this notion when he writes, "Given the complexity of language functioning, it is unlikely that any single construct of information processing theory is sufficient to fully capture the nature of a child's language or processing limitations" (p. 64).

With the caveat that we exercise caution, what are some of the concepts from information processing theory that deserve revisiting at this time? Box 5-7 contains a brief summary of each of the concepts outlined in the following sections.

The Concept of Mental Models. Montgomery (2002) uses the term *representation* to refer to "the symbolic coding and storing of information in long term memory" (p. 63). Lahey and Bloom (1994) talk about mental models as private representations of ideas in an individual's head. Language rules (linguistic competence),

BOX 5-7

Information Processing Theory Concepts Relevant to Language Learning Disabilities

Mental Models
The more background knowledge or experience that a child brings to a task, the "easier" or more manageable that task should be. For example, if a child internalizes the rules for creating stories, he or she can process and generate other stories without as much dependence on external cues.

Competing Resources
When the demands of a task exceed the child's abilities, something must "give" to free up the necessary resources to complete that task. For example, a child presented with new content in a textbook that is packaged in a literate language style of complex syntactic constructions and unfamiliar vocabulary may be too overloaded to comprehend the information.

Automaticity
The more a child performs a specific task, the more "expert" he or she becomes and consequently the less energy or attention he or she must devote to completing that task. For example, when an individual moves from being a novice to being an expert driver, the individual frees up resources so that he or she can do other things (such as talking on a cell phone) while driving.

story grammar structures, and background knowledge of a topic are examples of mental models. The more background knowledge (or experience) a child/student brings to a task, the "easier" or more manageable that task should be. More stable, or elaborated, mental models lead to less dependence on context or contextual support and more reliance on the information in long-term memory (Lahey & Bloom, 1994). For example, when a child is able to tell the story "The Three Pigs" (and other stories) without verbal prompting from his clinician or without using the pictures from the storybook to remind him of the events, his improved performance suggests that a more stable mental representation or mental model is operating for (or beginning to operate for) story structure. In other words, the "skeleton," or rules for creating stories, if internalized, enables our child to process and generate other stories without as much dependence on external cues. Clinicians might think in terms of mental models as they develop their language intervention goals. Connecting background or old knowledge—what a child/student "comes with" to a task—with new knowledge (a new language form, a well-formed personal narrative, a written expository piece, etc.) is an important and useful construct.

The Idea of Competing Resources. There are times when it is difficult for individuals to "walk and chew gum at the same time." When the demands of a task exceed one's level or ability, it might be said, to use another metaphor, that all eggs have to be put in that one basket to succeed. Recall Lahey and

Bloom's (1994) example (see p. 64) of learning to drive a manual transmission car. Because the task requires one's full attention and alertness, the new driver cannot talk, listen to the radio, and move the gearshift and pedals into their appropriate places *at the same time*. All resources must be focused on the task (shifting gears) at hand. Similarly, an intermediate skier who ends up on a double black diamond trail (a very advanced slope) will not be listening to her iPod while skiing (which she normally does) because all her efforts must shift toward survival (and finding that mental model from her last ski lesson to apply to that trail).

Likewise, our student with LLD who has to study the Roman Empire (see Chapter 3, p. 46) is faced initially with the task of mastering difficult content. As noted, our student may or may not bring much background knowledge to this subject matter. Add to the mix the reality of textbooks. Textbooks are usually written in expository text that is packaged in literate language, complex syntactic constructions, and unfamiliar vocabulary words. To put it simply: *Something has to give.* Poor performance is likely because resources are so "split" for attention. If the student has weakness in all areas, that is, in content and linguistic knowledge, he is on an academic double black diamond trail. In addition to sifting through the text, he also has to respond to his teacher's demands related to the subject matter. Windsor (2002) makes the point that task complexity is a critical factor when looking at the performance of children and adolescents with LLD. She reminds us to consider how much processing has to occur on multiple levels for our students to complete tasks. Windsor (2002) wrote the following:

> Task complexity, that is, the number of mental operations in a task [may be] a more important variable than the specific nature of the task to be performed. More complex tasks will consume more of available resources than less complex ones. (p. 51)

The concept of competing resources helps clinicians to think about which variables they will control in intervention so that their students can use resources for exploration and practice with new language forms (Lahey & Bloom, 1994). Thus telling a coherent story, a new skill for some children, may start with content that is very familiar to them (see JG's goals in Chapter 3, Box 3-7). Montgomery (2002) reiterates these ideas when he cautions clinicians about piling on too many difficult things at once, similar to the example given earlier about the curricula requirements attached to learning about the Roman Empire. He stresses the mental model/competing resources connection. He notes, for example, that when students have to deal with sentences with unknown words, expressed in complex grammatical forms, the majority of attentional resources have to go somewhere. Thus the available resources may be allocated to trying to sort through the less familiar content, leaving few resources to process the entire sentence correctly, especially when lexical or syntactic aspects of language are weakly or incompletely stored in one's mental model (Montgomery, 2002).

The concept of competing resources has promise as we look toward creating meaningful goals and objectives for our students. Successful intervention should stress the connections between prior knowledge and new knowledge across a variety of language situations, purposes, and discourse types (Gillam et al., 2002). Adding to the special needs of school-age students with LLD, Gillam and colleagues (2002) also encourage use of students' textbooks as the main backdrop for intervention because they will be required to have discussions around the topics in their books in their classrooms. Our introductory discussion of curriculum-based intervention in Chapter 4 brings some of the pieces together. This is an area we will revisit throughout this text.

The Role of Automaticity. Many researchers, including the ones mentioned previously, have discussed the phenomenon of automaticity. If we go back to Lahey and Bloom's (1994) example of driving a manual transmission car, we can say that when one moves from novice to expert as a driver (and as a skier), one no longer has to use the amount of energy or attention required to complete the task of shifting gears. Consequently, resources are "freed up" so that the driver can now talk on her cell phone, listen to the radio, and attempt to apply her lipstick while shifting seemingly *automatically.* Thus, notes Windsor (2002), when we're good at things, we spend little time focusing on them, leaving sufficient time to focus on what we need to do to complete a task. If a student is "good at" sports topics, the student can spend more time tackling the organizational requirements of writing an expository piece. Fewer resources have to be allocated to learning the sport's lexicon.

Thus part of the intervention picture includes finding ways to help students develop various levels of automaticity in both nonlinguistic and linguistic domains. For example, our clinician's French-Canadian experience with the Monopoly game presented her with an automatic (old) skill, that is, knowing the routine and rules of the game, and a less automatic (new) skill, that is, the French language, which came together in a noncompeting fashion. More resources could be allocated to attending to and experimenting with the language because less time had to be spent on learning the rules and following the game. Thus embedding language intervention activities in situations that present fewer competing factors may be a path for future exploration and study. Indeed, it is our hope that "as children develop and get repeated exposure to and experience with language, the mental operations become increasingly automatic...and...the efficiency with which...resources are allocated increases, and language performance improves" (Windsor, 2002, p. 50).

Summary: Information Processing Considerations. The previous discussion, far from being exhaustive, highlights a number of concepts from information processing perspectives that may provide another way to evaluate the complexity of variables that come together in a language assessment or intervention session. The second language learning examples and case studies create a real-world connection to a number of complex theories of behavior and language learning. We still have a long way to go and are reminded by Johnston (1999) and others to exercise caution when applying information processing theory and others to children and adolescents with and without LLD. Nonetheless, they offer us promise as we try to be the most effective change agents for our students. Van Kleeck (1994) offers clinicians another opportunity to see children's language learning and disorders from a prism of changing views about definitions of language.

The "Meta-Link": Another Perspective into Language Performance and Language Learning Tasks. The study of metalinguistics is another area of research that offers clinicians and teachers valuable and relevant information for consideration. It is important for a number of reasons, including the following (Box 5-8):

■ Metalinguistic ability is believed to be connected to advancements in both language and thinking.
■ Metalinguistic ability is thought to be connected to, and interactive with, literacy acquisition, reading proficiency, and academics.
■ Metalinguistics is one of the most misunderstood areas in clinical and educational practice, as the cases in the previous section suggested.

In her now-classic and still-current chapter on metalinguistic development, van Kleeck (1994) discusses the concept of metalinguistics, introduced in Chapter 1 (p. 8). A definition is restated in her words: "*Metalinguistic skill*, or language awareness, refers to the ability to reflect consciously on the nature and properties of language" (p. 53). Building on the concepts addressed in the information processing section, van Kleeck (1994) says that metalinguistic ability—the ability to think about language and treat it as an object—"frees both language and thought from the immediate context and fosters the development of abstract, decontextualized thought" (van Kleeck, 1994, p. 53). Van Kleeck (1994) summarizes the long and gradual process in development that occurs across a number of phases and stages. She makes the following two general points that underpin her stage-theory discussion:

1. She makes an important distinction between *social* and *academic-like* situations for her readers.
2. She helps professionals to think about what children "may" and "may not" be able to do at certain points in development.

In relation to the first point, van Kleeck (1994) says that in social situations, including those related to casual conversations, relaxed kinds of communications such as reading a novel, and so on, speakers and listeners focus on the *meaning* of a message. The specific sounds, words, and sentences used are below the surface. In *proficient* reading, we are also focused on meaning. Ordinarily, we don't "stop to think" or analyze the individual pieces of language when we are listening to a speaker unless something happens that

---

BOX 5-8   *Importance of Metalinguistics*

Metalinguistic ability. . .
■ Is believed to be connected to advancements in both language and thinking
■ Is thought to be connected to and to interact with literacy acquisition, reading proficiency, and academics
■ Is one of the most misunderstood areas in clinical and educational practice

shifts us to the "meta-level." For example, students might become distracted by a professor's New York accent. If it is too pronounced, it may cause students to focus on the accent (the phonology/form) rather than the teacher's message. If we are reading a text that is easy or "pressure free" (e.g., a riveting, well-written novel, *People* magazine, the *Los Angeles Times* sports page, etc.), we do not stop to sound out every word or analyze every sentence or paragraph. Rather, we focus on getting the writer's message. Proficient readers do this with relative ease. Again, we stop to think when there is a need to do so. By contrast, reading something that is more like a "pressure text," for example, "The Beginnings of the Roman Empire," may require more "meta energy" and focus. Clearly, proficient language users and readers function on spontaneous and "meta" levels based on the communicative situation. Classroom instructions, assignments, and other instructional and learning tasks require both metalinguistic and metacognitive (thinking about thinking) awareness. *Metacognition*, a term that also appears widely in both clinical and educational camps, involves "insights one can have regarding internal mental actions or cognitive processes" (van Kleeck, 1994, p. 56). For example, one might reflect on what types of things he or she remembers best, the strategies that work for him or her, and why and how he or she plans to complete an assignment. Although there is some overlap between the two metas (and others discussed by van Kleeck, 1994), metalinguistic ability relates to focusing on the language code itself. In terms of language and meta advances, van Kleeck (1994) points out that for clinicians, the meta-link means moving children from social to instructional uses of language. Inherent in this progression is the assumption that clinicians (and teachers) understand why some tasks, such as those presented in the cases, are more difficult—or more meta—than they appear to be on the surface.

> Classroom instructions, assignments, and other instructional and learning tasks require both metalinguistic and metacognitive (thinking about thinking) awareness.

In her detailed discussion of the stages of metalinguistic development, van Kleeck (1994) summarizes a great deal of information. Within a Piagetian framework, she proposes the following two major stages (or phases) in metalinguistic development, while at the same time recognizing the overlapping nature of any stage/phase model:

1. Stage 1: Language is used to convey meaning.
2. Stage 2: Language is used to convey meaning, and language is an object in its own right.

Stage 1 children are between 0 and 6 years old. They focus on meaning and communication and can only handle one aspect of language at a time. (Our metaphor of not being able to "chew gum and walk at the same time" comes to mind.) Thus expecting a stage 1 child to use a new word or sentence *and* correct its pronunciation or syntax at the same time may be doing too much at once.

As mentioned in the case summaries, children in the earlier stages of metalinguistic awareness tend to use a "semantic approach" (logically following from the focus on meaning) to solve meta problems. The discussion of Sean's case (see p. 114) suggests a semantic approach when he responds that "lake-lake" are "different" because he has been to Lake Tahoe in California and Lake George in New York. He is using background knowledge and meaning to complete the task, which, in this case, requires a form/phonemic judgment.

Similarly, when young children are asked to judge whether "train" is a long or short word (a structural/form judgment), they tend to say that it is a short word because they think in terms of the way the referent appears in the real world (van Kleeck, 1994). Children may think that "The men wait for the bus" is not a "good" sentence because "children wait for school buses and men take cars" (van Kleeck, 1994). Early stage 1 children may also have difficulty with various segmentation judgments, that is, separating words, syllables, or phonemes from the speech stream, for many reasons, one being, again, their focus on meaning rather than on individual segments. The acquisition of segmentation skills (see Troia, 2004; this chapter, pp. 114–118; Chapter 6) is part of metalinguistic development and is reflected in both Sean's and Jane's cases.

Although stage 1 children are at the beginnings of what will become complete metalinguistic awareness, van Kleeck (1994) reminds her readers to recognize that children *can* be "meta" in their early years. They do indeed start playing with language and shifting to judgments about language form before they come to school. But this recognition that children have some metalinguistic awareness in their preschool years must come with the reminder to be cautious. Clinicians and teachers must ask themselves, At what level can children demonstrate their awareness? For example, are structured phonics programs too "meta" for some children in kindergarten? (The answer is clearly yes.) The early "glimmers" of meta awareness may provide us with additional insights into children's future language learning experiences. They may also provide us with useful guidelines about the complexity of tasks that are assumed to be "easy," as we saw in Jane's case. Chapter 6 will provide additional information in this area.

In stage 2, according to van Kleeck (1994), children are between 7 and 11 years old. In this stage, they continue to use language to convey messages. Now, however, they also become aware that language is an entity or object in its own right that can be manipulated consciously. Two threads in development occur: (1) children can focus on double meanings; and (2) they can manipulate language form while, at the same time, maintaining its meaning. Van Kleeck's (1994) bottom line is that advancing metalinguistic awareness in this stage leads to an understanding that (1) language is an arbitrary conventional code and (2) language is systematic. This knowledge, in turn, gives rise to many other skills that become solidified between ages 7 and 11 years. Abilities related to figurative language (e.g., appreciating that "bat" has several meanings, understanding idioms and metaphors) and understanding ambiguity and synonomy (e.g., appreciating humor and text coherence) are outgrowths of this awareness of the arbitrary nature of language codes. Phonological awareness (segmenting words, syllables, and phonemes), making syntactic and other form judgments (such as the phonemic judgments required on auditory discrimination tasks), and aspects of reading and writing, including editing one's work, are examples of the advances that are derived from the awareness that language is systematic.

The study of metalinguistics arms clinicians with an excellent framework for evaluating the children they serve, the sequences they choose, and the tasks and techniques used in language intervention. Applying this information to commonly used tests and intervention tasks is the next step for practitioners. Consider the following tasks and ask what they have in common:

1. "I am going to say some words, phrases, and sentences. You point to the picture that I say. (The choice is three or four pictures.) Ready? Point to..."
   Boy
   Pushing the cart
   Rained
   The boy pushes the girl
2. Circle all the pictures that begin with the /b/ sound:
   Bat
   Car
   Birthday
   Mop
   Bell
3. Do these words sound the same or different?
   Rope-robe
   Thief-leaf
   King-ring
   Lake-lake
4. Provide a definition for these words:
   Unhappy
   Enthusiastic
   Scary

These tasks are familiar to many SLPs, other specialists, and classroom teachers. We could add many examples to the list. We engage children and adolescents with LLD in metalinguistic tasks every day. In some instances, clinicians and teachers must heighten their own awareness about the tests and tools they are using and for what purposes. Suffice it to say that the tasks have one commonality: they are also metalinguistic in nature. Although task 1 may be less demanding than task 4 (see van Kleeck's [1984] landmark work), and although tasks 2 and 3 tap different levels of phonological awareness, they all take language out of its natural context and ask students to think about language on a more conscious level.

School-age students with LLD certainly need to develop "meta" awareness on many levels. The question becomes, Do we strike an appropriate balance between levels of spontaneous and reflective language in our assessment and intervention choices? Again, we have much to learn in this area, but we have also learned a great deal. For example, the next time we see blocks being manipulated to represent nonsense words, a student correcting his ungrammatical sentence, a standardized test, or a story peppered with figurative language, we might ask ourselves the following question: What meta abilities are required to complete this task?

Keep the Conversation Going

The conversation will continue throughout this text and beyond. Wallach and Ehren (2004) reminded us to keep talking to ourselves and to our colleagues. They point out, as do Apel (1999), Kamhi (2004), and others we have mentioned in this chapter and in other sources, that we have to know "where we are coming from." Do our beliefs and daily practice form a match or mismatch with one another? This is a theme we will emphasize throughout this text. As a means of summarization, Box 5-9 is presented to operationalize some of the concepts addressed in this chapter. It takes the form of questions that professionals might reflect on themselves (as they evaluate their choices) or share with their colleagues. Box 5-9 provides a beginning way to open the discussion with colleagues about some complex issues related to information processing, metalinguistic awareness, and popular memes.

BOX 5-9

Questions for Self-Reflection

The following checklist can help in the creation of a shared knowledge base among all professionals who work collaboratively with students with LLD. The questions on the checklist are far from exhaustive. They provide a way to begin to operationalize some of the concepts covered in the chapter. The complex, overlapping, and interactive nature of the different areas should be kept in mind.

Information Processing Considerations
<u>Internally focused factors </u>(what does the student "bring" to the task or tasks? What does he or she "do?"):

1. What do you know about the student's background knowledge that relates to the task? How will you connect that knowledge to the new information or new learning task?
2. How do you define *strategy*? How does the student approach the task? What behaviors reflect the use of effective strategies? Does the student modify strategies to match tasks? How do you recognize and categorize strategies?
   (For example, does the student use context to "guess" when he or she comes to an unfamiliar word in a passage when reading or listening? Does the student use visual imagery strategies when the content calls for visualization? Does the student use "key words and phrases" such as "before/after," "by contrast," "unlike the previous point," and so on when the text or situation is more "heavily" linguistic?)
3. Does the student use familiar routines and scripts to help him or her deal with language? With new information? In what situations?
4. Is the student aware of the strategies he or she uses? Can the student tell you about the strategies he or she uses and why? (Overlaps with meta section.)
5. When you (or others) say that the student is "inconsistent," what do you (or they) mean? Is there a different explanation for the "inconsistencies?" What would you do to find out?
6. What language strengths does the student bring to the specific task (or academic requirement)? What weaknesses? (Overlaps with question 7.)

<u>External factors </u>(task analyses/materials/clinician's choices):

7. What do you see as the competing resources in this task?
8. If your goal is to improve an aspect or aspects of language, what have you done to control other aspects of the task/session/lesson, such as (a) its nonverbal aspects; (b) its content; and (c) the response required from the student?

Continued

(This question relates to which pieces of the task you see as being more automatic or needing less attention from the student.)

9. What is it about the materials you have chosen that may be making the task "easier" or "more difficult" for the student? Factors included might be as follows (focus is on connected discourse here*):
   a. Text's organization:
      ■ Is the text's macrostructure, or frame of reference, clear?
      ■ Are the micro aspects "above" or "at" a student's level (e.g., vocabulary, sentence structure, cohesive devices, etc.)?
   b. Text's content:
      ■ What does the student already know about the topic? (See also question 1.)
      ■ How many aspects of a topic are being covered?
      ■ What do you see as the major "roadblocks" to comprehending the content?
   c. Text's form/genre:
      ■ What similarities/differences do you see between connected and disconnected text in the student's performance? (Goes back to macro and micro interactions.)
      ■ If you control the content (the topic), does the student perform equally well on narrative and expository text? If not, hypothesize about why.
      ■ What form changes will help the student acquire the content?
10. Do you see this task as requiring a "top-down" or "bottom-up" approach? Why? How will this knowledge help your student?
    (Ask yourself whether this concept "works" in all situations. In other words, depending on "where you're coming from," you might see a task as "top down" and a colleague may see it as "bottom up." Discuss the different perspectives.)
11. If practice alone (or doing things over and over again) is insufficient to facilitate "real" language learning and learning in general, what techniques will you use to help the student develop more automaticity for some of the required language and academic tasks?
12. When the student fails to "get it" or when it doesn't "stick," how and why do you modify a task? What factors do you manipulate or change?

Metalinguistic Connections
13. What is your definition of metalinguistics? What does the "meta" connection mean to you? What is the relevance to your student?
14. What are the metalinguistic characteristics of the task/session/lesson?
15. How will you find out if the student has the "meta" abilities to complete the task?
16. Of the tasks the student completes in classroom, clinic, and resource rooms, are there some that are "more meta" (or more difficult) than others and why? There could be some discussion here about the nature of common tasks/programs/approaches used by teachers, SLPs, and other specialists, such as the following:
    a. LiPS program (Lindamood-Bell, 2003)
    b. Structured phonics activities

*The questions would be modified for micro issues (e.g., sentence, word level, etc.).

Questions for Self-Reflection—cont'd

   c. Visual mapping supports
   d. Auditory discrimination tasks
   e. CAP testing

Clinician's Beliefs (Popular Memes)[†]

17. Do you believe that children learn to talk by stringing together sounds?
18. Do you believe that improvements in children's ability to discriminate and identify speech sounds leads to improvements in speech and language abilities?
19. Do you think that CAPD and SID as disorders represent separate categories from each other and from language and language disorders?
20. Do you believe that you can treat CAPD alone without targeting language?
21. Do you believe that activities such as blowing whistles and others for exercising the speech musculature improve speech production?
22. Do you believe that children can be categorized as "auditory" or "visual" learners? If yes, how do you arrive at these categorizations?
23. Where do your intervention ideas "come from"? Why have you chosen to use a particular technique, approach, or program? Who says it's valid? Relevant? Research based?

[†]Questions 17 through 22 were inspired by Kamhi, A. G. (2004). A meme's eye view of speech-language pathology. *Language, Speech, and Hearing Services in Schools, 35,* 109. Questions 17 through 22 all target popular memes that represent inaccurate characterizations of language and language disorders.

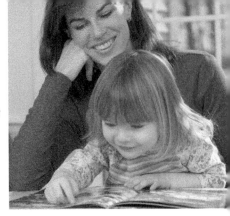

To be therapeutic, our language intervention experiences are designed to elicit and support specific language targets, to provide multiple opportunities for repetition and variation of the targets, to provide guided transfer or scaffolding that fosters independence, and to promote the metacognitive awareness needed to automatize strategies and behavior into skills and processes.

(Gillam & Ukrainetz, 2006, p. 68)

6 Integrating Spoken and Written Language

An Eye Toward Becoming Literate

SUMMARY STATEMENT ▬

The previous chapters put a face on the way language disorders show themselves across time. Through the discussions, checklists, and student examples presented, we developed an evolving framework for language intervention at school-age levels. Chapter 6, like the previous chapter, takes us in a slightly different direction. We will take a step back, albeit briefly, to the preliteracy and early literacy periods in children's language learning lives. We will consider the links among children's early language-based literacy experiences, later language learning, and school success. Chapter 6 weaves the concepts of social/communicative language experiences and academic language together with an eye toward helping children develop the language skills needed to become print literate, that is, to become readers and writers of the language. The chapter builds on the themes discussed throughout the text but considers additional ways in which speech-language pathologists and their colleagues can pull together goals and objectives that combine, rather than separate, spoken and written communication. Reminiscent of previous chapters, this chapter uses scenarios of children with and without language learning disabilities across time to highlight their changing needs. The chapter ends with a fast-forward to Grade 5 as we reconsider the challenges ahead. Among the topics covered in the chapter that speak to some of the concepts addressed earlier in the text are: keeping our eyes on the horizon when studying the early manifestations of language and literacy in the preschool period; operationalizing spoken-written language reciprocity in daily practice; and creating broader, more effective language therapy targets.

KEY QUESTIONS

1. What are some aspects of early reading routines that facilitate preschoolers' language and literacy and why might these experiences be important for future learning?

2. How can shared reading routines be structured to make them more effective for younger and older students with language learning disabilities?

3. What can preschool intervention teach us about school-age intervention?

4. Why is it important to revisit the concept of oral and written language reciprocity when trying to bridge the theory to practice gap?

INTRODUCTORY THOUGHTS

Social/ Communicative Language and Academic Language: A River and Highway Intersecting Across Time

The focus of this text has been on the language knowledge and skills, that is, the language underpinnings, related to and needed for academic success. In addition, the text's themes have emphasized the evolving and changing nature of language across the oral-to-literate continuum (see Chapter 2, pp. 35–37) and the reciprocal and integral relationship between spoken and written systems. Throughout this text, we have stressed the idea that language intervention is more powerful when we combine oral and written components and when we relate what we do with students to the "real world" of school. What becomes interesting at this juncture in our journey is to step back and consider some of the early manifestations of literacy and reflect on the ways that early reading routines, "home language," and the more socially based experiences that children have provide a foundation for, and insight into, the language challenges to come.

If we use the visual image of a river and highway going in the same direction on a parallel track, it may help us to think about times in development when social-communicative language and academic language seem a little removed from each other, that is, they seem to function on separate paths. Indeed, early communication (and literacy) experiences are usually embedded in interactional, naturalistic, and context-based situations, whereas academic language has its particular formal and decontextual style, as discussed throughout this text. If we return to our metaphoric river and highway, we can add that the river and highway do not remain separated forever. There are points in time when they cross and intersect. But as the river curves toward the road, a bridge or other supporting structures keep our drivers on the pavement, providing a smooth, and sometimes unnoticed, transition. Like our river and highway, socially focused and academically focused language also cross paths. The supportive structures that enable children to make smooth transitions from one path to another is the theme for this chapter.

Again, although the focus of this text is school-age language disorders, it is useful to consider some aspects of early literacy and reiterate what Fey and colleagues (1995) suggest—that we look at early language disorders with an eye toward "what they might become." Three intersecting areas are covered in the sections that follow: early reading routines; print awareness; and literature-based language intervention. The final section presents another example of school-age language disorders and integrates a number of techniques highlighted in the previous sections. The chapter ends and comes full circle by bringing readers back to the classroom to face the curriculum.

The Conversations in Early Reading Routines: A Social Experience Connected to Academic Success

CASE STUDIES

Scenario 1*

A 3-year-old child without language disorders and her mother are participating in a reading routine using the book *The Very Hungry Caterpillar* (Carle, 1979), as reported by De Temple (2001). The interaction progresses as follows:

Mother: "On Thursday, he ate through…? What are those?"

Child: "Strawberries!"

Mother: "How many strawberries?"

Child: "One, two, three, four."

Mother: "Very good. He ate through four strawberries, but he was…?"

Child: "Still hungry."

Mother: "Very good."

Scenario 2*

Another 3-year-old (again, without language disorders) is "reading" the same book, *The Very Hungry Caterpillar*, with her mother. An excerpt from this interaction is as follows:

Mother: "That night he had a stomachache. Why do you think he had a stomachache, [child's name here]?"

Child: "I don't know."

Mother: "Because he ate too much."

Scenario 3

A speech-language pathologist (SLP) is working with a 4½-year-old child with language learning disabilities (LLD). During the past 2 years, the child, Michael (not his real name), has made significant progress in expressive language, demonstrating improved syntactic, semantic (lexical), and phonological abilities. He is a reasonably good conversationalist with a lively personality and a growing awareness about how language can help you to "get what you want." He is still experiencing difficulties in comprehension and production of connected text (narratives); pre-literacy abilities are lagging behind his other language abilities, showing gaps in

---

*Scenarios 1 and 2 are taken from De Temple, J. M. (2001). Parents and children reading books together. In D. K. Dickinson & P. O. Tabors (Eds.), *Beginning literacy with language* (p. 37). Baltimore: Paul H. Brookes.

various aspects of phonemic and graphemic awareness, attending to book-reading routines, and producing coherent and "listener-friendly" early narratives such as accounts, recounts, and imaginary stories. He likes imaginary stories and prefers to engage in topics for which he has a specific interest—that is, mainly action stories such as *Spiderman* and *Star Wars*. Following is a treatment session excerpt, which fails to represent all of the intelligibility issues:

SLP: "You remember the story of *The Very Hungry Caterpillar?*"

(*Shows M the book.*)

M: "Can I tell you something? I have an Anakin suit."

(*M loves Star Wars and is going to be Anakin for Halloween.*)

SLP: "That's great...Let's look at this book first and then you can tell me about *Star Wars*. Tell me what you remember about this story."

(*The negotiating goes on for a few turns, but Michael is familiar with the speech and language intervention routine and joins the clinician-directed activity after a short time.*)

M: "Yea...He ate and ated it all. And then, he ate more things. Wait. Can I tell you something? I'm going to McDonald's after speech. And then, Halloween, it will happen after that soon..."

SLP: "OK. Let's get back to the caterpillar. You follow along with me. I want you to listen and answer the questions. I want to see if you can do the whole story by yourself when we're finished."

M: "OK." (*Looking a bit resigned to the situation.*)

SLP: "<u>Let's name</u> the things you see in these pictures as I turn the pages."

M: (*Pointing to the illustrations as the clinician turns the pages.*) "The caterpillar's over there. I see...um...what you call these...?" (*Clinician gives Michael the word, "pears."*) "OK...pears...plums...strawberries...oranges...watermelon...a leaf."

(*The naming focuses on identifying the "things the caterpillar eats." When M forgets a word, the clinician names it for him. Next, they review, without the book's pictures, some of the things the caterpillar has eaten.*)

SLP: "Now I want you to tell me '<u>what's happening</u>' in the pictures. I'll start and you'll finish. OK? And we'll use the pictures in the book as a reminder."

M: "A minder...What's a minder? Like your mind. My mind is evil. It's evil."

SLP: "A *re*-minder means to help us remember."

(*The SLP ignores the comment Michael makes about his "evil mind" at this time.*)

M: "OK. I get it. I get it."

SLP: "On Tuesday...and I want you to start with 'he ate.'"

M: "He ate one, two...he ate two plums." (*Says "plums" for "pears."*)

SLP: "On Wednesday..."

M: "He's still hungry so he asks his mom: 'Can I have three plums?'"

(*This goes on through the week recounting all the things the caterpillar ate. It ends up with a fat caterpillar who is building a cocoon and then becoming a butterfly.*)

SLP: "What is the caterpillar doing now? <u>What's happening?</u>"

M: "He's fat, so fat. He went to McDonald's and ate a big Mac."

SLP: "Did the caterpillar go to McDonald's? I think he's making a house. <u>What do you call</u> the thing he's making?

M: "A magical tent." (*Michael looks at the SLP for acknowledgment—or perhaps for the "real word."*)

SLP: "That's called a 'cocoon.'"

M: "OK. Cocoon. I can't remember that."

SLP: "That's good. I think you can remember that. So <u>what's happening</u> in this picture? Tell me the whole thing."

M: "He's ate so much so he's building a tent so he can be a big, fat, butterfly and it has a hole in it…because he's fat."

SLP: "OK. This is what's happening (*emphasizes this phrase*) in this picture. The butterfly is not hungry anymore. He's building a cocoon (*emphasizes the word*). He's going to turn into…"

M: "A big fat butterfly! Hurray! Are we finished now?"

SLP: "I want to ask you one more question. Then I want you to tell me the whole story of *The Very Hungry Caterpillar*."

M: "Ohhhh. Do I hafta?"

SLP: "<u>Why do you think</u> the caterpillar got a stomachache?"

M: "Because he threw up the oranges and the cake."

SLP: "I think that the caterpillar got a stomachache because he ate so many things."

M: "Yea. OK. He ate it all. Are we done yet?"

SLP: "<u>Do you think the caterpillar was silly</u> to eat so many things?"

M: "No, he was hungry."

SLP: "Yes, but maybe he ate a little too much."

M: "But he likes chocolate and cake, right?"

SLP: "Can eating too much chocolate give you a stomachache?"

M: "Yep. I love cupcakes."

SLP: "<u>Did you ever have a stomachache?</u>"

M: "Yea…I'm sick now. Gotta go to the doctor. I'm really sick." (*Puts his head on the desk and pretends to be sick, a role he likes to play.*)

> (*The reading routine continues with the book used as a scaffold for the story telling. Future sessions would aim toward using fewer external cues such as the book's pictures and the clinician's language/prompts to elicit the story.*)

NOTE: For an update 2 years into the future when Michael is in Grade 1, see Chapter 10.
NOTE: The <u>underlined portions</u> represent predetermined questions or comments that the SLP has chosen for the reading routine portion of her language intervention session.

What the Scenarios Say to Us. What can we learn from the scenarios? Following are some of the lessons illustrated:

1. The reading routines shed light on some of the ways in which children's preschool experiences with literacy and literacy-related activities influence their later language learning and school success.
2. The scenarios demonstrate ways to facilitate spoken language within a context that has the added bonus of facilitating written language.
3. The shared reading experiences provide us with insights into the ways that adult scaffolds and materials influence what children "look like" as language users.
4. The routines help us appreciate the preschool manifestations of school-age language disorders.

The first two scenarios from the longitudinal work of Dickinson and Tabors (2001) and their colleagues provide us with information about the patterns and progressions of early reading routines. Studying children at different points in the preschool period (from 3 to 5 years old), this team of researchers observed the ways that parents and children read books together. They considered both the type of language used by parents to stimulate conversations about the books and the ways that different books, at different periods of time, influenced children's responses to their parents or other adults who read to them.

De Temple (2001) points out that scenario 1 demonstrates "here and now" language. She calls this *immediate talk*. In immediate talk, adults direct children to focus on and respond to what they are actually seeing and hearing in the text. Thus when the parent asks, "What are those?" in scenario 1, an illustration of strawberries is right in front of the child. The parent and child can point to the picture and label it at the same time. Similarly, the caterpillar is still looking for food (he's still hungry) as a prompt for the next question. By contrast, scenario 2 has an example of *nonimmediate talk*. In nonimmediate talk, "the text or the illustrations [serve] as a springboard for recollections of personal experiences, comments, or questions about general knowledge or for drawing inferences and making predictions" (De Temple, 2001, p. 37). When the parent asks the child "why" the caterpillar has a stomachache in scenario 2, she is asking her to go beyond the text and make an inference (Box 6-1).

Although somewhat different in their level of questioning, the first two scenarios remind us that adult readers who provide scaffolds for children encourage interaction among the reader, the child, and the text. Further, the scenarios and the research behind them suggest that early "being read to" experiences introduce children to more literate forms of language, encourage inferential comprehension abilities, and provide a foundation for potential success in reading in the beginning elementary grades (Dale et al., 1996;

Adult readers who provide scaffolds for children encourage interaction among the reader, the child, and the text.

| BOX 6-1 | *Immediate versus Nonimmediate Talk* |

Immediate Talk

The reader is directed to focus on and respond to what he or she is actually seeing and hearing in the text. *Example:* "What are those?" (referring to a picture).

Nonimmediate Talk

The reader is asked to go beyond the text and make inferences based on recollections of personal experiences, comments, or general knowledge. *Example:* "Why did the caterpillar have a stomachache?"

Dickinson et al., 1992; van Kleeck & Vander Woude, 2003; van Kleeck et al., 2006; Westby, 1994).

Before leaving the first two scenarios, which are examples from children without language disorders, it is important to mention that one's choice of materials (in addition to the kinds of questions parents pose to children) may have an influence on the type and amount of language elicited. De Temple (2001) notes that books such as *The Very Hungry Caterpillar* may encourage more immediate talk whereas nonfiction books such as *Elephant* (Hoffman, 1984), two books used in studies by Dickinson and Tabors (2001) and their colleagues, may encourage more instances of nonimmediate talk. The choice of imaginary and factual books may be another variable to consider, but, of course, adults can structure their questions to provide a balance among a text's familiarity, the level of question, and the child's linguistic abilities. Controlling what *we* do so that children can accomplish what they need to accomplish is reminiscent of the information processing concepts discussed in the previous chapter. In other words, we might choose a familiar and often-practiced text so that the child can experiment with more complex language, such as engaging in nonimmediate talk. (See Westby [2004, 2005] for additional suggestions about choosing children's books.)

This brings us to scenario 3—the clinician working with a preschool child with LLD. What is observed in this reading routine? From the first interchange between the child and the clinician, the assumption we might make is that the child has heard the story of *The Very Hungry Caterpillar*. At this time, however, we do not know how many exposures he has had to the story. Let us assume for the moment that Michael, our child, is quite familiar with the book and has practiced going through its pages with the SLP several times across 3 to 4 weeks. If this practice schedule is accurate, we might then conclude that the clinician believes that Michael has achieved a reasonable level of familiarity with the story and can handle its basic content (like Lahey & Bloom's [1994] suggestions). Next, we should consider the questions the clinician is asking Michael. The underlined portions represent predetermined questions or comments that the SLP has chosen for the reading routine portion of her language intervention session. We might note that the progression is one that moves from encouraging immediate talk to practicing with nonimmediate talk. Questions that involve naming the items (e.g., "Tell me what the caterpillar is eating") and answering "What's happening?" (in the picture) encourage immediate talk. They are focused on the "here and now," especially when the pictures are present. Questions that ask "why" (e.g., "Why do you think the caterpillar gets a stomachache?"), encourage an evaluation (e.g., "Do you think the caterpillar was silly?"), and ask for a connection to real-life experiences (e.g., "Did you ever have a stomachache?") encourage nonimmediate talk.

We might stop to ask the following question at this time: Where does the sequence of questions used by the SLP come from? It is certainly reminiscent of De Temple's (2001) discussion of immediate and nonimmediate talk. Looking further, we would find that the SLP's choices are inspired by Westby (1994). In her chapter, Westby (1994) provides an excellent summary of the classic work by Snow and Goldfield (1981). Studying parents from different socioeconomic backgrounds and reading levels, Snow and Goldfield found that parents from both higher and lower socioeconomic groups read to their children and provided scaffolds for them, that is, they asked questions and interacted with their children while reading. Following these parents over a period of 2 years, however, the researchers observed a different patterning of questioning between the two groups of parents. The parents from the higher socioeconomic group started with more concrete and literal questions—such as the immediate talk questions—and moved to more abstract and inferential questions—such as the nonimmediate talk questions. By contrast, the parents in the Snow and Goldfield study who had less education and who were not strong readers themselves tended to focus on the literal, immediate talk questions with their children with little or no time spent on inferential questions.

In a more recent study, van Kleeck and Vander Woude (2003) found that the pattern of focusing mainly on literal questions (and not advancing to inferential questions) during reading routines was also a pattern evidenced by some parents of children with language disorders (van Kleeck & Vander Woude, 2003). The results of these studies, among many others, suggest that preschool children who have more practice with a broad range of comprehension questions during early reading routines tend to have an advantage over those children who have not had the same comprehension "practice" when they come to school. And while there are many factors that contribute to success in reading, it is clear that early reading routines are an important part of the road to literacy (e.g., Dickinson & Tabors, 2001; van Kleeck & Vander Woude, 2003).

As reported by Westby (1994) from the observations of Snow and Goldfield (1981), the following types of scaffolding questions form a sequence from "easier" to "more difficult" questions as reflected in scenario 3. These are presented in Box 6-2. Numbers 1 through 3 are literal questions; numbers 4 through 6 are inferential questions. They mirror some of the questions used by the clinician in scenario 3.

Van Kleeck and colleagues (2006) reiterate the significance of incorporating reading routines into language intervention goals but add that proceeding with sequences that help children move from concrete to abstract language use is often missing in early intervention programs. They point out that because reading comprehension exists along a continuum (as do many aspects of language,

Preschool children who have had more practice with a broad range of comprehension questions during early reading routines tend to have an advantage in school.

BOX 6-2   *Continuum of Scaffolding Questions as Reflected in Scenario 3*

1. Labeling	Questions such as, "What is this?"
2. Item elaboration*	Questions such as, "What kind of food is this?" "What color or shape is this?"
3. Event description	Questions such as, "What happened?" "What is the caterpillar doing?"
4. Reason/cause	Questions such as, "Why does he have a stomachache?"
5. Reaction	Questions such as, "Is he silly to have eaten so much?"
6. Real-world relevance	Questions such as, "Did you ever a stomachache?"

Data from Westby, C. E. (1994). The effects of culture on genre, structure, and style of oral and written texts. In G. P. Wallach & K. G. Butler (Eds.), *Language learning disabilities in school-age children and adolescents* (p. 184). Boston: Allyn & Bacon (see also Westby, 2005). Based on the observations of Snow, C., & Goldfield, B. (1981). Building stories: The emergence of information structures from conversation. In D. Tannen (Ed.), *Analyzing discourse: Text and talk.* Washington, DC: Georgetown University Press.
*The SLP in scenario 3 did not use any item elaboration questions.

as noted throughout this text), our early interventions should include exposure to *both* literal and inferential comprehension. In an 8-week, one-on-one intervention study, van Kleeck and colleagues (2006) asked whether book-sharing experiences would improve both the literal and inferential language of Head Start preschoolers with language disorders. The intervention phase involved twice-weekly 15-minute sessions in which adults read books to the children in the treatment group and asked them both literal and inferential questions. A control group received no intervention during the study's time frame. Scripts were predetermined and embedded in two storybook texts used in the study.

There were a number of "steps" the adult readers were taught to use to elicit and encourage language interaction with them about the storybook texts, as follows:

1. Adults asked both literal and inferential questions determined by the researchers (see the following paragraph).
2. If a child was unable to respond adequately, the adult provided scripted cues or prompts that were practiced so that they sounded as "natural" as possible and occurred as part of the book-sharing experience.
3. If the child still could not respond adequately after steps 1 and 2, the adult modeled the appropriate response or responses, which were also scripted. Responses modeled for the children included literal as well as inferential types.

The two storybooks used by van Kleeck and colleagues were *Mooncake* (1987) and *Skyfire* (1990) by Frank Asch. Adapting the hierarchy developed by Blank and colleagues (1978) and used currently in their *Preschool Language*

BOX 6-3   *Four Levels of Questioning*

Literal Questions
These questions are similar to immediate talk and to numbers 1, 2, and 3 in Box 6-2.

Level 1
Questions such as, "What's that?" (pointing to a particular item from the text).

Level II
Questions such as, "What's the bear doing here?"

Inferential Questions
These questions are similar to nonimmediate talk and to numbers 4, 5, and 6 in Box 6-2.

Level III
Questions such as, "How do you think Bear feels because his friend Little Bird is leaving?"

Level IV
Questions such as, "What do you think Bear's gonna do with his arrow with the spoon on it?"

Data from van Kleeck, A., Vander Woude, J., & Hammett, L. (2006). Fostering literal and inferential language skills in Head Start preschoolers with language impairment using scripted book-sharing discussions, *American Journal of Speech-Language Pathology, 15*, 85-95.

6

Assessment Instrument (PLAI)-2 (Blank et al., 2003), four levels of questioning, similar to those mentioned in the previous sections, were developed; these are summarized in Box 6-3.

Van Kleeck and colleagues were encouraged by the findings of their study, although they remained cautiously optimistic about what could be said at this point in time. Nonetheless, they found that the preschoolers in their treatment group made progress in both literal and inferential comprehension. The children's receptive vocabulary also improved significantly after the 8 weeks of scripted shared book reading. Although the children's literal skills still exceeded their inferential skills (as measured by the PLAI-2; Blank et al., 2003), van Kleeck and colleagues (2006) note that they have "accrued some evidence" that shared book reading had a positive effect on *both* aspects of comprehension. Looking more closely at the items used in the scripted routines, van Kleeck and colleagues (2006) point out that most discussions surrounding the books were on literal levels (70% literal vs. 30% inferential) so that additional research might show a different result if the percentages were reversed or equalized.

Recognizing that inferential skills are still more difficult for preschoolers with and without language disorders, van Kleeck and colleagues remind practitioners to explore the different possibilities offered by shared book-reading

Some evidence suggests that shared book reading has a positive effect on both aspects of comprehension—literal and inferential skills (van Kleeck et al., 2006).

experiences that have the potential to introduce preschoolers to complex language in more socially friendly ways. Adding this dimension to early intervention speaks to keeping our eyes on the horizon of Grades 3 or 4. Indeed, we might ask the following question: Can preschool experiences provide a stronger bridge that links early (socially based) and later (language-based) paths? As van Kleeck and colleagues note, we know that there are children with LLD who have specific reading comprehension difficulties that exist apart from decoding problems. Considering the work that has been done with phonological awareness and early intervention (covered in an upcoming section), they wrote the following:

> We have done much in becoming proactive in providing preventative interventions for phonological awareness skills for pre-schoolers with language impairments to facilitate their ability to engage in decoding. Taking proactive steps to prevent later comprehension difficulty is an equally important endeavor that warrants a greater research focus. (van Kleeck et al., 2006, p. 92)

(Appendix A provides a copy of van Kleeck and colleagues' [2006] scripts at each level used in the book-sharing intervention. Modifications for school-age children by using topics from their curriculum requirements as a backdrop and following the different levels of questioning should also be considered.)

Although optimistic about the study's potential value, van Kleeck and colleagues point out—as readers to this book already know—that there are challenges attached to engaging children, especially children with LLD, in book-sharing experiences. Van Kleeck and colleagues (2006) reference Pena's (2000) work with culturally and linguistically diverse children. Pena (2000) also found that considerable effort was needed to keep children who had less evolved language abilities willing and able to participate in shared reading experiences. As reflected in scenario 3, the SLP had to find ways to keep Michael, a delightful and motivated child, involved in the story. We saw how Michael tries to change the topic, provide humorous responses, or ask the SLP directly if he can do something else. While the excerpt also shows some of Michael's evolving strengths, including his growing metalinguistic awareness, the doubled-edged sword of keeping him engaged in the story to facilitate his language abilities, as well as helping him "stick" with a task to prepare him for kindergarten, remains an intervention reality. On the other hand, Michael's growing "word" awareness, reflected in his asking "what 'remind' means," coupled with his "mind as evil" and "I'm sick" statements (ones he has used previously) to get a reaction from his clinician, are all positive trends. They demonstrate Michael's unfolding understanding that language has segments and that language can be "used" and "manipulated" in particular ways (as discusssed by van Kleeck, 1994, Chapter 5, pp. 129–132, this text).

As van Kleeck and colleagues (2006) note, another direction for research is to look at the kinds of materials, situations, and parent/clinician feedback that facilitate engagement in shared reading materials. Although additional research is always recommended, the three abridged scenarios that provided us with snapshots into reading routines at home and in the clinic suggest ways that language intervention targets, such as moving children from immediate to

Considerable effort is required to keep children with less-evolved language abilities willing and able to participate in shared reading experiences (Pena, 2000).

nonimmediate comprehension, can be embedded into a meaningful activity. Likewise, incorporating aspects of metalinguistic development by, for example, helping children become more aware of word segments (e.g., Michael's spontaneous "what does 'a minder' mean?") is another way to structure shared reading experiences to meet intervention goals. Our SLP in scenario 3 could choose a number of ways to introduce word awareness and segmentation into her session. As inspired by van Kleeck's earlier works (1994, 1998), the SLP could say things such as, "I said 'caterpillar,' that's a long word; I said 'the,' that's a short word," and so on. She could also add, "When I put them together, I say two words, 'the caterpillar.'" There are any number of ways to combine oral, written, and meta aspects of language into our intervention sessions as we build bridges to literacy and academic success.

Print Awareness: Another Bridge to Literacy

CASE STUDY

Scenario 4

Two SLPs (C and A) are working with two preschoolers with LLD. L is 4.6 years old, and K is 4.4 years old. They are both diagnosed with specific language impairment (SLI). Both boys are believed to have average (or a bit above average) cognitive abilities. They both are energetic, playful, and engaging children with some attention and mild behavioral issues. L's issues are focused mainly in the expressive language area (including morphological, syntactic, and phonological delays); K's issues are also focused on language production, and he is slightly more unintelligible than L. Both boys are easier to understand when the topics are constrained and highly contextualized. When they change topics and talk outside of contextually based situations, it becomes more difficult to understand them.

In general, K had more significant language delays (across receptive and expressive domains) when first seen in the clinic 2½ years ago. Both boys have some very basic emergent literacy skills at this time. They have been read to, there are many literacy artifacts in their homes (books, letters on the refrigerator, all kinds of writing materials, etc.), they know that words are in books, and they have some primitive letter awareness (e.g., they recognize the first letter of their first names and can name some letters). But both children have limited letter-sound awareness and phonological awareness at this time. It might be said that they fall more within van Kleeck's (1994) semantic stage of meta development (see Chapter 5, pp. 130–131, this text) and the *logographic* stage of reading; that is, they recognize stop signs, McDonald's signs, and so on (Frith, 1985, in Catts & Kamhi, 2005f). They have both made excellent progress and are participating in the current session together for a peer-peer experience, as follows (their phonological errors are not shown in this excerpt):

SLP-C: "OK. We're going to play the McDonald's game now."

L and K: *Clap and smile and give the SLPs "high five" slaps.*

(*The boys have participated in the role-playing game at other times and have also experienced going to the real McDonald's. They enjoy the "group" experience, which is an occasional departure from their one-on-one therapy.*)

SLP-A: "I'm going to pretend I'm taking you to McDonald's. I'm going to eat with you. C is going to be working at McDonald's. She'll take our order and get our food."

L: "We gonna drive the car?"

K: "Yea. I wanna drive the car—fast—my brother drive fast!"

SLP-A: "We're going to walk. Let's go outside the room and then pretend we're coming into McDonald's."

(*The three "customers" go outside of the therapy room. A sign with the word "McDonald's" is on the door. Beneath the large sign with the name and the arches behind it are additional words in smaller print that read: "Welcome. Come in."*)

SLP-A: "Let's make sure we're at the right place. What does this say?"

(*SLP-A points to the large McDonald's sign.*)

<u>SLP makes a request about the print.</u>

L and K: (*Laughing and with enthusiasm, speaking almost simultaneously*) "McDonald's!"

SLP-A: "Great! Wait, there are more words. I'd better see what they say, too. Right?

L: "They say: 'Hamburgers,' right?"

K: "They say: 'French fries.' I want some!"

(*The boys are familiar with the "ordering" routine and have practiced with the names of many foods.*)

SLP-A: <u>(Points to the print. Comments about the print.</u> Then <u>Tracks the print)</u>. "There are three words here...one...two...three. It says: 'Welcome. Come in.' Let's point together and say the words together. You help me."

<u>SLP makes a request about the print.</u>

L: "Let's go inside."

K: "Yea. I'm hungry."

(*They both point and repeat the phrases with the SLP.*)

(*Inside there is a counter with many plastic replicas of the McDonald's foods, a toy cash register, spoons and forks, and other fast food props. There is a whiteboard with several food names written on it with the cost next to the items.*)

SLP-C: "Welcome to McDonald's. Come in. What would you like to eat? Do you see what we have today?" <u>(Points to the items on the board.)</u>

K: "I want a hamburger. French fries, too."

L: "Me, too. And ice cream!"

SLP-A: "OK. Let me see what else you have. What does that last one say, please? I don't have my glasses with me."

SLP-C: (<u>Pointing to the printed word</u> where the "s" is a little smudged.) "That's supposed to say 'salad' but the 's' is messy. I'm going to fix it." <u>(Comments about print.)</u>

SLP-C: "Hey, guys, who can help me make that 's' letter for 'salad'? I want our customers to be able to read this!"

L: "I can do it!"

K: "I do it, too! I can make the letter good!"

(*They both take turns trying to fix the 's' with the* SLP's *help.*)

SLP-C: "OK. My computer is broken today so I have to write down what you want. And then I'll bring the food to you. OK?"

SLP-A: "Guys. What did I want? Do you remember? Can you see the word on the list?" <u>(Request about print.)</u>

L: "It's there. You want salad. Why you didn't get a hamburger?"

SLP-A: "I'm on a diet! I don't wanna get fat. I'm going to eat a nice salad."

K: "A nice salad. That's silly." (K *thinks it's all funny.*)

SLP-C: "OK. Hurry and order. People are waiting."

SLP-A: "Let me get my credit card out. L, you go first. What do you want for lunch?"

K: "Hamburger, French fries."

L: "Me, too, ice cream. I want chocolate ice cream!"

SLP-A: (*A little turn-taking discussion occurs here.*)

SLP-C: "I'm writing this down. For K:" (*Writes his name.*) "Is that right? That's a K for [name here]." <u>(Comments about print.)</u>

(K *recognizes his name or at least the first letter of his name.*)

"K wants a hamburger...that's a hard word to write...French fries...Did I spell that right? Do you see an 'F' at the beginning of the words, guys? What do you think this says? I wanna get your order right."

<u>(Questions about print.)</u>

The session would continue with various targets covered for language production and for print awareness/print referencing. The print referencing is useful for literacy development, as well as for language production goals. As the McDonald's scenario continues, we would see the children change roles and take the orders, with appropriate language and contextual support from their SLPs.

Scenario 4 provides examples of what Justice and Ezell (2004) call *print referencing,* that is, "an evidenced-based strategy that may be used by speech-language pathologists and other early childhood specialists to enhance the emergent literacy skills of young children" (p. 185). Reiterating the notion that a *continuum* of change occurs across literacy domains, Justice and Ezell (2004) say that *emergent, early,* and *conventional* literacy are the three major terms we use to describe the developmental road to higher levels of spoken language, reading, and writing (p. 185). The children in scenario 4 are clearly at the emergent stage, but we can see how the print referencing technique can provide another way for SLPs to help preschoolers become more aware of print and the functions of print. Justice and Ezell (2004), among others (e.g., Ezell & Justice, 2000; Kaderavek & Justice, 2002), provide a number of excellent guidelines for their readers that have a strong theoretical and research base. As demonstrated in scenario 4 and as inspired by Justice and Ezell (2004), the SLPs provide a number of *cues* for the children during the McDonald's theme-based intervention session. Both nonverbal and verbal prompts are highlighted in scenario 4 (the prompts are underlined). The nonverbal references include (1) pointing to print while speaking and (2) tracking print. The verbal references include (1) questions about print, (2) comments about print, and (3) requests about print.

Justice and Ezell (2004) remind practitioners that "literacy is inherently the metalinguistic correlate of oral language" (p. 186). By increasing children's awareness of print in language intervention sessions and shared storybook reading routines, we are increasing their metalinguistic savvy, which can, in turn, have a positive impact on the ability to develop literacy. Taking readers through various stages of metalinguistic awareness as it relates to print literacy, Justice and Ezell provide a description both of metalinguistic milestones and of the skill areas attached to each stage. Figure 6-1 outlines the written language awareness achievements of children in the preschool period with the print referencing targets.

As seen in scenario 4, the two boys were working on *print interest* and *print function* levels. They will move slowly into the next stages, *print conventions* and *print forms*.

Expressing some of the notions also expressed by van Kleeck and colleagues (2006), among others, Justice and Ezell (2004) remind practitioners who work with preschoolers with LLD to think beyond working on oral language alone, as follows:

> If storybook reading is incorporated [into preschool language intervention] emphasis is typically placed on using this context to promote language comprehension and production. However, with print referencing emergent literacy skills may be developed simultaneously using the same materials with a minimum of time and effort. (Justice & Ezell, 2004, p. 186)

Language Intervention within Literature-Based Frameworks: Pulling the Pieces Together by Linking the Forest and the Trees

CASE STUDIES

Scenario 5*

An SLP and a student with LLD are working on the creation of a semantic map as part of a prestory discussion (Gillam & Ukrainetz, 2006). They are talking about plants and animals that one would find in a forest and categorizing the plants and

---

*From Gillam, R. B., & Ukrainetz, T. A. (2006). Language intervention through literature-based units. In T. A. Ukrainetz (Ed.), *Contextualized language intervention* (pp. 76–77 [scenario 5], 80 [scenario 6]). Eau Claire, WI: Thinking Publications.

Metalinguistic Milestones   ## Skill Areas

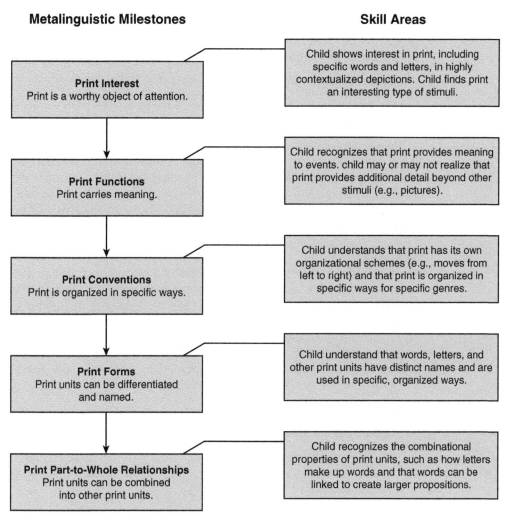

Print Interest
Print is a worthy object of attention.

Child shows interest in print, including specific words and letters, in highly contextualized depictions. Child finds print an interesting type of stimuli.

Print Functions
Print carries meaning.

Child recognizes that print provides meaning to events. child may or may not realize that print provides additional detail beyond other stimuli (e.g., pictures).

Print Conventions
Print is organized in specific ways.

Child understands that print has its own organizational schemes (e.g., moves from left to right) and that print is organized in specific ways for specific genres.

Print Forms
Print units can be differentiated and named.

Child understand that words, letters, and other print units have distinct names and are used in specific, organized ways.

Print Part-to-Whole Relationships
Print units can be combined into other print units.

Child recognizes the combinational properties of print units, such as how letters make up words and that words can be linked to create larger propositions.

Figure 6-1 ■ A suggested sequence of print awareness and print referencing. (*Redrawn from Justice, L. M., & Ezell, H. K. [2004]. Print referencing: An emergent literacy enhancement strategy and its clinical applications.* Language, Speech, and Hearing Services in Schools, 35, *185–193.*)

animals into a big and small arrangement. This activity relates to one of the significant story concepts:

SLP: "Can you think of a big plant that lives in the forest?"

Student: "A tree?"

SLP: (*Writes "tree" under the category* PLANTS *that is written on a board; has two categories under* PLANTS: *big and small.*) "Yes, a *tree* is a *big plant* that lives in the forest." (*Points to the words as she writes them on the semantic map.*) "Can you think of a small plant that lives in the forest?"

Student: "Well, grass is small, right?"

SLP: (*Writes "grass" under the category of* PLANTS/*small on the board.*) "Yes, grass is a small plant that lives in the forest. What are we saying about trees?"

Student: "Trees are big. They're plants. And they live in the forest."

SLP: "Yes, trees are big plants that live in the forest." (A recast of the student's utterance into a more literate, relative clause sentence.)

The session would continue with a discussion of big and small animals that live in the forest. The SLP and the student would be looking at the printed words and the semantic map as a frame of reference for the discussion. The clinician might work to highlight the similarities and differences they are mapping. Depending on the age of the child or student, she would talk more explicitly about relations. She might also review with the student the reasons why they are completing various activities.

Scenario 6*

The SLP and the student are in the middle of a shared reading experience. They have worked on the semantic mapping (as per scenario 5) and they have also looked through the book and created their own descriptions and discussions based on the illustrations. Thus there is some familiarity with the book and its basic content. The excerpt that follows, also from Gillam and Ukrainetz (2006), is what they call "the heart of the intervention." The clinician reads the story to the student and then asks a series of comprehension questions. The questions and scaffolds used are geared toward the clinician's goals for her individual students:

SLP: "Tell me what we know about the ant." (Prompt.)

Student: "The ant was soaking wet."

SLP: "Yes sir. We know the ant was wet." (Recast into a more complex complement structure.) "What else do we know about the ant?" (Broad question; more *inferential*.)

Student: (*Hesitates and does not say anything.*)

SLP: "Think about how the ant treated the other animals." (Prompt.)

Student: "Mad. Mean?"

SLP: "Was he mean? How was he mean"? (Narrower question.)

Student: "Cause just a little space for him, so um…"

SLP: "There was just a little space for the ant under the mushroom, so…" (Semantic and syntactic expansion plus a prompt.)

Student: (*No response.*)

---

*From Gillam, R. B., & Ukrainetz, T. A. (2006). Language intervention through literature-based units. In T. A. Ukrainetz (Ed.), *Contextualized language intervention* (pp. 76–77 [scenario 5], 80 [scenario 6]). Eau Claire, WI: Thinking Publications.

SLP: "Does he share his space with any of the other animals?" (Narrow the focus with an elaboration question.)

Student: "No."

The session continues with various discussions about what the ant did for the other animals in the story. The illustrations in the text serve as a reminder for the events. Various facilitation techniques would be used to help the student comprehend and respond to inferential questions, while at the same time expanding his language.

Scenarios 5 and 6 are abbreviated examples from Gillam and Ukrainetz (2006) that show language practitioners how to use book reading and book discussion as contexts into which their goals and objectives can be embedded. To bring background knowledge and context into what the SLP and the students are talking about in the scenarios, one might ask about the story they are using and why it was chosen. The story used by Gillam and Ukrainetz (2006) is *Mushroom in the Rain* (Ginsberg, 1974). It is a story about an ant who hides under a mushroom in the forest's clearing to take shelter in a rainstorm. The mushroom is rather small at the beginning of the storm but there is enough space for the ant. As the storm continues, a sequence of animals—including a butterfly, a mouse, a bird, and a rabbit—ask if they can share the space under the mushroom to get away from the storm. At first the ant refuses to let each animal under the mushroom, but, eventually, he allows all the other creatures to share the space. The story reaches a conclusion when, thanks to the frog's prompting, the ant realizes that the mushroom has grown during the storm.

According to Gillam and Ukrainetz (2006), the story represents a reasonable choice because its structure adheres to story grammar elements in a number of positive ways, including having the added benefit of repetition, which occurs in each major episode. Each episode contains the same *initiating event* (getting wet in the storm), *attempt at action* (each animal requests a spot under the mushroom), *complication* (the ant doesn't let them in because there isn't enough room), *another attempt* (requesting that the animals already under the mushroom squeeze together), and *consequence* (the request for shelter is granted). There is one "unique" episode where the animals hide the rabbit from a fox.

What, specifically, might scenario 5 demonstrate for us? Gillam and Ukrainetz (2006) use semantic mapping for a number of reasons. They point out, for example, that research suggests that visual displays such as those in the form of semantic maps can provide students with LLD with useful scaffolds and tools for improving reading comprehension. They also write, "We employ graphic organizers in a variety of formats to provide students with a visual representation of the relationships between key ideas in a story and to highlight important vocabulary" (Gillam & Ukrainetz, 2006, p. 75). In scenario 5, we see how semantic mapping, a popular technique that is sometimes overused or used inappropriately, can be placed into a meaningful context. As Gillam and Ukrainetz (2006) suggest, we see the SLP and the student working on concepts and vocabulary that will have *relevance* to one of the stories they will use in their literature-based unit. One of the key issues of the *Mushroom in the Rain* story has to do with the size of the different animals in relation to the mushroom, which, as noted, starts out small (with just enough room for the ant) but grows larger during the course of the rainstorm. (See Singer & Bashir [2004] for a discussion of less effective uses of semantic maps; see also Chapters 9 and 10, this text.)

Scenario 5 also represents the first phase of what can become an entire unit. (Scenario 6 represents a later phase.) Gillam and Ukrainetz (2006) outline the following five areas that form a sequence of literature-based activities that can be modified for preschoolers, as well as school-age students with LLD:

1. Prestory knowledge activation (scenario 5)
2. Shared reading of the entire story
3. Post-story comprehension discussion (scenario 6)
4. Focused skill activities
5. Book as a model for a parallel story

Each of these areas builds on the other. For example, as seen in scenario 5, practice with the key concepts and vocabulary that are a core part of the story can provide a base of knowledge and familiarity that enables a clinician to "push" the child further with language in the phases that follow. Many different facilitation techniques, such as those presented in Box 6-4 later in this chapter and discussed in the sections that follow, can be used during this phase of language intervention, depending on students' needs.

In between scenarios 5 and 6 would be Gillam and Ukrainetz's (2006) *shared reading of the entire story*. As noted previously in the introduction to scenario 6, there would be additional practice before the actual reading of the story by the clinician. In the second aspect of the literature-based intervention, there could be additional prestory discussions. For example, the clinician and student might discuss the shelters that animals could likely fit under, how rain helps plants to grow, and other related questions that encourage the activation of real-world knowledge and logic. The child and the clinician would also "step away from the printed text and create their own oral descriptions to match the illustrations in the book" (Gillam & Ukrainetz, 2006, p. 78).

The *focused skill activities* (area 4) could involve any number of semantic, syntactic, narrative, or pragmatic targets depending on, again, a student's individual needs. Phonological targets could also be integrated into the literature-based sessions for children with co-occurring intelligibility issues. We see examples of the way a focused skill might be embedded into the sessions in scenarios 5 and 6. For example, we see a number of *relative clause recasts* by the SLP in scenario 5 when she uses variations of the following statement: "Yes, a tree is a big plant *that lives in the forest*." We see a similar recast with the complement sentence in scenario 6 when the SLP says, "*We know that* the ant was wet." In these examples, complex, literate syntactic forms are targeted or embedded within the literature-based intervention session.

Finally, *book as model for a parallel story* (area 5) can also have a number of pieces to it. There can be a review of the original graphic organizer and story. Another story with similar but related concepts can be added or the earlier story may be revised. (See Appendix B for a detailed outline of Gillam & Ukrainetz's [2006] Sequence of Literature-based Activities.)

As the quote at the beginning of the chapter suggests, language intervention has to be intense and targeted, among other aspects mentioned. The two scenarios (5 and 6) in this section highlight some of the language facilitation devices that can be used in the storybook units. They are also evidenced in the previous scenarios. Gillam and Ukrainetz (2006) talk about the following three types of facilitation devices:

1. *Linguistic facilitations* are adult modifications of the form or content of a child's immediate utterance.
2. *Response facilitations* are adult questions or other kinds of support that encourage the child to say (or do) something.
3. *Regulatory facilitations* are things an adult says (or does) to raise a child's/ student's awareness of a targeted language skill.

According to Gillam and Ukrainetz (2006), regulatory facilitations have a special function. They can lead students toward understanding what is critical or significant in an activity. Regulatory functions can make background knowledge more explicit and connected to current knowledge, and they can help children/students evaluate their own learning. Gillam and Ukrainetz recommend that at least 40% to 60% of utterances directed to students should employ any or all of these facilitation devices. Box 6-4 outlines the facilitation devices discussed by Gillam and Ukrainetz (2006).

BOX 6-4

6

Facilitation Devices Embedded in Oral Interactions Around Storybooks

Linguistic Facilitations
1. *Syntactic expansion:* A contingent verbal response that makes the student's utterance grammatical.
   Student: "That bird gonna ask him come in."
   Adult: "Yes, the bird is gonna ask him to come in."
2. *Semantic expansion:* A contingent verbal response that adds new, relevant information to the student's utterance (also called an *extension*).
   Student: "Then him fell all over that."
   Adult: "Yea, the kangaroo fell into the bear's swimming pool."
3. *Recast:* A contingent verbal response that retains the semantic information from the student's previous utterance but alters the syntactic structure.
   Student: "That board picture was from Jason."
   Adult: "Yea, Jason drew that picture on the board."
4. *Prompt:* A comment or question that induces the student to complete a thought or to change an ungrammatical utterance.
   Student: "Him's going to run back home."
   Adult: "Who's going to run back home?"
   Student: "He's going to run back home."

Continued

Facilitation Devices Embedded in Oral Interactions Around Storybooks—cont'd

5. *Elaboration question:* A question that induces the student to expand on what he or she has said.
   Student: "He was scared of that dinosaur."
   Adult: "Why was he scared?"
   Student: "He thought the dinosaur might chase him and bite him."
6. *Vertical structure:* The clinician asks a question to obtain additional information; the student answers it; then the clinician puts the original utterance and the response to the question together to form a more complex utterance.
   Student: "That moose holding up a hammer."
   Adult: "What would happen if he dropped it now?"
   Student: "It would hit his toe."
   Adult: "If the moose dropped the hammer, it would hit his toe."

Response Facilitations
1. *Model:* The clinician models the target word or form.
   Adult: "Little Grunt is very sad because he doesn't think he'll ever see his dinosaur again."
2. *Questions to elicit a new utterance:* The clinician asks a question or makes a statement designed to elicit the target structure.
   Adult (points to picture): "Tell me how each person in the Grunt family feels about what the chief said and why each person feels that way."
3. *Prompt:* The clinician pauses, repeats the student's utterance, or provides a partial response to encourage the student to use the target structure.
   Adult: "Little Grunt is very sad..."

Regulatory Facilitations
1. *State the goal or target:* The clinician tells the student what he or she will be working on.
   Adult: "We're going to look at the book again, and we're going to focus on talking about how the characters feel about what happens."
2. *Compare or contrast:* The clinician highlights the similarities or differences between related words or grammatical structures.
   Adult: "Little Grunt is sad about having to tell his dinosaur to go away. But Chief Rockhead Grunt is happy that the dinosaur is leaving because he was too big to live in the cave."
3. *Informative feedback:* The clinician tells the student whether something he said was right or wrong and explains why.
   Student: "Everyone was happy that the dinosaur left."
   Adult: "Not Little Grunt. Little Grunt was sad when the dinosaur left because the dinosaur was his pet."

From Gillam, R. B., & Ukrainetz, T. A. (2006). Language intervention through literature-based units. In T. A. Ukrainetz (Ed.), *Contextualized language intervention* (pp. 69–70). Eau Claire, WI: Thinking Publications.

The clinician in scenarios 5 and 6 uses recasts to expand the child's syntactic repertoire for relative clause and complement sentences while keeping the semantics constant in both. She uses prompts in the form of broad and narrow questions in both scenarios; she also uses a sentence completion prompt with a *syntactic and semantic expansion* (linguistic facilitation) in scenario 6 when she says, "There was just a little space for the ant under the mushroom, so..." Toward the end of scenario 6, we also see an *elaborated question* (a linguistic facilitation) when the clinician asks, "Does he share his space with any of the other animals?" Although we do not see any regulatory functions used explicitly in these abbreviated scenarios, both *compare-contrast* and *stating the goal or target* are mentioned at the end of scenario 5. Although more indirect at this point in scenario 6, the SLP is providing the student with some *informative feedback* when he incorrectly identifies the ant as "mean." One can see that she begins directing him with her prompts and questions to a more accurate and appropriate answer.

Summary Points from the Scenarios

Early Reading Routines, Print Awareness, and Literature-Based Frameworks Meet on the Road to Literacy. The six scenarios presented thus far—two with average-achieving children and the remaining examples with children with LLD—highlight different aspects of shared reading routines as a context for language learning within an intervention framework. But as with other aspects of language intervention discussed throughout this text, the clinician must set the direction of intervention and know "where" he or she is "going" and where suggested sequences and techniques "come from." The scenarios presented address the ways that specific targets can be embedded into a broader, more natural learning context, the shared reading experience. We can see that the social-interactional aspects of shared storybook reading, starting with modeling and basic questions and prompts, offer tremendous potential as an intervention context.

Thinking in terms of "here and now" language and moving to "there and then" language is one way to think about controlling linguistic complexity. The *immediate/nonimmediate* language of Dickinson and Tabor (2001) and the literal/inferential questions of van Kleeck and colleagues (2006) put the prompts and questions we use for scaffolding into perspective (see pp. 142–145, this chapter). Again, familiarity with the content of a story can ease the "competing resources" dilemma (Lahey & Bloom, 1994; see Chapter 5, pp. 126–128). We are reminded by van Kleeck and colleagues (2006) that even though literal questions are easier for preschoolers with and without language disorders, we should incorporate inferential (nonimmediate) questions into our interventions with, of course, the appropriate supports and evaluation of background knowledge and familiarity with a story. Indeed, as mentioned earlier, research suggests that children who have been exposed to nonimmediate talk in the preschool period have better outcomes when they reach kindergarten and Grade 1 than children who have not been exposed to nonimmediate talk. Children with deeper and more elaborated shared reading experiences perform better on tasks involving story comprehension, emergent literacy knowledge, and receptive vocabulary (De Temple, 2001).

Print awareness/print referencing is another dimension of both early and later language intervention that was reflected in the scenarios. Justice and Ezell

(2004) offered practitioners many excellent ideas in this arena. Including print (and other aspects of written language) in language intervention sessions should not be thought of as "an *extra* thing to do" (a lament of some SLPs); it should be seen as "an *integrated* part" of language therapy. Although we focused on print awareness in scenario 4, one can see that print is a major scaffold in scenario 5 (and could be in the other scenarios as well). In trying to resolve some of the confusion about the role of SLPs, especially and in view of shared reading as a context for language and literacy intervention, Gillam and Ukrainetz (2006) wrote the following:

> Our primary goal with literature-based language intervention is not to teach... students [with language learning disabilities] to read. Rather, our goal is to improve the many aspects of language. . . that influence the ability to participate in, and profit from, instruction in general education classrooms in both oral and print modalities. (p. 60)

Finally, the Gillam and Ukrainetz five-part sequence described here and presented in Appendix B provides us with an overarching way to consider the many aspects of literature-based intervention. Their macrostructure begins where some of the earlier reading routines and early print awareness activities (i.e., the first two levels) leave off. But the specific facilitation devices outlined by Gillam and Ukrainetz (2006) can be seen as weaving their way through all the scenarios with different degrees of explicitness. In general, the closer to school age (Grade 1) children are, the more explicit and direct our intervention can become. Caution must always be exercised, however, when making statements such as the previous one about the explicitness of language intervention in relation to children with LLD.

Clearly, the dynamics of child, tasks, and materials are always present in language intervention decisions. All of the researcher-clinicians referenced in this chapter talk about the importance of choosing our storybooks (and other materials) wisely. Self-questioning becomes a tool to more effective intervention choices once again: are we looking for a repetition and simple plot (e.g., *The Very Hungry Caterpillar*), a strong but repetitive story structure (e.g., *Mushroom in the Rain*), a print-salient storybook (e.g., *Nine Ducks Nine* [Hayes, 1990]), or a text with figurative language (e.g., *Merry Christmas, Amelia Bedelia* [Parish, 1986])?

The Horizon Looms Large: Connecting Early and Later Literacy Experiences

Fast-Forward to Grade 5

Consider the following excerpt from a Grade 5 text, *Social Studies: The Early United States* (2000):

> Lincoln held back on declaring an *Emancipation Proclamation*, an order freeing the slaves. He feared that such a step might turn people in the border states, as well as some states in the North, against the Union. Lincoln's waiting made the abolitionists angry. William Lloyd Garrison wrote that Lincoln was "nothing better than a wet rag."
>
> As the war went on, Lincoln thought more and more about the question of slavery. Had the time come to write an Emancipation Proclamation? What would be the consequences if he made such a decision? (p. 513)

The passage from the Grade 5 social studies text, as with many of the other excerpts from the curriculum already presented in this text (as well as those to follow), serves as a reminder of the challenges facing students with language learning disabilities (and, perhaps, other students) as they move through the grades. As Westby (2005) points out and as Bashir (1989) noted in earlier writings, "young children use their oral reading skills to learn to read, while older children use their reading abilities to further their language learning—they read to learn" (Westby, 2005, p. 157). But again, as noted by Westby (2005), the phrase *reading to learn* carries with it many assumptions (Box 6-5). A student can *read* the Grade 5 text *to learn* about the war *if* he or she has experience with literate language styles, new and rare vocabulary words, and increasingly complex syntactic forms. In addition, writes Westby (2005), "reading-to-learn" readers must have knowledge about their physical and social word, understand why they are reading, and have some awareness of the ways that different texts (e.g., narrative vs. expository) work to convey information. The reading-to-learn phase of development (and we could also say the *listening-to-learn* phase) also includes active involvement on the part of the reader (and the listener). Good readers work at trying to make sense out of what they read just as competent comprehenders of spoken language work to make sense of what they are hearing. Meta-awareness and control of various strategies that can be used in different situations accompany the reading-to-learn individual, as we shall see in the chapters that follow.

Thus children bring their preschool experiences in language and literacy with them to school. Westby's examples in the previous paragraph that address "what it takes" to use reading to learn and her body of work (e.g., Westby, 1984, 1985, 1994, 2005, 2006) remind us that many aspects of later language ability can take root within the early reading routines that were discussed in the previous sections of this chapter. For example, children can experience and learn novel vocabulary words by listening to stories and answering questions about the stories (such as Michael's learning of "cocoon" and other words in scenario 4).

6

BOX 6-5   *Assumptions of "Reading to Learn"*

A student can *read* a text to *learn* the material if he or she has experience with the following:
- Literate language styles
- New, rare vocabulary words
- Increasingly complex syntactic forms

The student also needs the following to be a "reading-to-learn" reader:
- Knowledge about his or her physical and social world
- An understanding of why he or she is reading
- Awareness of the ways in which different texts convey information
- Active involvement
- An ability to make sense of what he or she is reading

Data from Westby, C. E. (2005). Assessing and remediating text comprehension problems. In H. W. Catts & A. G. Kamhi (Eds.), *Language and reading disabilities* (2nd ed., p. 157). Boston: Allyn & Bacon.

They can practice with and acquire more complex language structures (as noted in the relative and complement clause sentences in scenarios 5 and 6) and they can be guided to use background knowledge, as well as a text's information, to make inferences (as in scenario 2, among others). As we look back to the early literacy experiences of children, we can make connections, some direct and others more indirect, between what they learn in this period and what they may need to do to access the curriculum. Again, while not trying to overstate the case for a direct and clear-cut intersection between the river and highway of preschool and school-age acquisitions, a reasonable question that forms the theme of this chapter (and one that many researchers and practitioners pose) is, What are preschool children learning in the interactions occurring *before, during, and after* the shared reading routines that may help them later on? The previous sections provided examples of activities that addressed this question.

The Grade 5 excerpt speaks to those of us interested in language and literacy on a number of levels. Similar to points made in Chapters 3 and 4, we can see that it "takes" a great deal of presupposed knowledge and skill to absorb the content of this subject matter, the Civil War. Our students with LLD may not have the level of spoken or written linguistic ability (and experience) needed to access and hold onto the meaning of the text. Leaving the specifics of the Emancipation Proclamation aside for the moment, do they understand the meaning of "emancipate" (and its relation to "emancipation") or "to proclaim" (and its relation to "proclamation")? Is there anything in the vocabulary that surrounds the core content that might be confusing for students with LLD? For example, are words or phrases such as "declare," "consequences," "turn... against," or "as well as" known and understood? Likewise, is the excerpt's form (expository text) having an effect on the student's comprehension? In other words, how much experience has the student had listening to, reading, and writing expository text? Can the student handle the literate style of syntax reflected in the passages? For example, we might note the use of a complex complement sentence with an embedded/interrupting clause in the following statement: "He feared that such a step might turn people in the border states, as well as some states in the North, against the Union." In addition, the figurative language reflected in Garrison's statement that Lincoln was "nothing better than a wet rag" and phrases such as "held back" and "turn against" (mentioned previously) can be difficult for students with LLD. Indeed, the linguistic demands can make it virtually impossible for them to absorb the content of the Civil War unit from the written text—and, most likely, from spoken text as well.

Donahue and Foster (2004) would agree that a linguistic analysis of the social studies excerpt provides us with information that is useful for speech-language pathologists, teachers, and other professionals who work with students with LLD. They would also agree that preliteracy experiences can provide a foundation for academic success. Indeed, when children enter school for the first time it is assumed that they have come with intact language and early literacy skills. But Donahue and Foster (2004) would also remind us that "reading is social discourse" (p. 176). By this they mean that readers form relationships with the text, the authors, and the characters. In other words, readers bring more than their linguistic, metalinguistic, and metacognitive skills to the task of, for example, comprehending the Civil War passage. They bring with them their social values, attitudes, biases, and personal experiences about a topic. Proficient comprehenders go beyond decoding and reading fluently. They use their understanding of social relationships to pose questions to themselves about what an author's agenda might be, how accurate his or her point of view is, and whether the author should be believed. They may use their own experiences to empathize or identify with a character. As VanSledright (2002a) also points out, history is a content area subject that has many of these "socially based" attributes.

Continuing with this discussion, Donahue and Foster (2004) add that expert readers use a number of strategies to confirm their initial impressions of a text after reading. They may reread the text to confirm (or not) their first reading, check facts on a related Web site, or look up words they do not fully understand, among other checks and balances. Experienced and critical readers are on a search for answers and check their own goals for reading. They might ask themselves questions such as the following: Am I supposed to get and retain information? For how long? For a test only? Am I reading this for fun? To write a book report? And so on.

Bringing to mind, once again, the notion of a language learning continuum, Donahue and Foster (2004) write that "reading comprehension is a remarkably complex cognitive [and linguistic] ability that develops across the lifespan, in the same way that oral discourse abilities evolve as social/political contexts, roles, and agendas change" (pp. 176–177). They remind professionals that they can bring a social component to reading in the elementary grades and beyond using activities such as some of the ones described as part of the shared reading activities that come from a more social-oriented mode in the early stages of literacy. Conversely, as we look ahead to social studies texts and other curricular challenges facing students, we can also modify the activities chosen in the preschool period to make the social-information processing aspects of reading more explicit. While not differing significantly from other strategies that are useful for effective reading and learning, some of which have been outlined in this text and elsewhere (e.g., Ehren, 2005; Pressley & Hilden, 2004; Chapters 7 and 8, this text), Donahue and Foster (2004) encourage professionals to help students see how their own values and experiences intersect with the text. They point out that teachers and SLPs could work together to assess the social-information processing demands of texts. It is useful to make explicit the relationship between the reader (the student) and the text. Questions that involve developing a relationship with authors (What is he trying to say? What do you think he means?) and characters (Do you agree with what he is doing? Which character do you admire? Not admire? Why?) are part of bringing a more explicit social component to the reading/learning process.

The Grade 5 excerpt presented earlier, covering Lincoln's dilemma about the Emancipation Proclamation, offers an opportunity for discussion about students' understanding of the conflict (the Civil War) or conflicts in general, their knowledge and attitudes toward slavery (past and current), what they may know or believe about the Civil War, their empathy for Lincoln, and their attitudes and opinions about Garrison's statements. These areas of discussion and

Teachers and SLPs can work together to assess the social-information processing demands of texts and help make the relationship of the reader and text more explicit.

6

study could be part of a unit that brings the students' perceptions, biases, and knowledge to the table in the form of a social discourse.

The Continuum Revisited

Westby (2005), and also in her landmark works (Westby, 1984, 1985), presents another useful framework that begins the preschool period and continues to the later elementary grades. This hierarchy also speaks to the evolution of aspects of literate language. Using narratives and shared reading as a backdrop (see also Chapter 7), Westby indicates that goals and objectives can be created that keep an eye on "what's next" on the horizon. Many of the concepts discussed in the preschool reading routines, including the sequences suggested by Gillam and Ukrainetz (2006; see Appendix B), are inspired by Westby's work and vice versa. She offers the following, sometimes overlapping, stages and accompanying objectives and activities for consideration as we look across time. Rigid separations among stages and grade levels are not suggested in the examples. Rather, the examples represent aspects of literacy that build on one another that can be modified depending on the individual needs of children. Some of the suggestions have been adapted and modified from Westby's (1985) work for this chapter.

The Early Stage. This period encompasses preschool and the very beginnings of school: kindergarten and Grade 1.

> *Objectives:*   Provide exposure to literate language
> Structure interactions to facilitate reporting

The suggestions from the shared reading routines moving from immediate to nonimmediate (literal to inferential) language are all part of this stage of language-based literacy intervention. The Snow and Goldfield (1981) sequence of questions (see pp. Box 6-2, p. 144) is another tool for encouraging children to talk about different aspects of stories, moving from lower to higher levels of comprehension. Activities such as telling and retelling stories from wordless picture books, making books and drawing pictures about activities (similar to Gillam & Ukrainetz's [2006] suggestions), assisting children in relating personal past experiences, and providing opinions about characters' behaviors (as with Donahue & Foster, 2004) are among the activities that can help children acquire the language-based literacy skills that they will take with them to school. Westby (1985, 2005) encourages practitioners, as noted in earlier sections of this chapter, to choose books that match their goals and objectives. Children should be exposed to language style changes (from oral to literate) through books. They should hear and practice with structures that they will face in excerpts such as the Civil War passage. Structures such as *"if* I had," *"because* the elephant did this," and *"after* the caterpillar," and time words such as "yesterday" and "tomorrow," to name only a few, should be part of children's evolving repertoire. Modeling and exposing children to these forms in high context and familiar situations is the way to start. Using recasting and other techniques (see Box 6-5), as well as print referencing techniques, can be integrated into interventions at this stage depending on a child's age and needs.

The Middle Stage. This period encompasses Grades 2 through 6.

Objectives: Facilitate understanding of relationships among
                  characters' traits, emotions, and events
                  Require the child/student to structure the narrative

In this stage, Westby (1985) encourages practitioners (much like Donahue & Foster [2004] did more recently) to help students think beyond what the text says. Clearly, given the large gap between Grades 2 and 6, the activities and demands made on students have to be evaluated carefully. But activities such as identifying emotions in pictures (those that might be relevant to the upcoming story), sharing personal experiences children have had that relate to a character (times when they were mad, happy, sad, scared, etc.), reading books emphasizing traits (good, bad, brave, etc.), predicting what characters would do in certain situations, evaluating one's predictions, and discussing the behavior of a character all speak to developing inferential comprehension, as well as integrating the social processing aspects into intervention.

The Advanced Stage. This period encompasses aspects of Grade 6, overlapping with the ending portions of the previous stage, and going beyond it.

Objectives: Facilitate comprehension of more complex narratives
                  Facilitate more sophisticated meta-awareness skills

In this advanced stage, students are encouraged to tackle difficult topics embedded in complex structures. A good deal of language practice, experience, and skill underlie this aspect of language intervention because implicit relations are made explicit. For example, students may have some knowledge of story structure (having practice in shared reading routines and other intervention activities), but now they are asked to discuss the story grammar elements of theme, plot, and moral in more detailed ways than they have done in the previous stage. For example, they are encouraged to talk about (and find) other stories that might have similar themes, plots, and so on. They are guided to tell (and write) stories from the perspectives of different characters in a story or read different versions of the same story. At this stage, students are exposed to books that have stories that go in several possible directions or that have stories embedded within stories. The advanced stage toward literacy brings students' analytical and metalinguistic skills into the forefront of their literacy-based activities. Through all the stages of intervention, we look back and look ahead to gain a better understanding of what will help our students achieve literacy and academic success. Van Kleeck and her colleagues (2006, pp 143–147, this chapter) in language and VanSledright (2004, Chapter 4, this text) in curriculum development, among others, reiterate the sentiments of looking back and looking ahead. They remind us to see the beginnings of "advanced stage knowledge" in the earlier phases of development. Van Kleeck and colleagues (2006) talked about introducing inferential language and meta-awareness to children in the late preschool period and VanSledright (2004) talked about the importance of "partially educating children" in history before the fourth and fifth grades.

Looking Ahead Once Again and Pulling the Pieces Together

CASE STUDY

Scenario 7

An SLP is working with a fifth grader with LLD. He is covering various topics in his social studies curriculum. The focus in his grade is on the early United States. Tim, at 11 years old, has had a history of school problems, including behavioral (attentional difficulties and acting out when frustrated) and academic difficulties. He is described as having "better" (but slow) decoding skills than reading comprehension skills. His reading abilities are generally 2 to 2½ years below his peers. His report indicates that he had moderate receptive and expressive language problems as a preschooler and was left back in the first grade. He is currently in the mainstream class but falling behind and having difficulty keeping up with the curriculum. He has been in and out of speech-language services for most of his school years. While written language, particularly reading comprehension, is a major concern, he clearly has ongoing oral language problems that manifest themselves as processing difficulties, "immature" and limited vocabulary, word-finding difficulties, and problems with connected discourse (keeping stories clear and coherent and managing expository text). The SLP has consulted with Tim's teacher and has, as one of her tasks, looked through the social studies text with the teacher to gain an insight into the world and expectations of Grade 5 (as per Chapter 4). She alternates working with Tim in a one-on-one situation (that follows), a group situation (similar to the ones described in Chapter 3, pp. 47–48), and a team teaching situation within the classroom.

The SLP's goals include helping Tim manage the language of the curriculum and develop more effective comprehension strategies. She would like him to become more familiar with the patterns and peculiarities of academic text. The intervention is on a "meta" level, bringing techniques to the surface that Tim can use across the curriculum. The SLP has chosen to use the social studies textbook as a backdrop for part of her intervention with Tim. The session has a threefold purpose, as follows:
1. Reviewing a mapping activity that is part of the one-on-one therapy routines to help Tim manage expository text and its accompanying vocabulary
2. Identifying key words or phrases that signal meaning and others that may be misread or misinterpreted by Tim
3. Helping Tim develop a better understanding of why he's reading, what he can bring to the text, and what the author is trying to say
  Some of the concepts discussed by Donahue and Foster (2004), Gillam and Ukrainetz (2006), Justice and Ezell (2004), and Westby (2005) are applicable here and are modified to be relevant to school-based issues and Tim's specific language needs. The information processing principles discussed in the previous chapter also guide the clinician.

> SLP: Remember a little while ago when we worked on this compare and contrast map? (*The clinician points to the interlocking circles, a Venn diagram, that represent a prior discussion about two baseball teams, the Angels and the Yankees.*)

> *Tim:* "Yep! I said I hate those Yankees. I remember I had you laughing because you're from New York."

SLP: *(laughs)* "Yes, I thought that you and I had a *conflict* about how we feel about those teams." (SLP *writes the word "conflict" on a white board.*)

(They had been working on the notion of having two different points of view and how these views can be compared and contrasted. The use of a familiar and loved topic for Tim provided a way to begin to dissect expository text and introduce some techniques to facilitate more effective spoken and written comprehension. The SLP also wants to explore "where" Tim's coming from in terms of understanding conflicts [large and small], presenting opinions and arguments to make cases, and using appropriate and more literate structures to make ideas clear on the printed page.)

Tim: "It was like a mini war just like we talked about."

SAMPLE TITLE FOR MY TOPIC:

Comparing the Angels and Yankees **(Facts and Details)**

Why I Hate the Yankees **(Opinions and Feelings)**

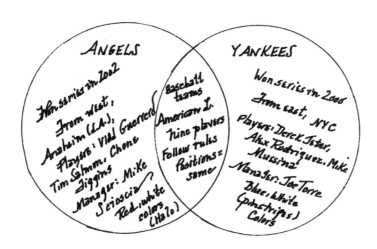

Sample Sentence: *The Angels who play in Anaheim won the World Series in 2002.*

Linguistic "Glue" Words (like Scioscia and Torre)

Different, alike, although, on the other hand, compared

with, rather than, same, similar, but, still, instead of . . .

A compare-contrast diagram using a sports topic as a model for learning about expository text.

SLP: "Well, you could say that. We would certainly continue to *disagree* or have a *disagreement* about the teams and our love for the teams. I like the way you used 'mini' because it gets the idea of what you're really saying in a good way." (*The* SLP *writes the words "disagree" and "disagreement" on the board.*)

Tim: "Right. Because I'll always love the Angels and you'll always love the Yankees."

SLP: "Do you think if you grew up in New York, you'd be a Yankee fan? Do you think I'd be an Angels fan if I grew up here?"

Tim: "You should be because you live here."

SLP: "Maybe you're right. But let me go back to my first question: Do you remember what I asked first?"

Tim: (*Hesitates for a while.*) "What was it?"

SLP: "If you grew up in New York, do you think you'd be a Yankee fan today?"

Tim: "No way! I'd be a Mets fan. I'd still hate the Yankees!"

SLP: "You're probably right, so we'll probably not find an easy way to *resolve* this disagreement. But at least it's about sports and not too serious." (*Writes "serious" and "resolve" on the board.*)

Tim: "Some sports fans are crazy and they think it is serious...Their team loses and they go crazy."

SLP: "True! As you know, I went crazy when the Red Sox beat the Yankees! But, really, it wasn't a serious thing like a war!"

Tim: "Yeah. You were funny about the Sox."

SLP: "OK. Don't remind me. (*They laugh.*) OK. Let's go on and use some of the ideas we talked about in the baseball topic with a social studies topic. Some of the maps we've used, and the words, and sentences we've made up can help with history."

Tim: "Not as much fun as baseball!"

SLP: "But you know a lot of things that you can *use* to help you understand and remember history. That's why we're doing these things with the maps and the key words, and reading and talking about subjects. I want you to use these *strategies*."

(*Tim does not look totally convinced but he's willing to go with it at this point. He likes the idea that his SLP knows about sports and he enjoys the one-on-one attention.*)

SLP: "I want you to use some of the things practiced in our sports talks when you have to study social studies. Let's look at our compare-contrast circles as a start. Then we'll use our cause-effect map the next time. We'll talk about how two wars—or conflicts—are alike and how they're different. I know you've studied the American Revolution in class. You'll be studying the Civil War in a few weeks." (*Points to circles and points to names as she reads them.*) "Let's look at the board first."

(They talk about the meanings of some key words: conflict, disagree/disagreement, serious vs. minor, resolve/resolution. They also discuss ways of resolving conflicts and disagreements. Tim and the SLP share personal experiences with disagreements and conflicts they have had at times, including the Angels-Yankees disagreement. This aspect of the prereading brainstorming can be elaborated on or can be abbreviated.)

SLP: "Could we say that the American Revolution and the Civil War were both serious conflicts?"

Tim: "Yep…because they're big wars, George Washington and all that other stuff."

SLP: "That's good. Keep George Washington in mind…actually, I'll write it on the board, because we'll come back to him. First, let's write 'serious conflicts' in the middle of the circles."

SAMPLE TITLE FOR MY TOPIC:

Two wars in the United States   **(Facts and Details)**

How I feel about wars   **(Opinions and Feelings)**

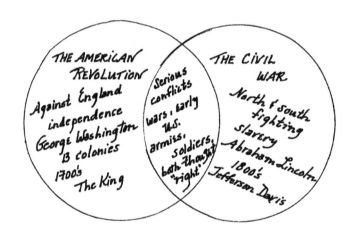

Sample Sentence: *The American Revolution and the Civil War are similar because they were serious conflicts.*

Linguistic "Glue" Words

Different, alike, although, on the other hand, compared

with, rather than, same, similar, but, still, instead of . . .

A compare-contrast diagram using Grade 5 social studies as a backdrop for learning about expository text.

(Tim and the SLP alternate writing.)

SLP: "What else might be alike about the two wars?"

Tim: (Hesitates; the SLP waits to give him time to respond.)

SLP: "Think of the teams in baseball. What word would be used to talk about the people who would be fighting?"

Tim: "Oh, OK, the soldiers would fight each other."

SLP: "That's good and we could also say that in both wars, the *army* fought the battles."

Tim: "Right. The armies fight each other and they have soldiers in 'em!"

SLP: "Terrific. The American Revolution and the Civil War *(while pointing to the circles)* are similar because they both had armies that fought one another. Wow! That's a *looong* sentence. What should we write now?"

Tim: "'Have armies.'"

SLP: "Let's say a long sentence that we'll put in the box here as an example."

Tim: "The wars, we could say they're alike because they both have armies with soldiers."

SLP: "Yep. The American Revolution and the Civil War are alike because they both had armies and soldiers who fought."

(The SLP lets Tim know she made a couple of changes. He thinks the changes are "good.")

The session would continue along these lines. The SLP would use the baseball model to remind Tim about the various components of the compare-contrast activity. For example, they would talk about different "linguistic glue" words that occur frequently in compare-contrast text. These words help to hold the ideas together (e.g., Wallach, 2004; Wallach & Ehren, 2004)—the way that Mike Scioscia and Joe Torre hold the Angels and Yankees together. One could move to a comparison of the North and South and their different opinions about the war and other aspects of the Civil War conflict that could serve as a backdrop to help Tim and students like Tim develop a comfort level with expository text structure. A problem-solution or cause-effect map might be used as well to help students negotiate the texts in which their social studies content is embedded (Westby, 2005). At some point in the session or in a future session, Tim's SLP would take a longer version of the Grade 5 excerpt presented on page 158 (or another part of the text) and complete a reading, questioning, rereading activity similar to some of the aspects of the shared reading routines but, obviously, focused on a higher level involving literal and inferential comprehension. Scenario 7 reminds us that language disorders at school-age levels have many layers. We see how brainstorming, reading and writing, discussion, and other techniques (e.g., recasting), in combination with topics that go from familiar (baseball) to less familiar (early American history), come together to provide a more unified and integrated language intervention approach.

Indeed, SLPs have a unique role to play in the education of students with LLD. Chapters 7 and 8 will elaborate on these concepts.

In Closing For Now

As we analyze and dissect the curricular challenges facing students with LLD, we might ask ourselves what we can do to prepare students for the long road ahead. As noted throughout this chapter and in the works of those mentioned, among others, our preschool interventions will be far more powerful if they are pointed in the direction of the horizon as Fey and colleagues (1995) suggest and if oral and written language are seen as reciprocal elements of a communication system. Indeed, Gillam and Ukrainetz (2006), who encouraged us at the beginning of this chapter to think about language intervention in very specific ways, remind us yet again:

> Intervention that targets language comprehension and production in the context of listening to, reading, and talking about stories [and expository text] enhances [both] the development of interpersonal oral communication and cognitive/academic communication in students with language impairment. (p. 62)

There is certainly much work to be done, but everything is possible if we allow ourselves to see the possibilities.

6

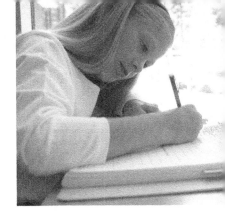

Once formal schooling begins, children may be expected to listen and retell stories, relate personal experiences to parents and teachers, follow directions, and provide factual descriptions or explanations of events. These different types of discourse present children with different spoken language challenges and reveal conditions under which language production problems arise.
(Hadley, 1998, p. 132)

7 Seeing the World Through Connected Text

Bringing Structure and Content,
Macro and Micro Pieces Together: Part 1

SUMMARY STATEMENT

The reality of a fast-moving curriculum that is content loaded and embedded in complex structures presents challenges to practitioners who work with students with language learning disabilities. This is the recurring and oft-repeated theme of the text. The added challenge—the transmission of information largely through print coupled with the requirements of school, which demand that students demonstrate what they know via writing—has also been a focus of our discussions. This chapter continues to explore these interwoven themes. Following from the previous chapter, Chapter 7 continues to present ways of balancing what a student knows with what he or she "has to learn." Using the curriculum as a backdrop for language intervention, as inspired by Ehren (2000, 2006a),

The following graduate students from the Department of Communicative Disorders at California State University, Long Beach in Long Beach, California, are acknowledged for their excellent contributions to this chapter: Aileen Beck and Carly Knoll for their presentation on BP, our student writer for the Mars piece, and their superb discussion of "curriculum-based intervention" in the 2006 spring semester; Irene Seybold and Tiffany Wong, for their research on the language of science; and Charlene Geddes and Alyssa Fukumoto, for their original and ongoing research in discourse sampling, which is summarized in this chapter.

written and spoken language are fused once again. The importance of considering what we really mean by "comprehension" is revisited as we consider the complexity of connected levels, or *macrolevels*, of discourse (e.g., narrative and expository text) and ways to help students "get there." The less connected levels, or *microlevels*, of discourse (e.g., sentences and words) are seen through the lens of how they relate to the "bigger pieces" of text. As with all the chapters, the questions of "where to begin" and "what to do" always remain in the forefront of the discussion.

KEY QUESTIONS

1. What are some of the key concepts related to connected discourse, and why are they important for language intervention and academic success?

2. In what ways can narratives serve as a bridge to mastering the more complex and abstract expository text of school?

3. How do content and structural knowledge interact across discourse genres providing authentic opportunities for collaboration between speech-language pathologists and teachers?

4. What can the language of science teach us about connected discourse and the importance of creating curriculum-relevant intervention programs?

INTRODUCTORY THOUGHTS

The Importance of Looking Across Genres of Connected Text

Figure 7-1 illustrates a sample from a Grade 4 student (BP) from Beck and Knoll (2006). The assignment was to "write a detailed summary for the unit we have just covered about the planet Mars."

The student who wrote the piece is suspected of having a "learning disability," but he has not been diagnosed and is not receiving any special services at the time of this writing. BP is reported to have had preschool language disorders, but the nature of those difficulties was unknown to his teacher. BP has been referred for an assessment, although, interestingly, "language" is not believed to be a top priority (or major problem) for him. Depending on the philosophy of his school and the professionals' backgrounds and perceptions about language, he may (or may not) see a speech-language pathologist (SLP) as part of the initial assessment. (Recall the issues surrounding definitions and perceptions of *language* vs. *learning* vs. *reading* disabilities in Chapter 2.) The comments on BP's paper were as follows: "Needs 3 paragraphs and complete sentences. Follow the pencil points for organization." The teacher provided some scaffolding with the pencil points (arrows and numbers) that led the student to possible paragraph breaks such as the following:

■ What are we talking about (Mars, the Red Planet)?
■ What did the scientists send to Mars (the Mars Rover that "wheeled around" the planet)?
■ What did they find (e.g., there could be life, it's like earth, etc.)?

Readers evaluating this sample might be asking themselves a number of questions, such as the following:

■ Where was BP from kindergarten to Grade 4?
■ How did he get this far without intervention? Can he make it through Grade 4 with some additional and very specific support?

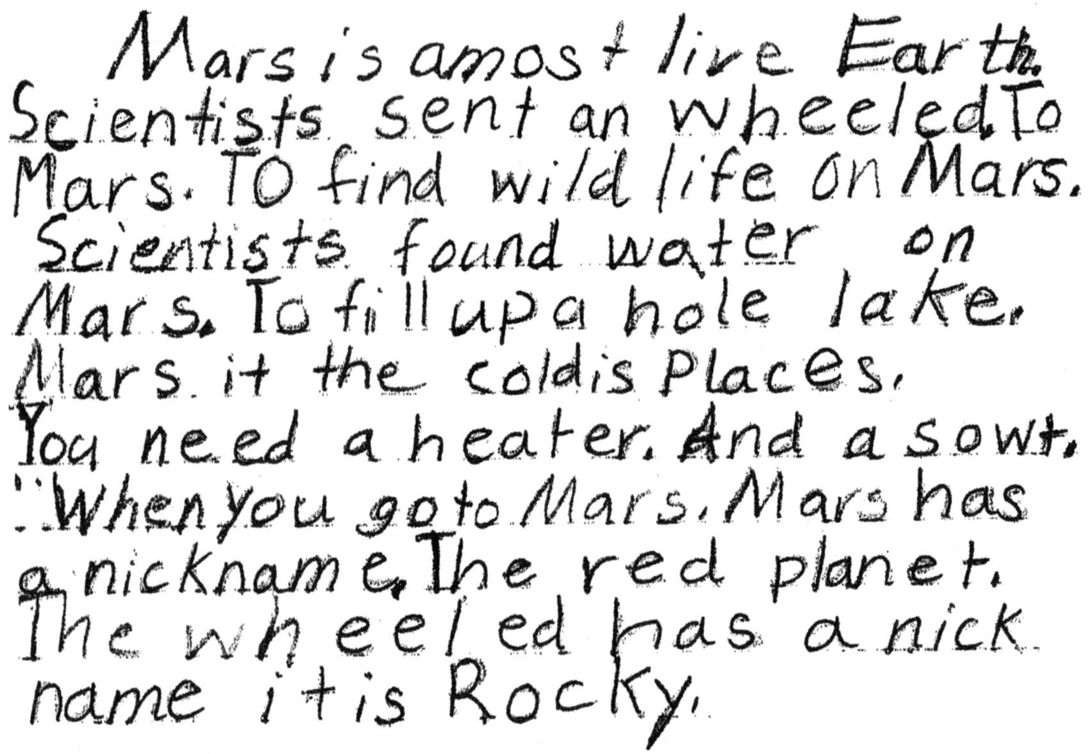

Mars is amost live Earth.
Scientists sent an wheeled To
Mars. TO find wild life On Mars.
Scientists found water   on
Mars. To fill up a hole lake.
Mars. it the coldis Places.
You need a heater. And a sowt.
"When you go to Mars. Mars has
a nickname. The red planet.
The wheeled has a nick
name it is Rocky.

Figure 7-1 ■ A written-language sample on the topic of Mars written by a Grade 4 student. *(From Beck, A., & Knoll, C. [2006, May].* Curriculum-based and collaborative language intervention. *Paper presented to the Department of Communicative Disorders at California State University at Long Beach, Long Beach, CA.)*

- Is this sample reflective of ways that early language disorders manifest themselves at school-age levels (suggested by Bashir and colleagues [1992, 1998])? Or is BP's difficulty mainly one involving writing?
- Have the demands of the curriculum in science (as reflected in the written example) and other core subjects exceeded his language skills and ability?
- How can we help BP (and students with language learning disabilities [LLD]) perform more effectively?
- How can we help him navigate through the complex maze of science and other subjects?
- What are the macro and micro skills that might help BP create a more coherent and accurate summary of "The Red Planet," among other assignments he has to complete?

There are any number of ways we can proceed to begin to unravel the complexity of connected discourse and help students such as BP survive and thrive in their classrooms. Although we still have much to learn, many practical and theoretically sound suggestions appear in the literature (e.g., Culatta & Merritt, 1998; Culatta et al., 1998; Dickinson et al., 1998; Justice et al., 2006; Ukrainetz &

Ross, 2006; Westby, 2005). This chapter will take a closer look at some of these suggestions, among others, in our continued effort to arm students with the skills, knowledge, and strategies needed for successful learning.

Shifting Gears in Language Assessment: A Small "Step One"

Hadley's (1998) quote at the beginning of this chapter reminds us that helping students manage connected discourse across several genres forms a significant long-term goal of language intervention at school-age levels. What can we do before students such as BP are faced with the demands of Grade 4 expository text? Indeed, it is important for clinicians and teachers alike to consider how the activities they choose, especially when they involve working on "smaller pieces" of language, relate to *connected language* across multiple discourse genres. For example, SLPs sometimes focus on helping students acquire syntactic-grammatical proficiency and other aspects of form. They may focus on helping a student become more proficient at using complex and literate-style sentences, past-tense markers, pronoun usage, and so on through recasting and additional activities that bring the rules and patterns of language to the surface (to the level of metalinguistic awareness).

These targets involve microstructure aspects of language that are part of the internal structures used in narrative and expository text (Justice et al., 2006). Microtargets in intervention become more relevant when they are connected to the "macro" aspects of narrative and expository texts—those genres that will be especially challenging for students with LLD. We can see in BP's piece that *one* of the issues that may be interacting with his ability to write a coherent paragraph is his limited use of complete, complex, and elaborated sentences. Hadley (1998) and other researcher-clinicians address the need to consider the ways in which macro and micro aspects of language influence one another. Expanding on this notion, Justice and colleagues (2006) point out that "there could be trade-offs in the extent of syntactic precision as children produce language that is conceptually advanced" (p. 178). They go on to say that when children attempt to produce more complex narratives, one might see a reduced complexity in some of the microstructures (e.g., syntactic and/or lexical entries). The reverse is also true: narrative organization and structure may suffer when children use more advanced micro forms (Justice et al., 2006). In addition, although not mentioned in Hadley's opening quote, there may also be trade-offs when children move from spoken to written language tasks.

> When children try to produce complex narratives, the microstructures may be reduced in complexity; in contrast, narrative organization and structure may suffer when children use more advanced micro forms (Justice et al., 2006).

Clearly, we want to help our school-age students develop language proficiency in a number of areas. Hadley's (1998) work, among others', reminds us to keep the language demands dictated by the different genres in mind. She talks about three variables that should be considered for assessment that also apply to intervention. The variables reiterate a number of concepts that relate to the oral-to-literate continuum, information processing, and "meta" concepts discussed in the previous chapters, as follows:

1. The first variable relates to the amount of *planning required* for a discourse.
2. The second relates to the *"size of the discourse"* (p. 132).
3. The third and last relates to the *level of contextualization*.

Hadley (1998) reminds us that conversational discourses function in a *less planned* and organized manner when compared with narrative and expository text. Narrative and expository text function in a more *planned* way. As Westby (1994) also noted, the more planning involved, the more difficult it may be to manage a text, particularly for students with LLD. The majority of suggested activities in this text and in the Bibliography require *planning and organization*. When we talk about the size of the discourse, we think about the amount of information needed to send a message. We can transmit meaning on the sentence level, the word level, and, in some cases, even at a sound level. Speakers and writers must make informed decisions about how much or how little to say or write. Hadley (1998) writes that the *utterance level*, which is closer to the sentence level, requires that the speaker or reader plan one sentence at a time. Although we see some utterance/sentence-level work being completed in school, absorbing the key elements and events of social studies, literature, science, and even aspects of math requires the mastery of *text-level* discourse. And text-level discourse "requires speakers to plan, organize, formulate, and monitor their ability to communicate a coherent sequence of events or details to a listener [or reader]" (Hadley, 1998, p. 132).

When speakers and writers participate in extended discourse, they have to consider a number of things, as follows (Hadley, 1998):

■ They have to figure out which *ideas are "major"* or significant and which ideas or points are less significant.

■ They have to consider how they are going to keep particular objects, characters, events, or ideas *clearly connected*.

■ They have to decide how much background knowledge needs to be included.

■ They have to think about what perspective they will take when relating the story, explanation, and so on to others.

When we review BP's expository selection about Mars, we can see that some of these principles might be made explicit before he attempts to write the piece. In other words, he needs help developing strategies (including self-questioning) that include "getting ready for reading" (or writing) and thinking about what's happening "during" and "after" reading (and writing) (Neufeld, 2006). For example: What do you want readers to know about Mars before you write about the planet? And what do you really want to say about Mars and the roving machine? What are the main points you need to make about Mars and how will you connect them (e.g., by linking words, by adding another sentence, by having three topic sentences)? Does this passage say what you want it to say? Written reminders in the form of a K-W-L outline (what I *know*, what I *want* to know, what I *learned*) from Ogle (1986, 1989) could accompany these organizational points, as shown later in this chapter in Box 7-7.

Pragmatically speaking, it is also interesting to note that teachers are often the sole readers (or audience) for many pieces written in school. This reality creates an interesting gap between the writer and his or her audience. A teacher-only routine restricts one's audience, which may restrict some of the reasons for writing more elaborately. Clearly, many students "get it." They learn that "the more I write and the better I write, the higher my grade." Some students, however, may require more explicit instructions and support to perform well on this

---

Conversational discourse = less planned and organized. Narrative and expository text = more planned. The more planning is involved, the more difficulty students may have managing a text.

K-W-L outline (Ogle, 1986, 1989):
K = What I *know*
W = What I *want* to know
L = What I *learned*

less-than-authentic level. Clarifying the purposes for writing and the length and elaboration needed are aspects of composition that have to be mastered by novice and problem writers. Indeed, we might think of ways of expanding our audiences for our young, evolving, and troubled writers, as well as making the rules and nuances of writing understood by students with LLD.

A Useful Discourse Protocol. There is certainly agreement among researchers and practitioners that mastering extended, text-level discourse is critical for school success. With this in mind, Hadley (1998) created a useful language-sampling protocol for school-age children. She developed the protocols to help SLPs obtain a picture of their students' language in an extended-discourse format. According to Hadley (1998), sampling connected discourse is important for the reasons already mentioned, but it is also important because connected discourse tends to "push the language system" to its limits (Lahey, 1990). In addition, notes Hadley (1998), it is useful to sample across conversational, narrative, and expository text genres. We may see different language patterns in children with each genre or see linguistic gaps that cut across genres.

The two main types of sampling used in the Hadley (1998) protocol are (1) an interview format and (2) a story retelling/generation format. These elicitation techniques were chosen because of their ability to encourage the use of more advanced language structures. Both interview format and the story formats help diagnosticians look at various aspects of both macrolevels and microlevels of text, including the text's overall organization, the syntactic and semantic complexity, and lexical diversity. Likewise, the decontextualized nature of the interview format (talking about experiences without pictorial and other nonlinguistic supports) also offers interesting insights into what children can and cannot do. In the interview format, both personal narratives and expository text are targeted with two or more opportunities to discuss selected topics in a decontextualized situation.

The Hadley (1998) protocols offer sampling guidelines to clinicians that encourage extended discourse in their students. The protocols can be used as suggested, or they can be modified based on the ages, language levels, and abilities of one's students. Writes Hadley (1998): "What is most important is that clinicians begin to consider ways to vary the discourse demands that are placed on school-age students during the collection of language samples" (p. 135). Appendix C provides examples of Hadley's "Conversational Interviews" and her "Story Retelling/Generation" protocols. Instructions are also provided by Hadley (1998) and appear in the appendix.

The Interview Protocol. This section consists of three blocks. It is recommended that the clinician spend about 4 minutes on each block. The purpose is to elicit conversation, personal narratives, and an expository sample. Hadley suggests using a conversational map technique—that is, the clinician models the behavior by telling the student about a personal experience, a favorite movie, and so on before asking him or her to do the same thing. Hadley suggests using the following topics in each block:

■ *Block 1* involves "You and Your Family." This block would encourage the telling of a personal story about the child and his or her siblings (conversation and personal narrative). It could also include a personal story about one's family pet (personal narrative).

■ *Block 2* includes "Favorite Things You Do." This block might include how the child spends his or her free time. The child would be encouraged to explain how he or she plays his or her favorite sport or game (expository text).

■ *Block 3* includes "Favorite Stories, TV show, or Movies." The child can be asked to summarize what his or her favorite movie or book was about. Various prompts accompany each block.

Hadley (1998) reminds clinicians that not all responses will qualify as being connected or extended samples of discourse. She notes that clinicians will have to use judgment about how many prompts are needed and which types of topics are more likely to encourage extended speech in their students with LLD. For example, for older students one might ask them why they like or dislike certain subjects or why they like or dislike certain classroom rules to elicit an expository sample (Hadley, 1998). The Yankees/Angels compare-contrast activity described in the previous chapter is another example of an expository text topic that can be used. Relating an experience at a memorable ballgame, by contrast, could be used to elicit a personal narrative.

The Story Retelling/Generation Protocol. This section of the protocol emphasizes "the role of explicit discourse planning in constructing oral texts" (Hadley, 1998, p. 136). This section begins with the child watching a 5-minute portion of a wordless video. Hadley (1998) used *Frog, Where Are You?* (Osborn & Templeton, 1994). Four steps follow:

1. The child retells the main events seen to the clinician.
2. The clinician asks a series of questions to determine whether the child has included the main elements of the story and provides prompts as necessary (see Appendix C).
3. The child is asked to generate an ending.
4. The child retells the complete story to a naïve listener (someone who has not heard the story).

According to Hadley (1998), one can consider the narrative ability of students with and without prompting or adult support, as well as evaluate how well a child can plan, especially when he or she has to tell the complete story to someone who has not heard it before. Clearly, the content and level of stories must also be modified when sampling younger and older students. Likewise, both spoken and written samples might be compared.

Geddes and Fukumoto (2005) used Hadley's (1998) protocol in a pilot study (and ongoing study) that included adolescents with and without language disorders. Although too early to report any conclusive results, their preliminary findings suggest that the personal narrative, narrative retelling, and expository sampling sections of the protocol were particularly sensitive to differences between students with and without LLD. They found that the Hadley protocol was helpful in guiding them through the sampling techniques. The protocol also provided them with insights into both the strengths and weaknesses that seventh- and eighth-grade students have with different types of connected text. Replicating aspects of others' findings (e.g., Scott & Windsor, 2000; Wagner et al., 2000), Geddes and Fukumoto found that (1) the students with learning disabilities performed similarly to their typically developing peers on the conversational discourse section and (2) personal narrative, expository discourse, and narrative retelling tasks differentiated the two groups. Overall, the typically developing students performed better than the students with LLD with, as mentioned, the significant differences occurring on the narrative and expository sections.

Geddes and Fukumoto (2005) used the following measures to compare groups:

1. For *conversational discourse*—vocabulary complexity (number of multisyllabic and less commonly used words; grammatical complexity (from simple, compound, to complex sentences); total number of words; total number of C-units (main clauses plus all connected subordinate clauses and nonclausal phrases); number of words per C-unit; syntactic errors

2. For *personal narratives and narrative retelling* (adapted from Gillam et al., 1999)—story productivity (total number of words; total number of C-units; total number of clauses; number of clauses within C-units); episode structure (complete or incomplete); story components (temporal relations; causal relations); added aspects to narratives (vocabulary complexity; dialogue for characters); grammatical complexity (from simple, to compound, to complex structures)

3. For *expository discourse* (adapted from Westby, 1994)—number of actions; number of details; number of connecting words; number of sentences; number of words

The conversational section of the protocol used by Geddes and Fukumoto, in which students are asked to talk about their lives—including providing information about their ages, birthdays, siblings, and so on—functioned more like a "warm-up" section in this study. But the authors were also interested in observing any differences between the groups that might surface. In general, they found that talking conversationally with students failed to yield significant differences between the groups within this sampling format (as per the measures mentioned earlier). The one exception occurred on the syntactic error measure. The students with LLD made more syntactic errors per C-units in the conversational sampling section than their typically developing peers who made no errors. Although the majority of the typically developing group took more of the initiative when communicating with the clinician and demonstrated fewer hesitations and repetitions than their counterparts with LLD, the groups looked more similar on the conversational part of the sampling.

Although not part of the study, Geddes and Fukumoto (2005) recommend that aspects of personality should be taken into account when sampling connected discourse. They note that it is important to remember that some students are reserved, whereas others are more outgoing. This natural personality difference could influence how comfortable a student might be (or not be) sharing information with an unfamiliar examiner. They encourage clinicians and teachers to consider personality factors, as well as other factors such as nature and severity of language disorders, when drawing conclusions about what students can and cannot do. Geddes and Fukumoto also noted that the nature of conversational exchanges, which function like *dialogues* rather than *monologues*, causes them to fail to have the qualities of connected discourse that are closer to school language. In other words, clinicians and teachers should be aware of the nature of conversational, narrative, and expository text differences; know what they are testing and why; and analyze their data accordingly.

In contrast to the conversational section, personal narrative, expository, and narrative retelling revealed preliminary differences between the two groups of seventh and eighth graders. In general, the students with LLD had fewer total number of words (and talked less time about a topic), C-units, and clauses than their typically developing peers. They also showed gaps in generating complete or elaborated episodes for their stories, using dialogue within their stories, and expressing clearly defined causal relationships. The students with LDD also used fewer complex sentences (subordinate–main clause, passives, etc.) and sophisticated or abstract vocabulary words in their narrative renditions. The expository results were also interesting. The typically developing students tended to provide a greater number of actions and details in their explanations. They also used a greater number of words overall, chose more abstract words to describe or explain concepts, and provided more organized explanations. When the number of sentences was the same in the expository samples for typical students and students with LLD, the complexity of sentences used by the typically developing students exceeded that of the students with LLD. These results are summarized in Table 7-1.

Table 7-1
Differences Between Seventh- and Eighth-Grade Students With and Without Language Learning Disabilities

Factor	LLD Group	TD Group
Personal Narrative Total number of words, C-units, and clauses	Fewer; talked less about topic	More; talked more about topic
Expository Text Elaboration, dialogue, causal relationships	Gaps in generating complete, elaborated episodes Gaps in using dialogue within stories Gaps in expressing clearly defined causal relationships	Gaps not seen with same frequency
Narrative Retelling Complexity of sentences and vocabulary	Fewer complex sentences Fewer sophisticated or abstract vocabulary words	Greater number of actions and details in explanations Greater number of words More abstract words More organized explanations More complex sentences

Data from Geddes, C. R., & Fukumoto, A. K. (2005, Spring). *Sampling adolescents' language abilities across conversational, narrative, and expository discourse genres.* Paper completed in the Department of Communicative Disorders at the California State University at Long Beach, Long Beach, CA.
LLD, Language learning disabilities; *TD,* typically developing.

The excerpts in the following sections provide examples of stimuli and student responses for three blocks of sampling:

- Block 1, the conversational and personal narrative section
- Block 2, the expository section
- Block 3, the narrative retelling section

These examples are presented to encourage readers to look across discourse types and think about ways they might modify and adapt this sampling approach using Hadley's protocol as a framework for elicitation. As noted in the statements that follow (designated with an asterisk [*]), adaptations will be made from Geddes and Fukumoto's (2005) pilot study as data are reviewed and the research continued. The excerpts are included here to provide readers with ideas about the topics that might be used and ways to begin to analyze the results.

The following is an excerpt from the conversational and personal narrative block (Block 1):

Block 1 Excerpt (Conversation and Personal Narrative)

Conversation*

Information about ages, birthdays, and siblings and their ages is discussed before this interchange about what actually happened (or will happen) on one's birthday.

Student with Language Learning Disabilities (LLD)

Clinician:	What are you going to do for your birthday? It's coming up in October.
Student with LLD:	Well, I don't really know. But but but we but we know we're having a ghost hunt. I really like ghost hunts 'cause they're fun. They're creepy but fun.
Clinician:	Do you do that every year?
Student with LLD:	Well, it, I first started it when I was ten years old. And then, we're starting to do it every year.

Typically Developing (TD) Student

Clinician:	Did you do anything for fun for your birthday? Tell me about it.[†]
TD student:	Well, we went bowling, I believe, and it was fun with my friends. We all went.

Excerpts from Geddes, C. R., & Fukomoto, A. K. (2005, Spring). *Sampling adolescents' language abilities across conversational, narrative, and expository discourse genres.* Paper completed in the Department of Communicative Disorders at the California State University at Long Beach, Long Beach, CA.

*Conversational discourse often looks awkward when transcribed. In addition, speakers do not always complete thoughts in "perfectly" grammatical structures as they have to do when writing a more formal report or summary. Written renditions would be an excellent addition to the sampling.

[†]A question and then another "question" (command) is used. One might consider modifying the language, especially for students with LLD. In addition, there is a difference in the two recounts requested that should also be noted. The student with LLD is providing an answer for *what is going to happen* or *might happen* in the future since his birthday has not occurred yet. By contrast, the TD student is recounting an event that *has happened* since her birthday has passed. These differences should be taken into account for future research and clinical application.

Continued

Block 1 Excerpt (Conversation and Personal Narrative)—cont'd

Typically Developing (TD) Student—cont'd

Clinician:	Was it like regular bowling or something else?
TD student:	…Um…just regular bowling. It was really fun. We just ate a lot and talked a lot. We were really bad because at first we didn't put up bumpers and we were really horrible and got horrible scores. And then, in the second round we put up bumpers. It was really fun.

Personal Narrative
Student with Language Learning Disabilities

Clinician's personal narrative:

> I have an older sister named Marilee. One time when we were little she convinced me that a tornado was coming. She told me that if I put my ear to the wall I would be able to hear it. I always believed my big sister so I put my ear to the wall and pretended that I could hear it too.

Clinician:	Have your brothers ever played any tricks like that on you?
Student with LLD:	Yeah, like like they played tricks on me, the tricks like there's an invisible monster around here and then he said. "Oh, my gosh, I can see him. Go, run, run." And I said: "Ahhhh!" (laughing).
(Clinician pauses a while, then prompts.)	
Clinician:	That's funny. What kind of monster was it?
Student with LLD:	He drew a picture of it. You know what it looks like? It looks like a one eye…um…alien thing.

Typically Developing Student

The clinician's personal narrative is the same one that was presented previously (about her sister, Marilee).

Clinician:	Have you ever done anything like that to your sister?[‡]
TD student:	Yes.
Clinician:	Can you tell me about it?[§]
TD student:	Umm…well. I did bribe her once. It was sort of funny. I had this huge toy chest and it was full of toys like knickknacks from McDonald's and stuff, just in this chest. And I wanted to see this movie really bad but she wanted to see another one. And my mom said that if we couldn't compromise we're just gonna go to see like this one movie she picked out. So, I decided to bribe her. I said: "Okay, if you pick the movie this time then you can have all the toys in this chest." And she's like: "Sure." And so we went to see my movie, and of course, the chest was rarely used again but it was…I got my movie…it was funny.

[‡]There's a difference in the personal narratives in terms of who's the "doer" and who's "getting things done to him or her." Because our first (LLD) student's brothers are older than he is, it was assumed (not necessarily correctly) that he's the one who might get tricked by his brothers (as was the case based on the monster story). Our second student is the older sibling so the opposite is assumed (she's the one tricking her sister into going to her movie). It is unknown whether these differences in perspective are significant at this time. But, again, this may be another factor to consider when sampling connected text.
[§]The question is phrased as an indirect request. This is something we may want to be cautious about for assessment, as well as for intervention.

Again, a written sample would complement the spoken samples. The following is an excerpt from the expository block (Block 2):

Block 2 Excerpt (Expository Text)

Expository Text
Student with Language Learning Disabilities (LLD)
Clinician's expository discourse sample (explaining a game she knows, can play, and likes):
My favorite game is Uno. In Uno you deal seven cards to each player. The cards all have different colors—red, blue, yellow, and green. When someone puts a card down, you match it either by color or number. The idea is that you want to get rid of all your cards. When you have one card left, you say, "Uno!" Whoever gets rid of all their cards first wins.

Clinician:	OK. So do you have a favorite game (or sport) you like to play? Tell me how to play.
Student with LLD:	OK. I like soccer. So you have eleven girls on the field, one goalie, defenders, mids, and forwards and the other team has the same players. And you have a ball and you have three refs, two sidelines and one in the center. And you just start playing.

(Clinician waits for the student to continue, then prompts.)

Clinician:	And what are you supposed to do? How do you play?
Student with LLD:	Kick the ball to each other and then make a goal.

Typically Developing (TD) Student
The clinician's expository sample is the same one—the explanation of "Uno."

Clinician:	OK. So do you have a favorite game (or sport) you like to play? Tell me how to play.
TD student:	I like playing Life.
Clinician:	Life? Can you tell me how to play that?
TD student:	It's kind of like Monopoly. You have money and you can buy your house with the money you have. And there's...you can either...you can either start college or just start with your career. And when you're in college you have loans and stuff like that so it's pretty much like life. And you can land on like life cards and stuff and you can get money for it and you...and there's stuff like if you don't buy your insurance there's like little spots where there's a tornado or something and your house gets wrecked or your car. If you don't have insurance you have to pay for it all over again.
Clinician:	How do you win?
TD student:	You win...well everyone wins. It's just that you count up all your money and at the very end of the game there's like a mansion, like a shack, and some other stuff. And whoever has the most money, that means you're like a millionaire or something.

Excerpts from Geddes, C. R., & Fukomoto, A. K. (2005, Spring). *Sampling adolescents' language abilities across conversational, narrative, and expository discourse genres.* Paper completed in the Department of Communicative Disorders at the California State University at Long Beach, Long Beach, CA.

The excerpts from Blocks 1 and 2, which cover the conversational, personal narrative, and expository pieces, serve as a beginning point (with other assessment measures) to help us form hypotheses about students' abilities to manage connected discourse. The excerpts give us a glimpse into the similarities and differences that may exist between typically developing students and students with LLD. Clearly, individuals' abilities to form clear, concise, and coherent monologues vary greatly within and across populations. But by sampling connected text, as Hadley (1998) and others suggest, we can learn more about the structural, pragmatic, and semantic gaps that influence and interact with academic success. Indeed, going beyond conversational discourse, as well as including "micro" aspects of sampling (e.g., word- and sentence-level analyses) within connected text formats, is particularly important in the older elementary and adolescent population. This focus on language sampling and intervention is relevant because it connects to instructional and textbook language as discussed in various sections of this text.

Some of the language patterns that join and separate typically developing students and students with LLD are reflected in the excerpts. All students were engaged in the activities and performed appropriately. We see some lexical and cohesive gaps in both groups of students and note that there is room for improvement. But the typically developing students' responses, while far from "perfect," were stronger, more informative, and more linguistically complex than the contributions of the students with LLD. For example, we might observe the way the students handle the request to explain a game or sport they play. The student with LLD creates a list when she names the positions of soccer players as a predominant part of the explanation rather than providing enough details about the rules of the game. Temple and colleagues (1993) discuss a similar pattern in young elementary grade writers, that is, they create lists, when attempting to provide explanations for something they know. The typically developing student profiled in the Block 2 excerpt provides an explanation for the game Life that also shows some missteps but gives the listener a better understanding of the core of the game. Both students could be directed to creating a better mental plan (what's the purpose of the game, key rules, sequence of events, players' strategies, etc.) for spoken and written language. Although both typically developing students and students with LLD required clinician prompting to continue or to wrap up their monologues, the students with LLD often needed additional scaffolding to pull the pieces together or add missing details to the pieces.

The excerpts presented thus far encourage us to ask another set of questions about the intermeshed variables, as follows:

- Do typically developing students have more background knowledge to apply to topics, in part at least, because they are better readers?
- Do they have more stable mental models (Lahey & Bloom, 1994) of narrative and expository text structures because they read, write, and have stronger metalinguistic and metacognitive skills than students with LLD?
- How does "micro" knowledge such as having the "connective tissue" or "linguistic glue" words, content-level vocabulary knowledge, syntactic proficiency, and so on influence one's comprehension and production of connected text?

■ And the key question: How do we help students with LLD manage the complex texts of school?

Although we have a long way to go, some excellent suggestions are available, some of which will be highlighted in this chapter and the next (see Chapter 8). (For one of the most thorough and excellent discussions of text assessment and intervention, see Westby [2005].)

Blocks 1 and 2 in Hadley's protocol provided us with guidelines for eliciting text-level language using an interview format. The last suggestion via Hadley (1998) encourages clinicians to engage students in a narrative retelling/generation task. As mentioned earlier, Hadley used a wordless video and various scaffolds to help children complete the story (see Appendix C). Geddes and Fukumoto (2005) included a narrative retelling test without the use of a video. They asked students to tell them the story of a movie or a book that they had recently seen or read (or had read to them). Students were also told that they could tell the clinician about their favorite movie or book. The level of decontextualization and planning required by this task certainly contributed to its difficulty.

The following is an excerpt from the narrative retelling block (Block 3):

Block 3 Excerpt (Narrative Retelling)

Narrative Retelling
Student with Language Learning Disabilities (LLD)
The clinician's narrative retelling of a movie:

I watched a movie the other day called *Men in Black*. In this movie, two secret government agents are responsible for saving New York City from an evil alien bug. They have to find the bug and kill it before it destroys the planet.

(Note: The clinician's rendition is rather abbreviated, which may be a factor to consider for future research.)

Clinician:	Have you seen any good movies lately? Or have you finished any books that you like?
Student with LLD:	I finished…um…Lemony Snicketts'.
Clinician:	Oh, *A Series of Unfortunate Events*.
Student with LLD:	Yeah.
Clinician:	Tell me about it.
Student with LLD:	Um…these three little kids, Violet, Klaus, and Sunny were…um…in their beautiful house with their mom and dad. But the mom and dad died in the fire and the three kids were orphaned. And…um…Mr. Poe is like their lawyer or some kind of thing. They had to have them go and stay with this relative. And…um…I can't remember his name but they didn't even know he was his relative. Um…this guy that played it was Tom Cruise. Is that right?
Clinician:	I'm not sure. I think it's Jim Carrey.
Student with LLD:	Yeah. Jim Carrey. And…um…he made him do all chores and like made food for him like really…

Continued

Block 3 Excerpt (Narrative Retelling)—cont'd

Clinician (pausing... *then says):*	Poor kids.
Student with LLD:	Yeah. And then they miss...um...he takes them to a train station where they can get killed. And Mr. Poe called them in the car and he found them driving the car and then he took them to a different place.

Second Example of Student with Language Learning Disabilities

The same clinician narrative retelling (*Men in Black*) is used.

(After the movie *choice is not used:)*	
Clinician:	Do you have a favorite book?
Student with LLD:	Um...*The Princess Diaries*.
Clinician:	What is it about?
Student with LLD:	About this girl, who's a, she's a teenage girl and she's just a regular kid. And she finds out that she's a princess, and her mom never told her that. And so she got mad.
Clinician:	The girl got mad or the mom got mad?
Student with LLD:	The mom got mad.
Clinician:	Why?
Student with LLD:	Why did the mom get mad? I meant, the, Mia, she got, um. She got mad as in the daughter got mad because her parents didn't tell her, for like, since she was little.
Clinician (after *pausing a while):*	What else happens in that book?
Student with LLD:	She likes this boy named Michael. And he goes to the same school as her and she has a friend named Lily. And that's Lily's, and Lily is the sister of Michael, her brother. And then she goes to Genovia.
Clinician:	Why does she go to Genovia?
Student with LLD:	Because that's where her grandma ruled the country and stuff.

Typically Developing (TD) Student

The same clinician narrative retelling (*Men in Black*) is used.

Clinician:	So have you seen any movies lately?
TD student:	Well, Friday, I saw *Ever After* with Drew Barrymore.
Clinician:	I haven't seen that one, what was it about?
TD student:	It's about a Cinderella story but it shows the beginning like how Cinderella becomes a stepsister and stuff.
Clinician:	Okay.
TD student:	And at the beginning...um...I forgot what her name is but it's not Cinderella. They call her that cause she sleeps near the fire. But, it's her mom who died and she's just with her dad. And her dad's always like out working somewhere else. And he comes home with a wife and two stepsisters. And then the next day he has to leave because he has to go

Block 3 Excerpt (Narrative Retelling)—cont'd

	on another business trip. And they all wait at the gate for him to wave because it's like tradition. But he falls off his horse and dies and he...um...before he dies like the wife's over there and the little girl is over there. And he tells the little girl that he loves her instead of the wife. So that's how she ends up like treating her like a servant instead of like how she's supposed to be, noble. And throughout the story she ends up like talking to the prince and stuff. And the stepsisters and the blond stepsister ends up trying to get married to the prince. But the other stepsister is seeing like how mean her mom is and ends up playing a trick on them to get them to come to the palace. It's really a good movie.
Clinician:	How does it end?

The story goes on for a while. The student provides the resolution of the story with Cinderella marrying the Prince (he proposes in front of everyone at a grand ball). Cinderella also resolves the conflict with her stepfamily. The student added many evaluative points along the way, including one at the end by stating, "It was a better deal for the sisters because they could stay in the palace, etc. but they had to serve Cinderella, the Queen."

Excerpts from Geddes, C. R., & Fukomoto, A. K. (2005, Spring). *Sampling adolescents' language abilities across conversational, narrative, and expository discourse genres.* Paper completed in the Department of Communicative Disorders at the California State University at Long Beach, Long Beach, CA.

7

What one may notice in the last renditions that involve narrative retelling is that narrative retelling can be a difficult task. Myers (2006) notes that first graders without LLD often have difficulty retelling stories sequentially and providing details without visual support. Thus, unlike the video format used by Hadley (1998) or a task that asks a student to retell a familiar story the student has just heard or has practiced with, the Geddes and Fukumoto (2005) task is quite decontextualized. As their research showed, it is far from "easy," even for later-grade elementary students without LLD, to produce a completely coherent, listener-friendly narrative as reflected in the samples. Lacking pictures and other visually oriented prompts to keep the structure and events of the story "in front of the student" contributes to the task's difficulty. But it also encourages the need to use explicit language so that the listener "gets it" (Masterson & Kamhi, 1991). Nonetheless, the students in the current study had to rely on their mental models of the stories to reproduce them (Lahey & Bloom, 1994). We can see from observing the samples and analyzing the data available that without pictorial or video support, verbal scaffolding, and other assistance, linguistic contexts have to provide some of the needed organization for Geddes and Fukumoto's students about where to "go" with the stories. The typically developing student talks for a much longer time and talks even longer with just one "minor" prompt, "Okay," and another at the end, "How does it end?"

Results suggested that the students with LLD required more prompting and scaffolding to keep the stories going. We can see in the Princess Diaries story, for example, that the clinician takes the student through a number of steps to glean more details about the story. Although not prompting her specifically with story structure elements (which she would do in an intervention session), the clinician tries to clarify some of the statements being made (e.g., "The girl got mad or the mom got mad?"), as well as move the story's plot along ("What else happens in the book?"). We do see the main theme expressed at the beginning of the student's rendition: a teenage girl finds out she's a princess. That triggers off events that follow. As listeners (or readers of this story), we are unsure what happens next, although some of the details are expressed by the speaker: the initiating event sets off a conflict with the girl's (the princess's) mother. But we don't know how the plot plays out, what the girl and her mother actually do, and how the conflict is resolved. Characters are mentioned—the regular teenager/"princess," whose name is "Mia"; Lily, her friend; Michael, the boy she likes; and grandma, the one who rules Genovia—but these characters need to be brought together in the plot lines. We have an initiating event and a response (the princess is angry, etc.), but goals, consequences, and the attempts at action are unspecified.

We could also consider the missing elements of the Lemony Snicketts piece and ask ourselves another question: How does one's background knowledge affect both production and comprehension of these two stories? For the speaker, perhaps seeing a movie many times (children often like to watch videos many times, memorizing the dialogue of their favorite characters) or reading a book more than once (or having it read to you frequently) could have an impact on the results of a story retelling task. Recall, for example, Lahey and Bloom's (1994) notions that automaticity in one area frees up "space" in other areas. Students who are very familiar with a story's content might perform better at putting it into a coherent and complete structure. Likewise, clinicians who are familiar with one or both of the stories will be better prepared to help students through the maze of pulling the pieces of theme (a problem or conflict or event that affects the main character[s]) and plot (the attempts and actions of the characters to resolve the conflicts) together.

The *Ever After* story from the typically developing student also has some gaps. But we might also observe the "longer chunks" of talking he engages in without interruption or the need for many prompts from the clinician (Geddes & Fukumoto, 2005). We see more detail and many of the key elements of the Cinderella story present, including the "happily ever after ending" (not in the transcript). This occurs when the Prince asks Cinderella to marry him and live in the palace. In this rendition, the resolution of the conflicts occurs when Cinderella allows her family to stay in the palace as long as they obey some ground rules that she sets. But in the end, Cinderella vows to be nicer to her stepfamily than they were to her.

The student also provided some setting and background information about the nature of this story. He tells the clinician how Cinderella got into her well-known situation (mom dying and dad remarrying into a tough crowd). It provides more details about why the stepfamily became "mean" to her (e.g., her dad's dying words are that he loves her more than the stepfamily). And these dying words create a whole series of consequences for Cinderella, as most readers know. Overall, the student provides some of the beginning, middle, and ending pieces of the story. He also makes a number of evaluation statements ("It's really a good movie;" "It was a better deal for the sisters…"), which are sometimes said to be one of the characteristics of better readers who make inferences about what they read and go beyond the written (or spoken) text. Adding one's assessment to the facts and events demonstrates aspects of inferential comprehension and monitoring abilities (Ehren, 2005; Westby, 2005). By contrast, character identification (providing the names of the characters) and elaborating on the plot's development ("And throughout the story she ends up talking to the prince") require improvements. We might ask ourselves, for example, What's the trick the blonde stepsister plays on her mother? How do they get to the palace? Better use of cohesive devices might also be used to specify time, who-does-what-to-whom, and other clarifications that would improve this student's narrative.

The Geddes and Fukumoto (2005) study provided us with some interesting patterns to consider of connected text in both typically achieving students and students with LLD. The question of what clinicians and teachers can do to help students produce spoken and written narratives that are more organized in structure, content, and pragmatics—and how similar or different the scaffolding and supports might be—is a theme for current and future research (De Kemel, 2003c; McFadden, 1998; Ukrainetz, 2006b, 2006c; Westby, 2005). But, again, regardless of where research and practice may take us, we know that mastery of connected text is interwoven with mastery of the curriculum.

> Mastery of connected text is interwoven with mastery of the curriculum.

Thus expanding our notions of language sampling to include a broad sweep across genres in written as well as spoken domains offers promise as we search for more effective ways to evaluate connected discourse in students with LLD. Much more information is available, especially in the area of narrative assessment and intervention, as Hadley noted in 1998 and as Westby (2005), among others, noted more recently. Providing school-based clinicians with more effective, reliable, and time-saving ways to sample their students' discourse skills would be an enormous help. Hadley's guidelines offer some useful direction along with the clinical tool developed by Gillam and Pearson (2004; see also Justice et al., 2006). If, indeed, connected discourse is more likely than utterance-level (sentence-level) discourse to shed light on students' linguistic vulnerabilities, and since connected discourse is more connected to school text, one must wonder what BP's language sample (the writer of our Mars piece) would look like across spoken and written domains and genre types. More important, how might the information gleaned from the sample help us help him?

Knowing What We're Looking For: Another Step Toward Making Connected Text Connect to School

Expository text is the major text of school. Of course, students will be participating in many activities in language arts, English, and other subjects that require facility with narrative text as well. But in content subject areas such as history and social studies, science, and aspects of math (story problems), students will face different types of expository text. In addition, they will have to explain themselves clearly and concisely in both spoken and written genres. Grades 1 through 3 involve exposure to both narrative and expository discourses. By fourth grade, however, the predominance of expository text is established (Box 7-1). Students are expected to *compare and contrast* events, people, places, and ideas. (Recall the compare-contrast examples on pp. 165, 167 in Chapter 6.) They are expected to *describe* and summarize (e.g., the Mars piece) chapters they have read. They are required to think about and write about how and why certain events occurred. They will be asked to *list* the accomplishments of an author, the battles of a war, or the events leading up to independence for a nation. They have to manage both *cause-effect* and *problem-solution* types of texts, among the others mentioned, and they will be asked to provide opinions and *persuade* others. Knowing the realities of school, our question, once again, is how to "get kids there" who cannot do it on their own. How do narrative and expository discourse abilities intersect on the continuum of language and academic success? And how do we help students acquire proficiency in both genres?

Some Generalities about Text and Text Processing. Our discussion of information processing concepts in an earlier chapter (see Chapter 5, pp. 125–128) reminds us that both *internal* (what the student comes with to a task) and *external* (the task, materials, instructions, etc.) factors must be considered when evaluating what a student can and cannot "do" with connected text. In the samples presented earlier, we noted that the narrative retelling task (recalling a recently seen or read movie or book) certainly provided the clinicians with information that was useful, especially when compared with the other genres sampled. But eliciting the narrative retellings differently may have provided different results. For example, students may have performed better if they were asked to tell the story of a movie they have seen several times. On the other hand, just because a student has watched a video many times does not mean he or she has understood the core of the story or its nuances. Students may also have fared better if they viewed the movie with the clinician, who provided support while they were watching. But then again, "upping" the amount of contextualization, which changes the nature of the tasks, could inhibit, rather than create a situation where more elaborate language is required (Masterson & Kamhi, 1991;

BOX 7-1   *Specific Challenges of Students in Fourth Grade*

The predominance of expository text requires students to do the following:
- Compare and contrast people, places, events, and ideas
- Describe and summarize chapters
- Think and write about how and why events occurred
- List facts, dates, or accomplishments
- Manage cause-and-effect and problem-solution texts
- Provide opinions
- Persuade others

Wagner et al., 2000). Likewise, presenting different titles may also change the direction of a narrative performance. In fact, Cain (2003) found that title prompts did influence the type of narrative school-age students produced. For example, directed titles such as "How the Pirates Lost Their Treasure" elicited more goal-directed stories when compared with topic titles such as "The Farm," which were less specific. Consequently, there are any number of factors that may influence results, especially when sampling connected text. These considerations, which cut across many aspects of testing and intervention, should be kept in mind.

When trying to unravel the complexities of connected text—how we understand it, produce it, and learn from it—researchers make a distinction between *content knowledge* and *structure knowledge*. Content knowledge (sometimes called *content schema*) is the background information or experience an individual has had. It is the listener's or reader's world knowledge that he or she brings to the text. Structure knowledge (or textual schema), by contrast, is the listener's or reader's knowledge of the conventional structures of organization in various discourse genres (De Kemel, 2003c; Ohlhausen & Roller, 1988; Pantaleo, 2004; Snyder et al., 2002). In a number of classic studies (e.g., Beck et al., 1991; Carver, 1992; Fincher-Kiefer, 1992; Ohlhausen & Roller, 1988), investigators looked at the interaction between content and structure knowledge. Concerned mainly with reading, and observing both adults and school-age students, the results shed some light on this complex relationship. Some of the findings may help us consider modifications for students with LLD and also help us understand what we might do to help our students manage the complexities of the curriculum. These findings are summarized in Box 7-2.

Mastering the content of the curriculum, which occurs predominantly through teacher lectures and textbooks, assumes that students come with a certain degree of prior knowledge (Beck et al., 1991; Best et al., 2005; McKeown et al., 1992). In their studies observing fifth graders without LLD and the textbooks they had to use for social studies, Beck and colleagues (1991) went even further by stating that textbooks often assume an *unrealistic* amount of knowledge. They also observed that textbook language and structure did not always make it easier for students to absorb and retain new content in various social studies units. For example, Beck and colleagues (1991) discuss two of the fifth-grade topics being covered—the French and Indian War and the American Revolution. They found that students had a surprisingly limited understanding of the topics even after reading about them. Many facts were presented in the texts, but the way the facts were connected was not made as explicit as it might have been for the students. Again, keep in mind that Beck and colleagues' students were typically performing students. Consequently, it is assumed that by fifth grade students without learning disabilities are able to make inferences about what they read (or hear in a lecture). But as results suggested, even Beck and colleagues' (1991) fifth graders needed help to improve their comprehension and retention of curricular content.

Beck and colleagues (1991) found that "beefing up" background knowledge plus making the texts more readable by clarifying, elaborating on, and spelling out the critical relations contributed to students' comprehension (Wallach & Butler, 1994a). An example of a "beefing up" of background knowledge

Even typically developing fifth-grade students often need help improving their comprehension and retention of curricular content.

BOX 7-2

Results of Studies of the Interaction of Content and Structure Knowledge

- Proficient readers *use linguistic information* in a text to help them absorb critical points. For example, they might use phrases and words such as "by contrast," "the important finding was," "similarly," and titles and topic sentences to comprehend what they are reading.
- The use of structural knowledge is especially important if the *content is moderately or very unfamiliar* to a reader. In this case, the text's organization (structure) and its structural cues become even more important in facilitating comprehension.
- Readers *use background knowledge* when trying to comprehend what they are reading when they have it (i.e., when they are familiar with a topic or aspects of a topic). Background knowledge is most useful when the text is well structured so that the reader "can see the connections between text information and previous knowledge so that [internal and external] knowledge can be combined…to create a meaningful representation" (McKeown et al., 1992, p. 91).
- When a text is poorly written or poorly organized and fails to provide readers with explicit cues for organization (and readers have to do it "on their own"), comprehension will suffer.
- Comprehension (and retention of information) will be especially difficult to achieve if *both content knowledge* (one has little or no background knowledge about a topic) and *structural knowledge* (one has little understanding of the underlying organization of texts) are limited.

Data from Beck, I. L., McKeown, M. G., Sinatra, G. M., & Loxterman, J. A. (1991). Revised social studies text from a text-processing perspective: Evidence of improved comprehension. *Reading Research Quarterly, 26,* 251–276; Carver, R. P. (1992). Effects of prediction activities, prior knowledge, and text type upon amount comprehended: Using rayding theory to critique schema theory research. *Reading Research Quarterly, 27,* 165–173; Fincher-Kiefer, R. (1992). The role of prior knowledge in inferential processing. *Journal of Research in Reading, 15,* 12–27; and Ohlhausen, M., & Roller, C. (1988). The operation of text structure and content schemata in isolation and interaction. *Reading Research Quarterly, 23,* 70–88.

included developing units on the five geographical locations involved in the wars (North America, Britain, France, Massachusetts, and Boston) and discussing the identity of the key players and their relationships (e.g., the colonists were British but they split off from their native country). An example of improving on the textbooks included adding statements to passages within the texts such as who fought the war, why they fought the war, and what was Britain's conflict with the American colonies. Other modifications included using narrative genres to introduce students to concepts being covered in the social studies units before they read the "facts" in expository formats (see the next section). What is interesting to consider is how the complementary components of content and structure knowledge offer a natural route for collaboration between classroom and content-area teachers (the content component) and SLPs (the structural component).

The Narrative–Expository Text Connection. When we discussed the oral-to-literate continuum in Chapter 2 (see pp. 35–37), we talked about the idea that narratives could be thought of as falling on a hypothetical midway point on the continuum (Westby, 1994). Inspired by Westby's (1994) work, among others' contributions, we learned that narratives are the earliest monologues, they combine informal and formal language, and they are character and event driven, among other characteristics. As a universal genre, narratives can teach children many things. They can learn about time and cause-effect relations and how and why people (the characters) do things. They can observe simple and complex lessons of life (especially in stories that have a moral) and acquire new and rare vocabulary and literate language structures. Meta skills can be refined through narrative activities by planning what you might say in a story no one has heard, providing dialogues for characters, and clarifying relationships by labeling characters clearly and improving on one's choice of words.

Chapter 6 covered some of the benefits of the shared reading experience using children's stories as a foundation for academic learning and success. It was implied that the exposure and practice that children have with narratives may help them make the transition to the more formal and complex expository text of school. Pantaleo (2004) emphasizes the importance of both adult and peer exchanges as part of the early reading experience and notes that the oral language and socialization that occurs in these shared experiences cannot be underestimated. Indeed, we might ask ourselves: Have children had enough preliteracy practice as preschoolers? What knowledge do children bring with them from their narrative experiences that may make the comprehension and production of expository text a bit smoother? Again, although not suggesting that the line from narrative to expository text is a straight and direct one, keeping the horizon in mind—considering where narratives might lead—should remain in the forefront of our intervention decisions.

Westby (2005) provides us with an elegant comparison of narrative and expository text differences. She points out that "these texts represent different ways of knowing" (Westby, 2005, p. 161). The particular structure and focus of each text, however, presents the listener-reader and speaker-writer with different challenges. Table 7-2 summarizes Westby's (2005) narrative–expository text differences.

One important distinction between the two genres relates to their underlying organizational structure. Narratives, notes Westby (2005), function in a cause-and-effect relationship. Events connect to one another in a particular way so that there is, in effect, a predictability to stories *when one knows the structure*. The term *story grammar* is often used to describe the structure of narratives in Western cultures. As noted by Westby (1994), although narratives are a universal genre, the way people tell and organize stories varies across cultures. (See Westby [1994] for a fascinating discussion.) By contrast, expository text has a number of functions that drive the text's organization. We talk of expository text in terms of whether it is a description of something; an enumeration (a list); a procedural text (instructions); or a compare-contrast, problem-solution, cause-effect, or persuasive text. Although many examples appear in the literature (e.g., Culatta et al., 1998; Merritt et al., 1998; Ukrainetz, 2006a, 2006b), Westby's (1994) visual representations of the underlying structure of narrative and expository text provide an excellent reference point for text analyses. Her graphics are represented in Figures 7-2 and 7-3.

Table 7-2
Text Differences

Narrative	Expository
Purpose to entertain	Purpose to inform
Familiar schema content	Unfamiliar schema content
Consistent text structure; all narratives have same basic organization	Variable text structures; different genres have different structures
Focus on character motivations, intentions, goals	Focus on factual information and abstract ideas
Often require multiple perspective taking—understanding points of view of different characters	Expected to take the perspective of the writer of the text
Can use pragmatic inferences (i.e., inference from similar experiences)	Must use logical-deductive inferences based on information in texts
Connective words not critical—primarily *and, then, so*	Connective words critical—wide variety of connectives (e.g., *because, before, after, when, if…then, therefore*)
Each text can stand alone	Expected to integrate information across texts
Comprehension is generally assessed informally in discussion	Comprehension often assessed in formal, structured texts
Can use top-down processing	Rely on bottom-up processing

From Westby, C. E. (2005). Assessing and remediating text comprehension problems. In H. W. Catts & A. G. Kamhi (Eds.), *Language and reading disabilities* (2nd ed., p. 162). Boston: Allyn & Bacon.

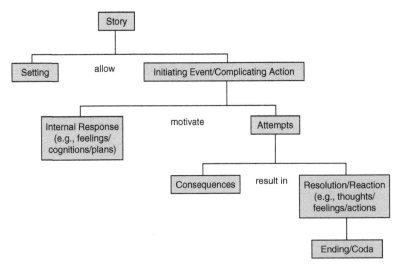

***Figure* 7-2** ■ A visual representation of the components of narrative structure. *(Redrawn from Westby, C. E. [1994]. The effects of culture on genre, structure, and style of oral and written texts. In G. P. Wallach & K. G. Butler [Eds.],* Language learning disabilities in school-age children and adolescents *[p. 191]. Boston: Allyn & Bacon.)*

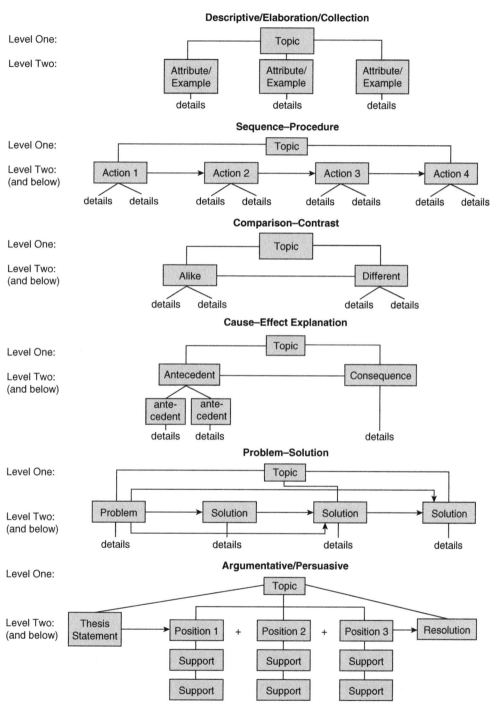

Figure 7-3 ■ A visual representation of the structures of expository text. *(Redrawn from Westby, C. E. [1994]. The effects of culture on genre, structure, and style of oral and written texts. In G. P. Wallach & K. G. Butler [Eds.],* Language learning disabilities in school-age children and adolescents *[p. 192]. Boston: Allyn & Bacon.)*

The story grammar structure of narratives as seen in Figure 7-2 includes a number of elements that are familiar to the readers of this text. Stories have *settings* that usually frame the beginning of a narrative. The setting is followed by an *initiating event* that the main character reacts to in some way, ultimately forming a *plan* or *goal* to deal with the event or situation. What follows are *attempts* a character or characters take to reach the goal, resolve the conflict, get out of a tough situation, and so on. The attempts result in *consequences* in the form of a *resolution* (or not) to the original event or conflict that sets the plot in motion. Westby (2005) points out that although the order of events can be modified, it is sometimes difficult to follow a story when events depart too far from a narrative's ordered structure. Film buffs who may have seen the movie *Memento*, some of David Lynch's films, or selected Harold Pinter plays understand how difficult it is to process a narrative when beginning, middle, and ending pieces are organized in less conventional ways. For example, the main character in *Memento* has an unusual short-term memory problem. He can't remember anything for more than a few minutes at a time. As a result, he is constantly disoriented and confused about what is happening around him. A murder and many other circumstances (e.g., "good" and "bad" characters helping or chasing him, but he's never sure who is who) complicate the narrative. Cleverly, the filmmaker creates short-term memory gaps in his audiences by starting the film at the end and reworking scenes out of sequence. Piecing the scenes together is quite difficult even after seeing the movie several times. Perhaps a visual scaffold or diagram would help solve this manufactured comprehension problem. Analyzing its unique structure, that is, "beefing up" structure knowledge, might be facilitative. Knowing the theme and core of the storyline, that is, developing familiarity with the story's content, might be another route to take to facilitate comprehension. Most adult language users would likely be able to weave their way through the tricks of directors, screenwriters, and others who play with a narrative's more predictable structure. Proficient language users will piece things together and make inferences about the events presented. They will search for organization by using the mental models they have in their heads for narrative structure. For students with LLD who have limited structure or content knowledge, every day may be like watching *Memento*.

Expository text functions differently from narrative text. According to Westby (2005), available research suggests that expository text is generally more difficult for students to comprehend and master than narrative text, although we still have much to learn about both development and disorders in this area. As Westby's (1994) Figure 7-3 shows, expository text has different "grammars," or organizational structures for the different subtypes of exposition. We can see that descriptive passages are somewhat different from sequence-procedural passages, which are different from compare-and-contrast passages, and so on. Thus unlike narratives that have a structure that usually works across diverse story themes (*Memento* notwithstanding), expository text has more structural variability (Westby, 2005). Westby (2005) also notes that with narrative text, speakers and listeners (and writers and readers) tend to use a "macrostructure" approach. Both content and structure knowledge facilitate students' abilities to hold on to what Westby (2005) calls the gist, or the theme of the story. They then make the details or subplots of a story "fit into" the story's main point. In other words, a "bigger-picture" strategy tends to operate

Recalling the movie Memento, in which the main character has a short-term memory dysfunction and is constantly disoriented and confused, may give us an idea of what it is like to comprehend a narrative when the structure eludes us.

when processing and producing narratives. This is what Westby means when she writes that one can use "top-down processing" for narratives (see Table 7-2).

Expository text, on the other hand, "involves dealing with the passage content at the level of individual facts" (Westby, 2005, p. 163). Usually, one has to process the individual facts and then organize those facts into a structural pattern. Hence, according to Westby (2005), expository text relies more predominantly on "bottom-up" processing. The ways facts and themes are developed in expository text is not as predictable as it is in narrative text. For example, there is no rigid order about the way facts have to be sequenced in the Yankees-Angels compare-contrast passage outlined in Chapter 6. Obviously, we can create a logical progression, but, again, there is some variability about how two writers might develop the Yankees-Angels piece. According to Westby (2005), "this relative independence of content facts, content schemata, and text grammars marks a major difference between expository prose and stories" (p. 163). Thus the two types of text require diverse skills and abilities that relate to curricular content in different ways.

Westby (2005) expressed this idea as follows:

> In order to understand texts, one must understand the content ideas and relationships among the content ideas that underlie the text. For narrative texts one must understand human motivations and goal-seeking behavior. For expository texts one must comprehend a variety of logical relationships. (p. 164)

Clearly, students must develop proficiency with both types of texts and the texts' subtypes to be successful in literacy learning and academics. By studying the characteristics of each genre, clinicians and teachers are better prepared to create relevant language intervention programs and classroom lessons. Both narrative and expository discourses will challenge students with LLD (Box 7-3). As part of the school experience, students will be required to participate in a number of narrative-focused activities. They will be asked to produce and comprehend stories ranging from personal to fictional to nonfictional narratives; stories may range from simple to complex in terms of their structure as well as their content. They will be asked to summarize factual stories and relate significant facts to previous and future lessons. They will be required to write book reports, recounts of summer vacations, and original endings for stories (Merritt et al., 1998; Scott, 1994).

On the expository side, students will have to follow classroom, test, and homework instructions, negotiate the problem-solution text of science, manage the cause-effect and compare-contrast texts of social studies, and write descriptive pieces about the planet Mars, among other activities. And, as noted, expository text is the predominant text that delivers the curriculum. Indeed, as we learn about the many factors that facilitate the comprehension and use of both types of discourse, we are reminded, once again, about how much knowledge is assumed to be intact by the time students open a fourth-grade textbook. Although we recognize that narrative and expository discourse each have unique characteristics, as per our discussion and as highlighted in the language sample excerpts, narratives can teach children many things and they may help provide a bridge to expository text.

Consider the abbreviated example that follows from McKeown and colleagues (1992, p. 82). Students are asked to read a story (or have a story of this type read to them). After reading the story, they have a guided discussion about

---

Margin note:

Top-down processing may be more predominant for narrative text, whereas bottom-up processing may be emphasized for expository text; however, both choices are dynamic and ever-changing based on the situation and level of background knowledge (Westby, 2005).

7

BOX 7-3	*Challenges of Both Narrative and Expository Text*

Narrative-Focused Activities*
- Produce and comprehend stories
  - Personal, fictional, and nonfictional
  - Simple and complex structure and content
- Summarize factual stories and relate significant facts to previous and future lessons
- Write book reports, recounts of personal experiences, and original endings for stories

Expository Text Activities
- Follow classroom, test, and homework instructions
- Negotiate problem-solution text in science
- Manage cause-and-effect texts of social studies
- Write descriptive pieces

*Data from Merritt, D. D., Culatta, B., & Trostle, S. (1998). Narratives: Implementing a discourse framework. In D. D. Merritt & B. Culatta (Eds.), *Language intervention in the classroom* (pp. 227–330). San Diego: Singular Publishing Group; and Scott, C. M. (1994). A discourse continuum for school-age students: Impact of modality and genre. In G. P. Wallach & K. G. Butler (Eds.), *Language learning disabilities in school-age children and adolescents: Some principles and applications* (pp. 219–252). Boston: Allyn & Bacon.

the ideas and feelings expressed by the main character, a teacher named Samantha Stevens:

> My name is Samantha Stevens. I spent many years of my life getting a school going in our town and helping to teach the children…In Britain, only those who can afford it send their children to school. That used to seem fine to me. But here everyone goes to school—and I really think that is the way it should be. (Wallach & Butler, 1994a, p. 16, quoting McKeown et al., 1992, p. 82)

According to the authors (McKeown et al., 1992), changing the type of text used can make the concepts covered in the Revolutionary War more accessible to students. McKeown and colleagues (1992) used the personalized story of Samantha Stevens, among others, to present the point of view and feelings expressed by the colonists. Students learned about the nature of the conflicts in narrative formats before or in conjunction with studying the facts presented in the more formal, expository texts found in their history books. As Westby (2005) pointed out, one of the characteristics of narratives is their focus on characters' motivations, feelings, and intentions. This *agent focus* is absent in expository text. Further, because narratives often require that the listener-reader understand multiple perspectives (e.g., Samantha's vs. the British loyalists), narratives provide an opportunity to see both sides to the coin, a skill that will come in handy when reading and writing compare-contrast, problem-solution, persuasive, and other types of expository text.

It is impractical to think that every unit of every history text can be converted from expository to narrative text. The research merely suggests that the way information is presented to students, especially when they have content knowledge gaps, can influence what they comprehend and retain. Language learning disabled students, as we have discussed, may have both content and structure knowledge limitations coupled with reading difficulties that confound the situation. Fifth graders without language and reading problems have a tremendous advantage when compared with students who have LLD and, yet, many typically developing students also have difficulty negotiating the tough text of their textbooks. Language intervention, when relevant and curriculum based, can make a difference for students with LLD. Speech-language pathologists can, no doubt, see the logic of using history or science, for example, *as a backdrop* for their work with students with LLD.

If a student has difficulty comprehending and producing coherent and structured narratives, the questions one must ask (yet again) are, Why have I chosen to work on narratives? How do I see my "clinical" work connecting to that lesson on the Revolutionary War? Relating to school work in general? As Norris (1997) and Ehren (2000) have reminded us many times, the SLP's role is not to teach the content of the curriculum (e.g., the Revolutionary War); the teacher should be well trained to do that. Rather, the SLP's role is to help the student acquire the language skills needed to access the curriculum, as we have emphasized in this text. It is true, however, that choosing a story such as the one presented earlier about Samantha Stevens (a teacher in the colonies) to help a student with narrative discourse has the added bonus of exposing the student to some aspects of the content he or she might encounter in the classroom. But the focus for the SLP—who complements, not replicates, the teacher's role and responsibilities—would be to work on various aspects of narrative structure itself. The SLP might choose to work on both macro and micro components of narratives depending on the student's needs. She would facilitate awareness of and practice with story elements—such as the setting, complication or conflict, reaction or internal response, attempts at action to resolve the conflict, consequence(s), and resolution—as part of her macro component. In her micro work for narratives, she might help the student acquire and use various connecting words, such as "and," "then," and "so," moving to more specific and literate variations (that are predominant in and critical for expository text) such as "because," "before," "after,' "when," "if-then," "therefore," and so on (Westby, 2005; see Table 7-2). More literate syntactic form work, that is, work on adding more complex sentences such as subordinate-main and relative clause sentences to the student's repertoire (see the compare-contrast example on p. 167 in Chapter 6), might also be part of the micro component.

The clinician should think about ways to help students *use what they have learned* in the narrative intervention in different and expanded ways. For example, as students improve in their comprehension and production of narratives about the colonies or other topics, they should "practice with" expressing the same content in more complex forms. For example, an SLP might progress from the story of our colonial teacher (including covering the conflict that brought her there, her attempts and plan to go to America, what events led her to start the school, her feelings about the war, etc.) to helping the student write a compare-contrast piece about the colonists and the loyalists and how their differences set the stage for what became the American Revolution. This example shows that the clinician has moved the student to an expository text activity but controlled the content. (The content is still about the colonists and the loyalists.)

Again, the SLP's goal is not to cover the material in the American Revolution unit. (That's the teacher's job.) She should *not* be reinforcing or reviewing the core vocabulary words for that unit such as the names of the opposing generals; the dates of certain events; and the names, causes, and events of the key battles. It *is* the SLP's role to help the student develop the skills and strategies needed to comprehend and produce the structures in which the content is embedded. The SLP may be covering content knowledge (and that may be a bonus in terms of the background knowledge factor), but the focus should be on helping students acquire semantic knowledge that relates to temporal and cause-effect relations, among other broad concepts. In other words, time and cause-effect relations go beyond the specifics of the American Revolution; they cut across the curriculum. And temporal, cause-effect, problem-solution, and similar relations are concepts that one will encounter in narrative as well as expository text, although they are expressed in different ways in the two genres.

The SLP may also help students acquire proficiency with specific vocabulary items as part of language intervention, but, again, she should not be teaching the Revolutionary War's content. Her "therapeutic focus" (Ehren, 2000) should include working on those connecting words and phrases (*before, after, prewar, postwar,* etc.) and other linguistic and metalinguistic skills that are needed for comprehension and retention of the informationally heavy text of school (Wallach, 2004; Wallach & Ehren, 2004). (See the science example that follows in this chapter.) But, again, the important point remains that seeing the horizon of expository text and knowing the challenges that students will face put narrative intervention in the unique position of providing students with some of the foundational skills and abilities that will make the transition to complex text a little smoother.

Thus narratives serve many functions; they can entertain us and they can teach us things about the world. Falling midway on the continuum with their uniquely organized structure, narratives can help children acquire literate language and learn about how and why events connect to one another. Some of the early narrative-focused experiences that preschoolers participate in were discussed in the previous chapter in our discussion of the shared reading experiences. Many of these experiences and the techniques discussed set a foundation for the activities that predominate in the school-age period. And, of course, we would always evaluate the clinical and educational decisions we make for students with a strong understanding of when and why a student is "ready" for any number of language intervention activities, as discussed throughout this text.

Analyzing Narratives with an Eye Toward the Future. Adding to Hadley's procedures for eliciting a connected language sample, Westby (2005) and Ukrainetz (2006b), among others, provide excellent guidelines for analyzing narratives. Ukrainetz (2006b) points out that one of the ways we can think about stories is to divide them broadly into two main phases: (1) pre-episodic narratives and (2) episodic narratives. Generally, the pre-episodic period starts and evolves in the preschool period and the episodic period takes off in the school-age period. Ukrainetz (2006b) offers the following descriptions to guide us in our analysis based on some of the classic works by Applebee (1978), Peterson and McCabe (1983), Stein and Glenn (1979), and Sutton-Smith (1986). She also provides examples of each stage, which appear in Box 7-4.

Pre-Episodic Period. This stage consists of three types of stories: (1) descriptive sequences, (2) action sequences, and (3) reactive sequences:

1. *Descriptive sequences* tend to be a collection of labels. Children often talk about what catches their eye if looking at a picture or following along in a shared reading experience. Descriptive sequences may also be thematically connected.

BOX 7-4

Second-Grader Stories Based on the Covers of Mercer Mayer Frog Books

1. A Boy, a Dog, a Frog and a Friend (1971)
Descriptive Sequence
One day a boy and a dog and a frog and a friend were fishing. The boy caught one fish. The dog caught two. And the frog caught none.

2. One Frog Too Many (1975)
Action Sequence
Once there was a boy. He loved to play in the pond right across from his house. One day he was playing in the pond. And he found a frog. And he took it home and put it in his room and went to eat dinner. He went back to his room. And there were frogs jumping everywhere. And he kept all the frogs.

3. Frog, Where Are You? (1969)
Version A: Complete Episode
Once there was a boy, a dog, and a frog. Once the frog left. And he went into the forest. And the boy kept looking for him. And then finally the frog came out. And they all went home.

4. Frog, Where Are You? (1969)
Version B: Complex Episode
A boy had a frog. The frog jumped off. He went into some trees. In a minute he was no longer in sight. The boy called and called for him. And then he saw that his frog had took a scary path. So he decided to take the scary path. So he took the scary path. And it was very, very creepy. Then he saw something jumping. He grabbed it. And it was his frog.

5. Frog, Where Are You? (1969)
Version C: Complex Episode
There was a boy. And he had a frog. Then he lost his frog. He looked downstairs. Be he was not there. So he looked in his room. The window was opened. So he went outside. He did not find him. So he looked by a pond. Then he heard a sound. So he went to a hollow log. He found two frogs.

From Ukrainetz, T. A. (2006). Teaching narrative structure: Coherence, cohesion, and captivation. In T. A. Ukrainetz (Ed.), *Contextualized language intervention* (p. 203). Eau Claire, WI: Thinking Publications.

Ukrainetz (2006b) says that in descriptive sequences, the statements can be reordered without changing the overall meaning of the text. As Box 7-4 shows, there is a description of what's happening in the first story, that is, the characters caught fish.

2. *Action sequences* have a temporal relation structure. One can follow what the child is saying, and the order is important for the story's overall meaning. Children create their stories with a logical sequence of events. Causal relations, however, are not expressed at this point in narrative development. The second story follows the sequence of events of a boy catching a frog.

3. *Reactive sequences* express causal relations. The causal relations expressed, according to Ukrainetz (2006b), are automatic rather than being expressed as a character planning to resolve a complication. In other words, a character's goal-directed behavior is not present in the story at this stage. Goal-directed behavior occurs in the episodic stage of development. There is no reactive sequence presented in Box 7-4. An example of a more automatic causal relationship would be a statement such as the following: "The frogs were jumping everywhere and making a mess of his room." The two events are related causally, but we don't know what the boy will do to resolve the problem.

Episodic Period. This stage is the core of story analysis. Westby's (1994) visual representation of a narrative (see Figure 7-1) reviews these elements. An episodic narrative has the elements of a *complication or conflict* that a character encounters or has in his or her life. The character or characters *try to resolve* the issue. According to Ukrainetz (2006b), a complete episode consists of three parts: (1) a complication, (2) goal-directed behavior (the character responds to the situation and makes attempts to resolve the conflict, etc.), and (3) a consequence. There are many different episode types, a sampling of which are outlined in Box 7-5.

In Box 7-4, we see examples of complete and complex episodes in the stories of second graders. Although brief in length, story 3 has elements of episodic

---

BOX 7-5	*Example Episodes within Narratives*

- *Incomplete episode:* has a complication and an internal response or attempt to do something
- *Abbreviated episode:* has a complication and a consequence
- *Complete episode:* has a complication, an internal response or attempt to do something, and a consequence
- *Complex episode:* involves multiple attempts to resolve a complication or multiple complete episodes
- *Interactive episode:* involves multiple characters who have opposing complications and consequences

From Ukrainetz, T. A. (2006). Teaching narrative structure: Coherence, cohesion, and captivation. In T. A. Ukrainetz (Ed.), *Contextualized language intervention* (p. 203). Eau Claire, WI: Thinking Publications. Based on the work of Peterson, C., & McCabe, A. (1983). *Developmental psycholinguistics: Three ways of looking at a child's narrative.* New York: Plenum.

structure: the frog leaves the boy (complication), the boy attempts to find the frog (he has a goal and goes into the forest and looks for the frog), and the frog shows up and they go home (consequences). Although not as elaborate or explicit as the more complex episodes (shown in stories 4 and 5), we see the beginnings of a more structured and organized grammar that drives the story in story 3.

Westby's (2005) story grammar decision tree (Figure 7-4) is an excellent complement for the information that was summarized by Ukrainetz (2006b).

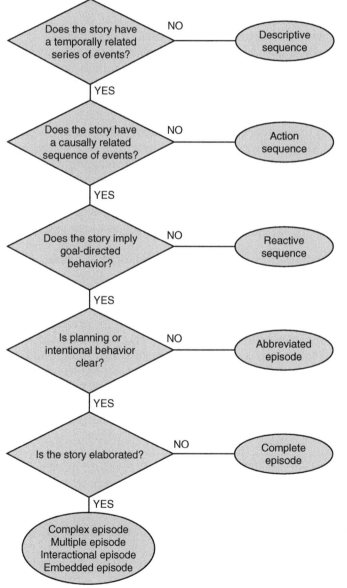

Figure 7-4 ■ A story grammar decision tree. *(Redrawn from Westby, C. E. [2005]. Assessing and remediating text comprehension problems. In H. W. Catts & A. G. Kamhi [Eds.],* Language and reading disabilities *[2nd ed., p. 181]. Boston: Allyn & Bacon.)*

The questions guide clinicians and teachers through the pre-episodic and episodic periods of narrative development. The chart is a useful tool for analyzing children's spoken and written renditions.

We can see that narratives have the potential to provide students with important structure and content knowledge that they can take with them as they progress through the grades. In addition to learning how to create a monologue, how to connect ideas that go beyond the sentence level, and how to pull those ideas together by using story grammar schema and more complex syntax, children will be exposed to many underlying concepts that are embedded in narrative structures. For example, children learn to comprehend and express temporal and cause-effect relations in narratives. They learn about many things through narratives, including learning about *physical states* (whether things are hot or cold; whether a character has children or not); *physical events* (a storm destroyed the ship); *internal states* (a character was angry because of some circumstance); and *goals* (a character wanted to accomplish something), among other things. They also learn that they may have to "read between the lines" to make connections among concepts. For example, there many be *reasons* why a character is angry that are not stated explicitly (Westby, 2005). These concepts gleaned from narrative practice will show themselves again in different form in expository text. Along with many skills, children learn new vocabulary and they learn how to describe events when listening to, producing, and reading stories, additional skills that are needed in the management of expository text. The concepts that ideas must follow logically and that events relate to one another in specific ways are pieces of the complex pie of connected discourse. And the road from narrative to expository text proficiency is a long and sometimes winding one.

As preschoolers move from the comfort of home and highly contextualized language environments to the less comfortable and decontexualized contexts of school, their narrative abilities, as we have seen in the examples presented in the current and previous chapter, evolve with them. Personal narratives, that is, recounting an event that has happened to them, set the tone for fictional narratives. And narrative proficiency influences expository text proficiency. Indeed, by being encouraged by adults to recount events in their world, young children learn about the elements of setting, characters, chronological sequences, complication, and resolution (Merritt al., 1998). They eventually apply this knowledge to less personalized stories. Likewise, by observing traffic signs, grocery store ads, and posted rules in parks and other public places, young children are gradually exposed to expository text (Hall et al., 2005). The early "show and tell" activities of Grades 1 and 2 provide expository text experiences for children, but Hall and colleagues (2005) argue that we have to do more to help children master expository text in the early grades. They write that "creating knowledge and understanding of concepts (i.e., same and different, time order, and problem and solution) [will] help create the beginnings of mental rhetorical structures that will support later understanding of text structures" (Hall et al., 2005, p. 196).

As we saw in Hadley's (1998) and Geddes and Fukumoto's (2005) sampling activities, sampling across discourse genres and spoken and written modes provides us with a more complete picture of a student's ability to manage connected text. To reiterate a key point: it is important to understand the strengths and weaknesses that children bring to each discourse and evaluate how proficiency in one discourse may influence proficiency in another discourse.

As we have said time and again, professionals who work with children and adolescents with LLD face as many challenges as the students they serve. They must understand the complexity of the tasks used when assessing and facilitating language, and they must look back as well as look ahead, as pointed out by Fay and colleagues (1995), when trying to understand and explore the nature of a student's language gaps and how and when to "fill" those gaps. Again, when students "fail" to comprehend, produce, or write a coherent story, "where" do we go to find out why, and again, what are the questions we might ask ourselves? As Westby (2005) notes, when narrative text is difficult for students with LLD, how will they manage the more complex and abstract nature of expository text? The double-edged sword of complex and unfamiliar content wrapped in more linguistically heavy text creates a maze of obstacles for students, especially students with LLD. But narratives can serve as one vehicle of transition when we keep our eyes on the horizon ahead and set our narrative goals and activities with the future in mind.

Back to Mars and the World of Science

Think of all the language learning, literacy experiences, and metalinguistic skills that precede the ability to write a coherent summary about something you have read. A complex combination of knowledge and skills underlies the success a student might have writing a piece about the planet Mars. Reflecting on the piece presented at the beginning of this chapter (see Figure 7-1), it is clear that we would need to learn more about the writer and how he arrived at this place in his academic career. We would certainly like to know more about his overall abilities to comprehend and produce connected text. It would be interesting, as mentioned earlier, to obtain a spoken language sample across genres, as well as evaluate other macro and micro language abilities across texts and modalities. Many questions remain unanswered about this particular sample. But among the things we do know is that Grade 4 science is tough. It gets even tougher by Grade 6.

Teachers are very familiar with the required textbooks that challenge their students in various subject areas. Speech-language pathologists and other specialists who work outside of the classroom are traditionally less familiar with classroom texts. But, clearly, understanding the language of the curriculum includes having, at the very least, a basic understanding of what students with LLD may face as they open their textbooks to absorb information about new and exciting—and complex—topics. Unfortunately, for children who have had little exposure to expository text or who have difficulty processing and producing connected text in general (including narratives), the ability to learn new content may be quite limited. As put by Hall and colleagues (2005):

> Children who have particular difficulty with expository text comprehension may be less prepared to learn new content knowledge or have difficulty learning from what they read [and further] children who can read expository text will outperform children without those skills in all of the content areas (e.g., science, social studies). (p. 196)

Figures 7-5 and 7-6 are examples from a Grade 4 science text and provide readers with a flavor of the complexity of the topics covered (the content) and the density of the language used (the structure). Some good supportive information, such as the pictures relating to real-life events and the "wrap-up" questions, provides a bit of context (which may or may not be helpful) and encourages students to engage in "meta" checks (review and critical thinking) for the unit. Figure 7-5 provides a reproduction of a page from the text. It is part of a unit about how matter changes states (changes from one form to another). Figure 7-6 reproduces a "Reflect and Evaluate" review of the unit. Clearly, the page reproduced in Figure 7-5 that covers *condensation* and *freezing* (with highlighted words in the text) is taken out of the broader context covered in the unit. Nonetheless, the example demonstrates the level of language (both spoken and written) needed to absorb information from paragraph to paragraph and from page to page. This expository excerpt has both description and cause-effect elements. The core of the unit is to understand how matter changes and the factors that create change—concepts that are complex. Given what was said earlier about content and structure knowledge, it may be that some prior experience with both descriptive and cause-effect text would be facilitative to comprehension and retention. Understanding how text works appears to be an important skill for students with LLD to acquire.

Looking further, using Figure 7-5 as an example, we can observe how the micro aspects of language (e.g., individual sentences) might interact with "getting" the overall meaning of the text. One of the topic sentences in the Grade 4 science unit about matter lets students know that this part of the discussion will be about water changing states. But the next statement—"this time in reverse order starting with water vapor"—may be especially difficult for students with LLD. It is assumed in the reference about "reversing order" that students remember that an earlier paragraph started with a discussion of water in its frozen state. Thus keeping the concepts expressed across text includes attending to the language that "links" concepts together.

Last, the literate-style syntactic forms (e.g., relative clause sentences, "if...then" structures) add to the text's complexity. Figure 7-6, "Reflect & Evaluate," reinforces the amount of information required by the Grade 4 science curriculum in one chapter. And although it is the teacher's role to teach the content (see "Word Power," for example), the SLP has much to do to help students with LLD manage both the macro and micro issues of the text's structure. For example, referring to Figure 7-6, SLPs might ask the following questions: Can the student handle the complex syntactic structures listed in the instructions? Do phrases and words such as *rather than, stands for, explain,* and *describe* confuse the student? What strategies does the student use when he or she doesn't know the meaning of a word?

A Closer Look at the Language of Science: What SLPs Need to Know

Many of the science texts available today, although understandably difficult for students with LLD, have made an effort to make the information more accessible

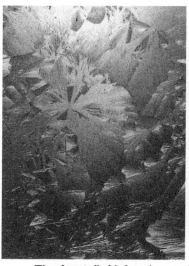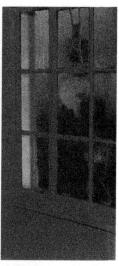

The frost *(left)*, fog *(center)*, and moisture on a windowpane *(right)* are all examples of condensation.

Let's take another look at water as it changes state—this time in reverse order, starting with water vapor. Suppose heat energy is taken away from water vapor. Then the particles that make up the gas begin to slow down and move closer together. If the particles lose enough energy, the gas changes to a liquid. **Condensation** (kän dən sā'shən) is the change of state from a gas to a liquid. In the activity on page B37, water vapor, an invisible gas in the air, condenses on the sides of a can.

Once condensation occurs, suppose that more energy is taken away from the liquid. Then the particles in the liquid slow down even more. If the particles in the liquid lose enough energy, the liquid begins to freeze. **Freezing** is the change of state from a liquid to a solid. ■

INVESTIGATION 2 WRAP-UP

REVIEW

CRITICAL THINKING

1. What kind of energy is involved when matter changes state?

2. What change of state occurs when boiling takes place?

3. Recall what you know about changes of state. Then explain which properties of HFCs help keep the air in a refrigerator cold.

4. Compare the behavior of particles of matter during boiling and during condensation.

Figure **7-5** ■ An example of text from a Grade 4 science text. *(From Science Discovery Works Series [2003]. [Grade 4, "Matter" unit.] Boston: Houghton Mifflin.)*

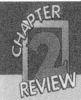

REFLECT & EVALUATE

Word Power

Write the letter of the term that best matches the definition. *Not all terms will be used.*

1. Matter that has a definite volume and a definite shape
2. The smallest part of an element that has the properties of that element
3. The change of state from a solid to a liquid
4. Matter that has no definite volume or shape
5. The ability to cause change
6. A kind of matter made up of two or more elements that are joined together

a. atom
b. compound
c. energy
d. gas
e. liquid
f. melting
g. solid
h. substance

Check What You Know

Write the term in each pair that best completes each sentence.

1. Material made up of only one kind of matter is (an element, a compound).
2. The change of state from a liquid to a solid is called (boiling, freezing).
3. Particles in a liquid move faster than those in a (solid, gas).
4. The chemical symbol I stands for (iodine, iron).

Problem Solving

1. Common table sugar is called sucrose. A molecule of sucrose has the chemical formula $C_{12}H_{22}O_{11}$. What does the chemical formula tell you about a molecule of sucrose?
2. Explain why frost forms on the inside of a window rather than on the outside.

Copy this drawing of the water molecule and label each atom. Then describe the makeup of a water molecule and write its chemical formula.

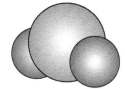

Figure 7-6 ■ An example of the review section from a Grade 4 science text. *(From* Science Discovery Works Series *[2003]. [Grade 4.] Boston: Houghton Mifflin.)*

to students. Improvements have been made about the way information is presented. For example, many chapters start with a common experience that relates to the topic that will be covered in the unit. A chapter might also start with an experiment that frames a question for the unit. In one sixth-grade text (Houghton-Mifflin's *Science Discovery Works,* Grade 6), children read a brief scenario about waiting at a bus stop. In the scenario, it's obviously a cold day. To complicate the situation, some of the children are carrying packages. The illustration shows heavy and lighter packages of different shapes. One package looks big and bulky, but the way the child is carrying it (on his head) sends a message that it is light and easier to carry. Another child is trying to carry a smaller package but it is weighing him down. It's smaller than the first package but it looks much heavier. The child is wearing winter clothes, but he's sweating. The scenario introduces the chapter on "Measuring Mass and Volume." In another chapter from the same text, children are making lemonade to learn how to "think like a scientist." They should know what they want to do, have a plan, use a recipe, check results, and so on. Colorful reminders such as those seen in Figures 7-5 and 7-6 are other ways that students are directed to important concepts that are being covered in the science curriculum. All these supports have the potential of helping students make better connections. But with all these improvements, science is still a difficult subject to master. Its "hands-on" component contributes to learning in a positive way (Pantaleo, 2004), but many students with LLD remain lost without language intervention that can help them navigate the many complexities of their textbooks.

What is it about the language of science that makes it so difficult? We have talked about how background knowledge, content knowledge, and structure knowledge interact to form a triangle of potential difficulty. We also know that a learner's particular strengths, weaknesses, and interests contribute to success and failure in mastering science. Halliday (1993) adds to the mix by pointing out that the language used in science texts has it own unique characteristics. He talks about this uniqueness as "scientific English." Among the characteristics of scientific English, according to Halliday (1993), are the following: (1) informational density; (2) nominalization; (3) technicality; (4) authoritativeness; (5) interlocking definitions; and (6) technical taxonomies. These characteristics contribute to the challenging nature of science and help us to understand the level of linguistic difficulty facing students with LLD (Box 7-6). By studying the nature of scientific writing, we can gain some insight into the language skills and abilities assumed to be intact and that serve as a foundation for managing the specific elements of a science curriculum.

Informational density is certainly evidenced in Figures 7-5 and 7-6. One observes the amount of content knowledge covered in these abbreviated examples presented in the figures. According to Fang (2004), the number of content words (e.g., nouns, main verbs, adjectives, and some adverbs) used in science texts far exceeds the number of content words, especially new content words, used in spontaneous speech. In spontaneous speech, the average number of content words per clause is 2 to 3 words. This number increases to 10 to 13 per clause in scientific writing. Thus the lexical density of science texts contributes to its uniqueness and its complexity. Further, the high density of information of

BOX 7-6	*Characteristics of "The Language of Science"*

- Informational density
- Nominalization
- Technicality
- Authoritativeness
- Interlocking definitions
- Technical taxonomies

Data from Halliday, M. A. K. (1993). Some grammatical problems in scientific English. In M. A. K. Halliday & J. R. Martin (Eds.), *Writing science: Literacy and discursive power* (pp. 69–85). London: Falmer.

Nominalization is conversion of verbs into nouns and adjectives and is an aspect of the language required for science learning.

science texts is typically coupled with more complex syntax (Fang, 2004). Another aspect of the language of science is *nominalization*. Nominalization involves the conversion of verbs into nouns and adjectives. Thus the verb *compress* becomes *compression*; the verb *vibrate* becomes *vibrating* particles. As a language process, nominalization is used to create technical terms, establish cause-effect relationships, and synthesize previously learned information (Fang, 2004; Unsworth, 1999). Although nominalization has useful functions, it also changes the grammatical layout of an event, creating some abstraction and ambiguity. Fang (2004) provides an example of the nominalized phrase, "the destruction of Brazilian trees." In this example, according to Fang (2004), information about who or what destroyed the trees (the agent) is obscured in the phrase as written, which can cause confusion when trying to comprehend its meaning. Clearly, the cause of the destruction can be explained further, but getting to the meaning means going across sentences and processing connected text.

In science language, definitions are often presented with one definition being dependent on another—called interlocking definitions by Halliday (1993).

Related to the aforementioned characteristics of science texts and science writing are the characteristics of *technicality, authoritativeness,* and *interlocking definitions.* The *technical* vocabulary used in science describes the physical world and its phenomena. Technical words and phrases establish categories, classes, and relationships among scientific phenomena (Fang, 2004), and, as noted, the concepts expressed in science are often abstract and difficult to visualize (Westby & Torres-Velasquez, 2000). Moreover, in scientific writing, information is presented generally in *objective and assertive tones* by *knowledgeable experts* (Fang, 2004). Consequently, science language tends to be more impersonal and less interactional, although, as mentioned, more personalized components have been added to current science texts. (See, for example, the Houghton-Mifflin *Science Discovery Works* series.) Science language is complicated further because definitions are often presented such that one definition is dependent on another. This is what Halliday (1993) calls *interlocking definitions.* For example, in a Grade 6 unit on "matter," matter is defined in terms of its physical and chemical properties. Physical and chemical properties are defined more specifically, and the reader has to keep all of these definitions in mind, as well as understand how they relate to one another. Some of these challenges were presented when we introduced Figures 7-5 and 7-6.

Finally, scientific language uses many *technical taxonomies* to express its content. According to Westby and Torres-Valasquez (2000), taxonomies are classification systems that categorize things into different groups based on their attributes and other abstract principles. Halliday (1993) adds that technical taxonomies are usually based on two semantic relationships: (1) superordination (animals vs. plants) and (2) composition (a leaf is part of a plant). Superordination involves an either/or relationship. Thus an animal is either a vertebrate or an invertebrate. Composition, by contrast, includes categories of attributes that can coexist with one another. In the case of composition, one could say that matter has both physical and chemical properties. Understanding the abstract principles by which things are categorized in a taxonomic classification system can be difficult for many elementary school children, including those with and without LLD.

In sum, the texts of school, including science texts, along with other content area subjects such as history and social studies, are more formal, syntactically complex, and linguistically dense. Scientific language, as suggested in the literature, has some unique characteristics that may have an impact on comprehension and retention of information. In addition to its linguistic characteristics, science is an inference-based curriculum (Best et al., 2005; Palinscar et al., 2000). Students have to make many connections "on their own" by integrating information across sentences and making connections among all the technical terms presented and the interlocking definitions that build on one another.

Clearly, background knowledge and experience will have an impact on a student's success or failure with any subject. Bringing existing knowledge into play through narrative practice with various subjects and other activities can facilitate comprehension. And, as mentioned, many science textbooks such as the Houghton-Mifflin series have added personalized experiences and activities at the beginning of chapters as a way to introduce complex subjects and make them more accessible. The availability of vocabulary acquisition strategies will also be part of the process of learning science (and other subjects).

Indeed, both content knowledge and structure knowledge, macro and micro components, come together to facilitate one's ability to learn from both spoken and written text. We can see, yet again, in the examples from both social studies and science that language facility cannot be separated from school learning. The linguistic skills and strategies needed for academic success are varied and multilayered. The horizon of comprehension and production of connected text and how we "get our students there" remains in the forefront for both speech-language pathologists and teachers. Our exploration of these interacting facets of language learning across genres and components is a complex business and will continue in Chapter 8.

Returning to Mars: What Questions Remain? We would exercise caution in drawing any conclusions about a student's abilities from written language samples alone. We would, however, form hypotheses from available information and develop strategies about where we might proceed in both assessment and intervention. We could ask ourselves what the piece suggests as a beginning step in our understanding of the student's language competence. The Grade 4 writer of the Mars piece may certainly "know more" about the subject than his written rendition suggests. Even in its abbreviated form, we can see that he has some information about the "red planet." Would our writer express himself in a more organized way in spoken language? Would he tell (or write) a more coherent or elaborate narrative about Mars by using characters and story events to make his points? Does he have sufficient syntactic knowledge to link thoughts together? Sufficient lexical ability for both content words and the smaller, connecting (linguistic glue) words and phrases such as *first, because, since, in order to,* and so on? As mentioned in an earlier section of the chapter, we would have to know much more about this child's spoken and written language abilities and academic performance across subjects, among other areas, to form a representative picture of his language and learning needs.

With caution always guiding us, we might ask ourselves what the Mars piece demonstrates about both macro and micro aspects of connected discourse and the possible challenges facing our fourth grader. Collaborative roles between teachers and SLPs are revisited briefly.

Background Knowledge. Does the student have enough information about the subject area? What has he really retained from reading or listening to the teacher's lecture? It would be helpful for us to observe some of the gaps that may (or may not) exist and provide our fourth grader with some practice and brainstorming activities (preferably done in the classroom) that may create a better foundation for what must be written. Mastering the subject's content falls within the realm of the classroom teacher. The SLP might work with the student on strategies for remembering names and for organizing what he wants to say (see next section on macro issues; Wallach & Ehren, 2004). The SLP might also work with the teacher in setting up the brainstorming activities. It could include using Ogle's (1986, 1989) classic K-W-L activity for encouraging discussion of subjects and taking a "meta" look at what one knows and needs to know. Box 7-7 is a modification of Ogle's original suggestion that might be useful in helping our student prepare to write his Mars piece.

Macrostructure. The written sample suggests that the student may need help organizing his thoughts in writing (and possibly in speaking as well). The K-W-L work (see Box 7-7) may provide a beginning step in the organizational process because the student verbalizes about what he knows (and wants to say) but also talks about what he wants his readers to learn by reading the piece. But the writer also has to know something about expository text and its organization. The Mars piece starts off as a possible compare-contrast piece (Mars is almost like Earth) and then moves to a more descriptive piece of an event involving an exploration of the planet. Many written works contain a combination of expository types. Our student may need some help in deciding which way to go and developing a keener awareness about how to signal changes for his readers.

The SLP might work with our Grade 4 writer in identifying the different types of text (shown in Figure 7-3) or focusing on one type of text depending on the student's needs and abilities. The SLP could work with the classroom teacher on follow-up activities involving the different types of texts and having her become a partner in reminding the student to use the different organizational

BOX 7-7	*Ogle Activity Sheet for Prewriting**

What I Know about Mars
It's a planet.
It has a nickname.
It's like Earth.
We sent a robot there.

What I Want My Readers to Learn about Mars
What's my purpose?
How is Mars like Earth?
Why was the robot sent?
What are some facts about the planet?

What I Learned
To prepare before writing
To use my writing map
To check whether my writing makes sense

Based on the framework from Ogle, D. M. (1986). K-W-L: A teaching model that develops active reading of expository text. *Reading Teacher, 39,* 564–570.
*Ogle's (1986) original K-W-L approach included three pieces: (1) what I *know,* (2) what I *want* to learn, and (3) what I *learned.* These three questions guided students in their metacognitive assessment of their knowledge about a subject or an activity.

structures (visual maps such as those proposed by Westby [1994] can be pasted in his notebook) when writing assignments are required. Westby (2006) also developed a reminder chart for expository types. The following is an example of descriptive and compare-contrast text in a modified version:

What Does the Text Want to Say?	**It's Called**	**Some Key Words***
What something is about	Descriptive	Is/are called; can be identified as
Where something is		
Who someone is		
How two things are the same or different	Compare-contrast	Different, same, alike, similar, although, but, on the other hand, yet, rather than

*Westby (2006) points out that there are no specific key words for descriptive texts. The SLP might pick connecting words that she thinks will help the student pull ideas together for descriptive pieces.

Microstructure. The Mars sample also suggests that some work on the micro aspects of language, that is, the sentence and word level (see the key words listed in the Westby [2006] example in the last section), might be integrated with macro work. The student attempts to express his ideas in more complex syntactic forms (e.g., You need a heater and a sweater when you go to Mars), but these attempts are minimal. The use of some of the connecting and more literate transition words is another area where improvements are needed. Although the teacher may be more concerned with punctuation and other writing conventions along with the length and organization of the piece as her comments suggest, the partnership between teacher and SLP is very appropriate for this child. The SLP's knowledge of syntactic acquisitions above age 5, and her understanding of "where the student may be" on the hypothetical oral-to-literate continuum, would offer the teacher (and the student) a way to develop the language abilities needed to produce a more coherent and grade-appropriate summary of the Mars unit.

Moving On

The comprehension and production of connected discourse in spoken and written forms is a complex business. This chapter continued our exploration of the multifaceted nature of text. It has also kept the curriculum within our focus, as school-age assessment and intervention must do. There is much to learn about this subject, which becomes a metaphor for how difficult retention and memory of complex topics can be even for more-than-proficient language users. We will continue our discussion of text in the chapter that follows. Reading comprehension and written composition will be the focus of Chapter 8, but we will shift back to spoken language as a reminder of the reciprocity that exists between systems. The road may be long and winding, but there is hope with each new roadmap that the literature provides.

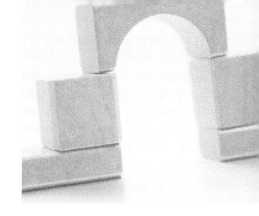

Being literate requires both interpretive and rhetorical skills; that is, readers must be able to interpret a text's meaning and importance beyond basic comprehension. Further, writers of content text must be able to predict what their audiences will know and believe and writers must use language and concepts in a way that persuades the audience to interpret their text in particular ways.

(Moje et al., 2004, p. 45)

8 Seeing the World Through Connected Text

Bringing Structure and Content, Macro and Micro Pieces Together: Part 2

SUMMARY STATEMENT ▰▰▰▰
The quest to unravel some of the mysteries of comprehending and producing coherent and meaningful connected text continues in Chapter 8. Weaving together strategies for writing as well as reading, we explore additional intervention ideas that will help students acquire and *use* strategies that work across curricular content. We also revisit general strategies for reading and writing that are believed to be effective in helping students with language learning disabilities have greater success absorbing and retaining class content. Taking the lead from Chapter 7, we will ask if and how

The following graduate students from the Department of Communicative Disorders at California State University at Long Beach in Long Beach, California, should be acknowledged for their help and support with this chapter: Aileen Beck and Carly Knoll for their research in the science area and Stephen Charlton and Julie Christie for their work on the history sections of this chapter.

well-documented strategies such as visual mapping, self-questioning, and summarizing might be modified to address the specific literacies required for different content areas such as science and social studies. From our discussion in previous chapters, we have seen that history and science have some unique and overlapping requirements in terms of how they communicate meaning. Looking across the speech-language, literacy learning, and educational literature, we find, yet again, much common ground. There is a call from all corners of study for more intense, consistent, and meaningful collaborative efforts (e.g., Yore et al., 2004).

KEY QUESTIONS

1. Can we separate content learning from language learning?
2. What do we need to know about fundamental and specific literacy skills, and how does this knowledge influence language intervention approaches?
3. What lessons can be learned from revisiting science and social studies, and how do these lessons influence language intervention at school-age levels?
4. How do we keep syntax-focused and microlevel intervention goals and objectives curriculum relevant and meaningful?

INTRODUCTORY THOUGHTS

Curricular Literacies Revisited: Is Basic Comprehension Enough?

We have talked about many things in this text thus far. A core goal of language intervention is to help students with language learning disabilities (LLD) get to a place where they have the linguistic skills and strategies needed to participate in class and the confidence to "do it on their own." Getting to the point where our students "get it"—that is, they are successful academically—is a challenging and complex business, as we have seen. Fortunately, the last several decades have been kind to those of us on the front lines of daily practice in schools. As we have seen throughout this text, many theoretical and practical guidelines provide us with clinical and educational options. Indeed, we have learned many things that we can take into our clinics, resource rooms, and classrooms. And although we still have much to learn, we are living in an era of rich and diverse research that has the potential to move us well beyond the "meme-based" approaches so eloquently described by Kamhi (2004) in Chapter 5.

Some Things We Know

Among the many things that we have learned are the following:

■ Content-area subjects such as social studies and science have a unique type of literacy that assumes the presence of strong foundational skills in language and basic literacy.
■ Basic or fundamental literacy forms a bridge to curricular literacies.
■ Language ability underpins many widely used reading and writing activities and instructional techniques. These topics guide the discussion that follows.

Content-Area Subjects: A Unique Type of Literacy. Many educators who study the curriculum and ways to improve both the what and how of curricular content have talked about the role of language in mastering content-area subjects (e.g., VanSledright, 2002a, 2004; pp. 99–101, this text). Although not necessarily talking about students with LLD, the themes weaved throughout the literature from our colleagues who write for *Reading Research Quarterly, The Reading Teacher, Reading Research and Instruction,* and related literacy-focused journals remind us to consider the following (Villano, 2005):

■ Students learn curricular content by reading and writing about it.

■ Mastery of basic comprehension strategies may be a start, but these strategies should be related to, and adapted for, the specifics of the genre (or the subject) being studied.

■ Students will be expected to absorb most of a subject's content through highly structured textbooks and classroom lectures.

■ A great deal of background knowledge is assumed to be intact when students are introduced to new topics.

■ Many textbooks are geared toward the "above-average" reader, which creates further challenges for both teachers and students.

In discussing directions in language and science education, Yore and colleagues (2004) make several additional points about the curriculum and its unique literacy requirements. First, Yore and colleagues (2004) point out that there are two types of literacy: (1) a fundamental literacy and (2) a derived literacy (Box 8-1). *Fundamental literacy* relates to being fluent in language, understanding the conventions of different discourses, and having a basic ability to handle the communication systems of science (and other subject areas). *Derived literacy,* by contrast, has more to do with the result of one's fundamental literacy, that is, one becomes knowledgeable and educated in science. Thus it might be logical to propose that students with LLD will have difficulty mastering a science curriculum without a reasonable level of fundamental literacy.

8

BOX 8-1   *Two Types of Literacy*

> ***Fundamental Literacy***
> ■ Being fluent in language
> ■ Understanding conventions of different discourses
> ■ Having a basic ability to handle subject-area communication systems
>
> ***Derived Literacy***
> ■ Is interactive with a person's fundamental literacy
> ■ Involves a person becoming knowledgeable and educated in a subject area

---

Data from Yore, L. D., Hand, B., Goldman, S. R., Hildebrand, G. M., Osbourne, J. F., Treagust, D. F., & Wallace, C. S. (2004). New directions in language and science education research. *Reading Research Quarterly, 39,* 347–352.

Thus language underpinnings of the science curriculum become significant targets for speech-language pathologists (SLPs) who are delivering language intervention to school-age students.

A second point that Yore and colleagues (2004) make is that although spoken language ability is an integral part of science and acquiring science literacy, *written* language is especially crucial for the scientist (and the beginning scientist). They go on to say that "scientists rely on printed text for ideas that inform their work before, during, and after experimental inquiries" (Yore et al., 2004, p. 348.). Making notes, keeping track of the steps in an experiment, and summarizing findings are all part of scientific literacy. Finally, Yore and colleagues (2004) point out that having a "critical stance" in science is important for developing a complete and deep understanding of science. A "critical stance" includes fusing old and new knowledge, comparing information across texts (sometimes called *intertextual ability*), and having the skills to evaluate theories and accompanying data.

> A "critical stance"—fusing old and new knowledge, comparing information across texts, and evaluating theories and accompanying data—is important to fully understanding science (Yore et al., 2004).

Along with critical stance is an appreciation for argument, another central feature of science. Understanding that one uses evidence in an organized way to "prove" (or disprove) theories by questioning, interpreting data, making claims, and so on includes a number of language-based skills. The student of science needs the words, sentences, and discourse abilities to express the relationships required to make an argument, as well as a general appreciation for science and its purposes. Yore and colleagues (2004) suggest that practice with genres such as description, directions, explanation, and argumentation enhances fundamental literacy, which, in turn, opens the way to acquiring derived literacy in science. With a strong language focus to their discussion, these authors believe that time has come for more direct and in-depth collaboration between the literacy and science education communities. We would hope that SLPs are considered part of the "literacy" community. And whereas teachers are generally focused on helping students acquire derived literacy, SLPs and literacy specialists are (or should be) focused on helping students acquire different aspects of fundamental literacy.

Pappas (2006) agrees with the idea that fundamental literacy is critical for learning science. She also talks about connecting science learning with language and literacy learning. But she adds the caveat that reading (and writing) science is different from reading other kinds of texts (e.g., narrative texts). As we noted in Chapter 7, science reading and writing have a unique discourse style. Thus although narratives may help students acquire aspects of fundamental literacy—some of which connect to science knowledge, such as learning about cause-effect relationships—narrative texts do not create a direct line to managing the language of science. Students still have to learn to handle the communication "quirks" of science directly. Pappas (2006) states that "because science is a particular discipline—a specific way of thinking and knowing—its concepts and ideas are realized in a distinctive social language or genre: learning science is also learning its linguistic registers" (Pappas, 2006, p. 246).

Sounding very much like a discussion of pragmatics, Pappas (2006) says that children have to learn the kind of language that scientists use; they read, write, and talk in a certain way. The "hands-on" activities in science certainly help students to talk in the "here and now," but they also have to link concepts and ideas logically and be able to explain what they are doing. Although other texts such as narratives may not provide enough fundamental literacy to crack science, Pappas (2006) recognizes that children's experiences "talking around books" is helpful because experiences that involve analyzing, explaining, and "collecting" facts in a systematic way may be useful in the ultimate quest to acquire scientific literacy. Speech-language pathologists are certainly well practiced in helping students with LLD understand the difference between narrative and expository text and among the subtypes of text in each genre (e.g., Scott & Windsor, 2000; Westby, 2005). They might also think about helping students learn about and express the differences among science, social studies, and other genres they will encounter in school.

VanSledright (2004), whose work was introduced earlier in this text (Chapter 4, pp. 99–101), agrees with the previous authors (Pappas, 2006; Yore et al., 2004). He reminds us that history also has its own form of literacy. He notes that while "general or global reading strategies" (such as self-questioning and summarizing) are helpful and can be applied to history, educators and specialists need to go a bit further and recognize that "one size may not fit all." Reading and comprehending history is still different from reading and comprehending science (Alexander, 2000). For example, notes VanSledright (2004), history presents an "ill structured" challenge for many students. By "ill structured" he means that understanding historical events can be elusive. This requires a great deal of inferencing about what really happened and then rethinking one's original assumptions. VanSledright (2004) adds that for many events there is a "thinness of evidence" so that historical events have a tendency to "remain open to repeated reinterpretation" (p. 343).

Recall the title used in one of our intervention sessions: "Christopher Columbus: How History was Invented" (Chapter 3, p. 47–48). The rewriting of the Columbus story is an example of what VanSledright is talking about when he says there is a "thinness of evidence." Further, history is tough because to appreciate history one has to be able to evaluate its source, the location of the text within the larger context of historical events, its possible subtexts or hidden meanings, and its collaboration with other sources (VanSledright, 2004). History involves reading and interpreting not only printed text but also interpreting other images such as timelines, photographs, and artifacts.

> To appreciate history, a student must be able to evaluate its source, the location of the text within a larger context of historical events, its possible subtexts or hidden meanings, and its collaboration with other sources (VanSledright, 2004).

VanSledright (2004) points out that even good readers have trouble with history. Clearly, comprehension strategies such as *rereading, summarizing,* and *figuring out word meanings from context* are necessary foundational skills students must bring with them to the task of mastering history. But his observations of middle school students who are not language learning disabled helps us appreciate "where" we might go beyond teaching basic comprehension strategies. Talking about what students may need to know in terms of the content-specific literacy of history, and drawing on the works of Barton (1997), Lee and Ashby (2000), VanSledright and Kelly (1998), and his own work, VanSledright (2004) wrote the following:

> They know little about the structure of the [history] domain, lack strategies for reading intertextually (corroborating evidence across sources), and have little

experience reading subtexts. [Students also approach the text believing] that the meaning is in the text, it is unmediated by the author, and it is their job to extract it correctly. (p. 344)

Thus students with and without LLD have much to learn about the language of history. VanSledright (2004) applauds the work of Beck and her colleagues (e.g., Beck et al., 1995; McKeown et al., 1992) as examples of ways that researchers have attempted to help students navigate the complexities of history and become more actively involved in the process of developing historical thinking (see Chapter 7, p. 196). We will provide additional examples of ways to link language learning and history later in this chapter.

VanSledright (2004) continues his discussion by reminding practitioners that Grades 4 and 5 are the times when the "hard-core," domain-specific aspects of history are introduced in most school systems. And as his words suggest, many fourth and fifth graders have "missing elements" (such as intertextual ability) in their comprehension and literacy backpacks. It is interesting to recall the findings of Bashir and his colleagues (e.g., Bashir et al., 1998), who have often said that Grade 4 is a tough transition point for many students with LLD. Indeed, as the demands of the curriculum change as VanSledright (2004) suggests for history, so, too, do the ways that early language disorders manifest themselves. VanSledright (2004) and other researchers in history and social studies education (e.g., Alvermann & Phelps, 2002; Villano, 2005) speak eloquently to the changing demands in social studies and history at Grades 4 and 5. They say that curricular requirements push students to the point where they not only have to understand more content but they have to do it with very difficult text and across texts.

In addition to the difficulties inherent in history, background knowledge enters the picture once again. It is assumed that students are "partially educated" in history at the point in their school careers when history becomes more demanding (Grades 4 and 5). Fourth and fifth graders have been exposed to history in Grades 1 through 3, but they have also learned history from home and from television. Educators also believe that most children have some knowledge about the history of their country by the time they reach fourth grade (VanSledright, 2004). Importantly, by Grades 4 and 5, the assumption that students are readers and writers of their language—and have evolving reading comprehension strategies—underpins the notion that they are ready to handle the complexities of history's literacies. The questions for readers in this text include the following: Do students with LLD come with a "partial education" in history? Do they have enough fundamental literacy to approach the linguistic complexities they will face in history?

Fundamental Literacies: Forming a Bridge to and Interacting with Curricular Literacies. Observing in classrooms, reviewing textbooks, researching state standards (see Chapter 9), and talking with teachers bring home the realities of how content loaded and structurally dense the curriculum can be. Learning about the curriculum helps SLPs understand why language intervention loses its viability and relevance without a connection to the curriculum. The horizon of Grades 4 and 5 provide us with a window into what might be ahead for our students with LLD. Not only spoken, but clearly, written language proficiency must be a key element in any language intervention program. The printed word transmits the curriculum to students. In turn, students must demonstrate what they "know" in writing. In addition to developing more general strategies for reading and writing, students have to develop additional literacy skills (such as comparing ideas across texts) that may be related, more directly, to specific curricular areas as discussed in the previous section.

Many descriptions of strategies for both reading and writing appear in the literature today (e.g., Bashir & Singer, 2006; Pressley, 2002; Pressley & Hilden, 2004; Singer & Bashir, 2004). Some strategies were outlined in previous chapters, and others will follow. These contributions from the research help us create more meaningful targets in language therapy and literacy learning. Knowing what we know about strategic reading and writing and acknowledging the complexity of the literacies required for science and history curricula, for example, encourage us to ask yet another question: How can we bring these two streams of literacy closer together? In other words, how do we keep our strategic language intervention goals and objectives from straying too far from the curriculum? And importantly for SLPs, what are the language foundations or underpinnings that relate to and interact with more general reading comprehension and written language strategies (Ehren, 2000, 2005b, 2006b; Wallach & Ehren, 2004)?

Some General and Popular Strategies Revisited. Thinking of both reading and writing as a complex interaction among the reader, the text, the activity, and the context reminds us to acknowledge the dynamic, complex, and ever-changing nature of this ability called "comprehension" (Ehren, 2005b; Snow, 2002). Ehren (2005b) presents an excellent summary of the state of the art as she looks for evidence-based practices in reading comprehension instruction. She reminds her readers that we still have so much to learn about "what works" for students without LLD. In addition, says Ehren, whenever we read about techniques in the literature, we should also ask ourselves the age-old question: What language abilities are assumed to be intact to use a strategy effectively? Again, many researchers in curricular development are asking a similar question about language and its relationship to different subject areas. As mentioned in the previous section, they are also asking the following question: What language abilities are needed to access science, history, and other content-area subjects? This coming together of a "language focus" is certainly encouraging. It opens the door to collaboration and developing a mutually beneficial and shared responsibility in literacy.

Ehren (2005b) looks at reading comprehension from a strong information processing framework. She outlines a number of evidence-based strategies. Some of the research she summarizes (Ehren, 2005b) was conducted through the University of Kansas Center for Research in Learning. The reading comprehension strategies that are outlined in this section should be part of a repertoire of strategies that students need to meet the challenges facing them in their content-area subjects. Ehren (2005b) pulls current thinking together by summarizing the available reading comprehension literature into three categories. The categories are based on the earlier work of Pressley and colleagues (1987) and include

(1) goal-specific strategies, (2) monitoring and repair strategies, and (3) higher-order sequencing strategies or packaging strategies. Box 8-2 summarizes each category.

Goal-specific strategies are all those techniques that readers use (or should use) to get and retain the meaning of the materials facing them. Among the goal-specific strategies that have been found to facilitate comprehension are activating prior knowledge, text analysis, self-questioning, visual imagery, and paraphrasing and summarizing. We have seen examples of these goal-specific strategies throughout this text; others will follow in this chapter. For example, in the previous chapter, we saw how the story about "Samantha Stevens" (p. 196) was used to activate fifth-grade students' prior knowledge about the colonists and the British before they faced the more difficult expository version of the conflict in their history texts. The use of a narrative text filled with characters, settings, and events that related to characters provided students with a stronger visual image of the colonies—where they were, what they looked like, and so on. And although it was recognized that visual imagery can take students only so far when complex and abstract concepts such as *freedom*, *independence*, and *tyranny* are part of the content, the use of narratives and visual images forms a starting point. Working on narrative-expository differences

---

BOX 8-2   *Categories of Reading Comprehension Literature*

Goal-Specific Strategies
Readers use these techniques to get and retain the meaning of the materials facing them.
   Examples: activating prior knowledge, text analysis, self-questioning, visual imagery, paraphrasing, summarizing

Monitoring and Repair Strategies
Readers use these tools to keep track of what they are reading and to stop and fix gaps or breakdowns in comprehension.
   Examples: going back to check out contextual cues, rereading paragraphs or chapters, taking notes, looking up words in the dictionary

Packaging Strategies
Readers use these higher-level abilities to pull information and knowledge together.
   Examples: planning what to do and how to do it, evaluating and revising strategies, switching strategies when needed

---

Data from Ehren, B. J. (2005). Looking for evidence-based practice in reading comprehension instruction. *Topics in Language Disorders, 25,* 310–321; and Pressley, M., Borkowski, J. G., & Schneider, W. (1987). Cognitive strategies: Good strategy users coordinate metacognition and knowledge. *Annals of Child Development, 14,* 89–129.

should follow as students learn to compare how the same content looks in a different form. Our Angels-Yankees and Revolutionary War–Civil War compare-contrast activity (see Chapter 6, p. 165) can serve to bolster a number of these goal-specific strategies. Brainstorming discussions before reading and writing, using visual maps to highlight structural concepts, summarizing the key ideas, and self-questioning are techniques that help students bring their knowledge about a topic to the surface. Ogle's (1986) K-W-L tool (see Table 7-3) is another way to activate prior knowledge, among the other goal-specific strategies mentioned.

Monitoring and repair strategies are those strategies that readers use to keep track of what they are reading and to stop and fix gaps or breakdowns in comprehension when they occur. Readers may ask themselves questions about a new word, a missed thought, an author's point, and other things when comprehension decreases. Readers try many things to keep comprehension going. They may go back and check out contextual cues, they may reread a paragraph or chapter, they may take notes, they may look up an unfamiliar word in the dictionary, and so on. Undergraduate students in speech-language pathology often say that they have to go back and reread paragraphs many times before they comprehend a speech science or advanced child language textbook. But, more often than not, they know when they're "not getting it," and they use various strategies such as listening more closely to a lecture before they read a complicated chapter to make their reading less painful. As per Pressley and colleagues (Pressley et al., 1985, as noted in Ehren, 2005b), the last example of students listening to a lecture before reading indicates that monitoring strategies increase a student's understanding of goal-specific strategies and the role they can play in facilitating and repairing comprehension breakdowns. Ehren (2005b) goes on to say that this aspect of reading comprehension—monitoring and repairing—can be particularly difficult for students with LLD. The examples from our adolescent student with LLD (see JG, Chapter 3, p. 73, this text) reflect his need to acquire more effective monitoring and repair strategies, a key element in his language intervention program. Singer and Bashir (2004) and Bashir and Singer (2006) provide additional examples of strategies in this area with a focus on writing. Their work will be highlighted in a later section of this chapter.

Packaging strategies involve those "higher-level" abilities that enable readers to pull it all together. According to Ehren (2005b), goal-specific and monitoring strategies should not be seen as techniques that are used in isolation. Rather, we should consider (and help our students understand) when and why we use strategies and the contexts in which particular strategies will work. Thus "the planning of what to do and how to do it, as well as the evaluating and revising of strategies, is what constitutes strategy use" (Ehren, 2005b, p. 317). Ehren (2005b) says that *constructively responsive reading,* a term coined by Pressley and colleagues (e.g., Pressley & Afflerbach, 1995), means many things: proficient readers know "where they're going," they use extensive self-monitoring, and they are very engaged in and actively involved with the texts before them. Proficient readers are far from passive. They pull strategies together when needed and switch strategies as necessary.

Proficient readers use self-monitoring and are engaged in and actively involved with the texts before them; in other words, they know what they are doing and where they are going.

Research suggests that although students with LLD are able to acquire language learning and reading comprehension strategies, they may use them less effectively than their typically developing counterparts (Ehren, 2003).

As research suggests, language learning disabled students may be successful at acquiring a number of strategies, but they may use available strategies less effectively than students without LLD (Ehren, 2003). When comprehension gets tough, they may rely on a single strategy, failing to employ alternative strategies if they have them. Lacking strategies or having difficulty "calling up" the appropriate strategy places the learner at a disadvantage. Ehren (2005b, 2006b) points out that although there is optimism about the role of strategy learning in academic success, clinicians and teachers must not only help students acquire a repertoire of strategies, but they must also teach them how and when to apply strategies to reading, writing, and curricular activities. She reminds practitioners to proceed with caution because the strategy research that is specifically related to students with LLD remains a work in progress.

Laing (2006) also discussed a growing body of literature that demonstrates the effectiveness of strategy-based comprehension. She notes that strategies such as questioning, summarization, and use of graphic organizers, along with monitoring and thinking-aloud strategies, are associated with helping children manage both narrative and expository text, points that were also made by Ehren (2005b, 2006b). Laing (2006) also says that teaching students multiple strategies, and how to use those strategies together and appropriately, is an important component of any reading comprehension intervention.

In a study of fifth-grade students with LLD, children participated in different strategy-based intervention sessions (Box 8-3). One group was assigned to the TWA approach (*think* before reading, think *while* reading, think *after* reading) (Mason, 2004); another group used an RQ (reciprocal questioning) format. The TWA program includes a number of the strategies discussed in the previous sections. Students were involved in using Ogle's (1986) K-W-L format and her RAP format (read a paragraph, ask yourself a question, what are the main ideas and details) (Ogle, 1989). Summarization activities were also included in the TWA section. Children in the RQ group were taught to ask self-generated questions and answer them. They were also encouraged to think about the purpose of reading and how their questions would help them get the information needed. Children were tested after an average of 11 to 15 sessions. Comprehension of expository passages was measured in a number of ways: reading the passages,

---

BOX 8-3   *Ways to Help Students Become More Strategic*

- TWA approach (*think* before reading; think *while* reading; think *after* reading)
- RQ (reciprocal questioning)
- K-W-L format (what I *know*; what I *want* to know; what I *learned*)
- RAP format (read a paragraph; ask yourself a question; what are the main ideas and details?)
- Graphic organizers

answering questions about passages, providing summaries, and restating the main idea.

Results showed that the students in the TWA training performed significantly better than the students in the RQ group. The quality and quantity of TWA students' main idea statements, summaries, and retellings were better than those found in the RQ group. Although more longitudinal studies are needed in this area, results suggested that intervention is most effective when multiple strategies are presented and used and when clinicians "help children recognize when they should use a strategy, when they [might] not use a strategy, and to know how to restore a comprehension breakdown when it occurred" (Laing, 2006, p. 20).

Laing (2006) talks about another popular technique to facilitate comprehension—the use of graphic organizers such as our compare-contrast organizer from Chapter 6. Many SLPs, reading specialists, and classroom teachers use graphic organizers for a number of reasons. They might be used to help students appreciate the structural differences between narrative and expository text to help students organize their written reports, among other possibilities. In a summary of the research to date, Kim and colleagues (2004) found that many different kinds of graphic organizers were generally facilitative to comprehension and organization of material. They pointed out, however, that it was important for graphic organizers to represent the skill that the student needs to learn. In other words, "a framed outline might be used to facilitate a child's ability to retell a narrative, while a semantic map that illustrates the relationships between science vocabulary concepts might be used to facilitate a child's ability to summarize information in expository text" (Laing, 2006, p. 20). Singer and Bashir's (2004) examples that follow in the next section (see Figures 8-1 and 8-2) illustrate the need to match graphic organizers more directly to the skill or ability being targeted.

Finally, in summarizing the graphic organizer research, Laing (2006), referencing Kim and colleagues (2004), says that results leave us with positive findings about their use with students in academic trouble. The graphic organizer research also leaves us with the following two additional points to think about:

1. When clinicians and teachers encourage children to construct their own graphic organizers (in addition to using teacher-generated organizers), there were slightly higher gains in comprehension.
2. Students with LLD are successful in learning how to use graphic organizers (and other strategies), but they do not always apply what they have "learned" to novel reading situations.

Finally, summarizing some of the current thinking about strategic reading comprehension intervention, Laing (2006) noted the following:

> One factor that is associated with the greatest transfer of the use of new strategies is explicit teacher instruction in the form of clear, sequential modeling, monitoring, and fading support for the use of the strategy…Moreover, almost any strategy that encourages children to think and understand more about what they are reading will result in improvements in comprehension. (p. 21, referring to the work of Resnick [1987] and Swanson [1999])

Language Abilities Underpinning Many Widely Used Reading Comprehension Strategy Activities and Instructional Techniques. Although the last sentence of the quote that ended the previous section may sound a little too optimistic, the research available has certainly provided us with many options to consider that address the specific processing, comprehension, and organizational difficulties of children and adolescents with LLD. We can see how fundamental and derived literacy concepts set yet another natural path toward collaboration among school-based professionals. The language-based nature of many of the strategies presented provides SLPs with many opportunities to help their colleagues find ways to operationalize the integration of fundamental and derived literacies in school settings.

In any intervention program with the goal of helping students acquire and use reading comprehension and other problem-solving strategies, both linguistic and metalinguistic skills and abilities must be considered.

Ehren's work, which has been referenced extensively in this text and elsewhere, takes us even further as we try to bridge the gap between fundamental and derived literacy. Her concept of understanding the "language underpinnings" of various school activities (see Chapters 3 and 4) reminds us that there are linguistic and metalinguistic skills and abilities that have to be "accounted for" in any intervention program in which the goals might include helping students acquire and use the strategies outlined in the previous section. In other words, Ehren (2004) would ask a question that she has asked speech-language pathologists many times: What language skills underlie goal-specific strategies, monitoring and repair strategies, and integrated reading comprehension strategies?

For example, Ehren (2004) would recognize that *paraphrasing* is a useful reading comprehension strategy. She would then ask SLPs to think about *what the language knowledge and underpinnings might be for this strategy.* Readers of this text might pause a minute to answer Ehren's question before continuing their reading. Among the language underpinnings of paraphrasing are various linguistic and metalinguistic abilities, including knowing that there is more than one way to say something, having a repertoire of synonyms, being able to manipulate a variety of syntactic patterns, understanding key ideas that form a sentence, being able to manipulate syntax without changing the meaning, and having knowledge of form-meaning differences.

Likewise, *what are the language underpinnings for monitoring comprehension?* Ehren (2004) says that metalinguistic awareness is related to having success with comprehension monitoring strategies. Among the linguistic underpinnings of monitoring strategies are having an awareness that comprehension (not just decoding) is the goal of reading, being able to judge one's own level of understanding of specific ideas in a text, and using self-talk when evaluating comprehension success and failure. *Comprehension repairs* (and editing one's written work) include additional linguistic and metalinguistic skills such as knowing that a breakdown has occurred, being able to formulate questions for clarification, and actively using a number of strategies. Finally, says, Ehren (2004), graphic organizers can be useful tools, if the student has the language savvy to choose appropriate words and syntax to express relationships, extract appropriate information from text and place it in an organizer, and put words and phrases into an accurate and sequentially meaningful hierarchy.

The implication of Ehren's (2004) and others' works is that SLPs have a significant role to play in helping students become strategic readers (and writers). Becoming a strategic reader and writer, in turn, provides students with the arsenal of language and literacy skills needed to manage the curriculum. By focusing on the language underpinnings of reading comprehension strategies (and other classroom requirements) in concert with using curricular content as a backdrop, SLPs build language intervention programs that connect to classrooms and textbooks.

More Strategic Language Work: An Example from the Writing Side of the Coin. Singer and Bashir (2004) take us in a slightly different direction. They provide us with additional guidelines for helping students acquire and use meta-based strategies for writing. Their EMPOWER strategy (see Singer & Bashir, 2004, and Bashir & Singer, 2006) takes students through a series of steps that "EmPower their writing." Based upon the earlier work of Englert and her colleagues (Englert et al., 1988), EmPOWER stands for *Evaluate, make a Plan, Organize, Work, Evaluate, and Rework*. Students answer a series of questions in each stage, follow guidelines, and become actively involved in a dialogue with their clinician or teacher. The talking that accompanies each step encourages the development of a heightened awareness of various language components and the process of writing in general. Eventually, of course, the goal is to have students use these strategies on their own. But, again, students have to be "language ready" (Ehren, 2004) to use these strategies effectively.

In the first step, *Evaluate*, students reflect on things such as "What is this assignment asking me to do?" and "How many parts will my paper need to have?" Singer and Bashir (2004) and Bashir and Singer (2006) provide some excellent ways to help students become more aware of how to read and decipher instructions for writing reports in this step. The *make a Plan* section includes a portion that encourages students to decide on what kind of a graphic organizer may help get them started and pull ideas together. They answer questions such as "What is the goal of my paper?" The planning section provides an excellent opportunity for SLPs to work on helping students understand the purposes and the structure of different types of texts. It is also important for clinicians and teachers to know what they are looking for, as the example that follows at the end of this section will demonstrate.

The *Organize* step is the actual mapping out of ideas and deciding if anything should be added to or subtracted from the graphic organizer or outline. *Work* asks students to order ideas and decide on topic sentences, and includes the writing of introductions, bodies, and conclusions. The amount of scaffolding needed will vary based on students' needs. The *Evaluate* step at this point in the writing process includes a checklist that helps students make improvements to their papers. Students are encouraged to get feedback from a teacher, a friend, or a parent during this preediting process. And, finally, the *Rework* step includes making any changes, reading the final draft to make sure it says what it needs to say, and printing out a final copy.

Bashir and Singer (2006) recognize the multifaceted nature of writing and the challenges that face student writers, especially students with LLD. They point out that "students with both language and executive function disorders may have difficulty regulating their language (e.g., oral and written comprehension and production) because the very systems that would allow them to recognize the need to use a given strategy in any given context are impaired. Given this, it is no wonder that many students with LLD have difficulty becoming self-regulated writers" (Bashir & Singer, 2006, p. 593). Thus although EmPOWER is only one way to guide students through the many assignments that will require a written product, its structure and its use of dialogue, graphic organizers, and other supports integrate some of the linguistic and "meta" components required for writing (Box 8-4). We might think back to how the EmPOWER strategies might have helped (or can help) the writer of the Mars piece presented at the beginning of Chapter 7 (p. 172).

An interesting point that Singer and Bashir (2004) make, among the many useful ideas they present, relates to the use of graphic organizers, which are part of the EmPOWER process. Laing (2006) makes a similar point about their use to help children organize their thinking: clinicians and teachers must match the technique or tool chosen to the desired outcome. Singer and Bashir (2004) present Figure 8-1 as a case in point. Figure 8-1 shows a graphic used with a third-grade student with LLD. The assignment for the student was to write a fictional story that includes some historical facts covered in a social studies unit. The story takes place in Plimouth Plantation in the year 1627. The graphic's purpose was to help the student preplan her writing by organizing some of the components of the story and its details. (So far, so good. The activation of prior knowledge and the use of narrative text may be good choices.)

Singer and Bashir (2004) believe that the graphic organizer used in Figure 8-1 fails to represent the narrative text's structure in an organized way. They believe that in its current form, this graphic might be confusing for the student. Although she has included many of the story elements, the graphic does not help the student create a clear mental model about the text's structure, not to mention that the graphic fails to help the student figure out how to put

BOX 8-4	*EmPOWERing Students' Writing*	
E	Evaluate	
mP	Make a plan	
O	Organize	
W	Work	
E	Evaluate	
R	Rework	

Data from Singer, B. D., & Bashir, A. S. (2004). EmPOWER: A strategy for teaching students with language learning disabilities how to write expository text. In E. R. Silliman & L. C. Wilkinson (Eds.), *Language and literacy learning in schools* (pp. 239–272). New York: Guilford Press.

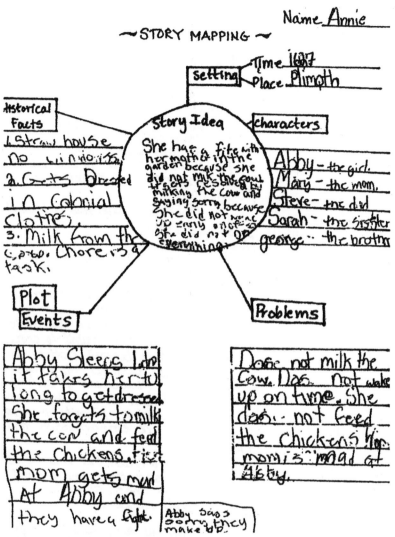

~ STORY MAPPING ~

Name *Annie*

Figure 8-1 ■ Graphic given to Annie, a third-grade student, by her teacher to plan a historical fiction narrative. *(From Singer, B. D., & Bashir, A. S. [2004]. EmPOWER: A strategy for teaching students with language learning disabilities how to write expository text. In E. R. Silliman & L. C. Wilkinson [Eds.], Language and literacy learning in schools [p. 253]. New York: Guilford Press.)*

these elements on paper. This type of semantic web might be more useful for vocabulary development and other aspects of word-concept relations.

Offering an alternative, Singer and Bashir (2004) show how a graphic organizing strategy, using a different tool, might be more helpful for the historical narrative activity. Figure 8-2 restructures the elements visually, providing a more direct roadmap to the assignment.

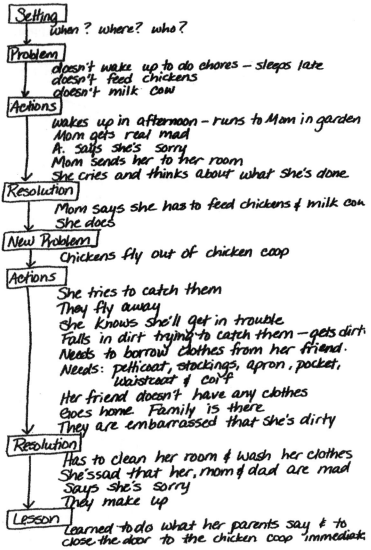

Setting
when? where? who?

Problem
doesn't wake up to do chores – sleeps late
doesn't feed chickens
doesn't milk cow

Actions
wakes up in afternoon – runs to Mom in garden
Mom gets real mad
A. says she's sorry
Mom sends her to her room
She cries and thinks about what she's done.

Resolution
Mom says she has to feed chickens & milk cow
She does

New Problem
Chickens fly out of chicken coop

Actions
She tries to catch them
They fly away
She knows she'll get in trouble
Falls in dirt trying to catch them – gets dirty
Needs to borrow clothes from her friend.
Needs: petticoat, stockings, apron, pocket,
        waistcoat & coif
Her friend doesn't have any clothes
Goes home. Family is there
They are embarrassed that she's dirty

Resolution
Has to clean her room & wash her clothes
She's sad that her, mom & dad are mad
Says she's sorry
They make up

Lesson
Learned to do what her parents say & to
close the door to the chicken coop immediate.

Figure 8-2 ■ Reconfiguration of the graphic shown in Figure 8-1 to represent a more accurate visual of the underlying text structure of a narrative. *(From Singer, B. D., & Bashir, A. S. [2004]. EmPOWER: A strategy for teaching students with language learning disabilities how to write expository text. In E. R. Silliman & L. C. Wilkinson [Eds.], Language and literacy learning in schools [p. 254]. New York: Guilford Press.)*

Meeting the Challenges of Evolving Concepts in Literacy: Keeping the Inferential Twist in Mind

We know that what we mean by literacy has changed over the past two decades, as noted in Chapter 2. We also know that clinicians and educators are caught in the middle of trying to meet the challenges of teaching high levels of literacy to too many children with too little time (Raphael & Au, 2005; Wallach & Ehren, 2004). Nonetheless, descriptions of literacy and explanations of what it means to comprehend written and spoken language continue to evolve as a result of national committees, literacy reports, and federal guidelines (Raphael & Au, 2005). As we mentioned, students are expected to read and absorb school content from many different types of text for many different reasons. And they are expected to reflect on what they read and write (Raphael & Au, 2005). Students are also expected to demonstrate intertextual ability by reading and evaluating information from various sources, and they are expected to show what they know in coherent and accurate written renditions. These are challenges for many students in our schools, not just those children with identified LLD.

Raphael and Au (2005) address many of the issues in literacy that are a concern for SLPs who work in school settings who are also faced with the realities of meeting state standards in an era of high-stakes testing. While addressing the needs of students from culturally and linguistically diverse backgrounds, these authors bring to the table many ideas that have relevance for students with LLD. Raphael and Au (2005) emphasize the need to create literacy programs that "foster the integration, interpretation, critique, and evaluation of text ideas" (p. 208). Within the context of these broader definitions of literacy and knowledge of the challenges facing students on state tests and in textbooks, these authors also ask practitioners to evaluate what they call the "misguided logic" of working on "lower-level skills" such as those related to decoding and word recognition at the expense of working on "higher-level skills" such as those related to strategic reading comprehension. They are not discounting the importance of decoding and phonemic awareness as part of the process, but they believe that teachers and specialists spend too much time on these lower-level processes without focusing on comprehension. Raphael and Au (2005) also say that, in some cases, there are stereotypic beliefs about what students can and cannot do. (Is this another case of the "rich get richer" mentioned in an early chapter of this text? In other words, do better readers spend more time on comprehension activities? Do poorer readers spend too little time on comprehension?)

These researchers ask us to evaluate the kind of comprehension instruction available to all children and encourage us to keep our eyes focused on the challenges that lie ahead. Indeed, SLPs might ask a similar question about the ways that "comprehension" goals and objectives manifest themselves in language intervention sessions. (Recall the "one-step, two-step, three-step commands" to enhance auditory comprehension.) Is what we are doing with students under the guise of facilitating "auditory or listening comprehension" or "auditory processing" focused in the right direction? Are our activities aimed at helping our students acquire the linguistic and "meta" knowledge and skills needed for

Raphael and Au (2005) question the "misguided logic" of working on lower-level skills (e.g., decoding, word recognition) at the expense of working on such higher-level skills as comprehension.

8

literacy learning and school success? Reminding practitioners who work both within and outside of classrooms that, to quote Bob Dylan, "times are a changing," Raphael and Au (2005) noted that

> within the next five years, approximately three quarters to four fifths of the questions on the NAEP [National Assessment Governing Board] reading assessment—[will] require students to use higher level thinking, such as making reader-text connections, or examining the content and structure of the text. (p. 207; National Assessment Governing Board, 2004; Donahue et al., 2003)

Moving instruction (and intervention) toward more strategic-based approaches is no easy task. Raphael and Au (2005) recognize that it is difficult to "make visible" the largely invisible and complex processes that drive both spoken and written comprehension. But they offer some suggestions that may help to make the implicit explicit and, at the same time, provide an organizational framework for teachers and specialists to consider. Using the question-answer relationships (QAR) format, the authors show how elementary school children from diverse backgrounds, including students with LLD, can benefit from some of the "meta" activities that relate to QAR. The QAR framework integrates background knowledge and textual information. The QAR format's aim is to help students appreciate the interaction between these two aspects of comprehension, as well as

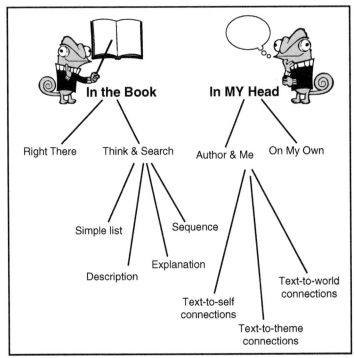

Figure 8-3 ■ The question-answer relationships (QAR) framework highlighting strategies for reading comprehension. (*Redrawn from Raphael, T. E., & Au, K. H. [2001]. Super QAR for test use for students:* Teacher resource guide, Grade 6 *[pp. 4–5]. Chicago: McGraw-Hill/Wright.*)

to help them become more active and strategic in their attempts to understand and retain what they read. Figure 8-3 provides an example of the QAR framework and its various subpieces.

The two "big" pieces—the macrostructure of QAR—are (1) *In the Book* and (2) *In My Head*. These two categories represent the idea that readers use information from the texts they are reading and their background knowledge to get an author's meaning. Clearly, there is a balance between the two sources of information, and that balance may change depending on the situation. The major aim in QAR is that students should be taught the importance of these two sources of information. Under the two major headings of *In the Book* and *In My Head* are the following, as shown in Figure 8-3: *Right There* and *Think & Search* and *Author & Me* and *On My Own*. When students are asked questions about what they have read (or what has been read to them), they have options that include looking through the text to find the answer (It's *In the Book—Right There*) or they can use background knowledge as a means to figure out what a reasonable answer could be. This is an *In My Head—On My Own* strategy.

Raphael and Au (2005) point out that too many times reading comprehension questions are limited to the *Right There* category. From their perspective, *Right There* questions fail to encourage enough strategic or critical thinking about a text. Although students have to learn when and how to use these different strategies for answering questions and checking comprehension, they should also learn that the "right answer" does not have to be found *only* in the text. The authors give examples of students becoming frustrated when they could not find precise answers to questions in the text, even when they had enough background knowledge to "figure out" an answer. But, caution Raphael and Au (2005), teachers and clinicians need to have some awareness of the level of students' background knowledge before they ask students to bring that knowledge into play. For example, using clues from books or chapter titles to predict what might be coming in the text, such as "Fall of the Roman Empire" and "Christopher Columbus: How History was Invented," which were seen in Chapter 3 (p. 47–48), can be a useful *In My Head* strategy. Using titles can encourage students to call on their background knowledge when approaching the text. Its success depends on what knowledge students actually bring to the task.

Raphael and Au (2005) provide a wonderful example of a student who said to his teacher, "I know it's 'In My Head' but I went to my head and there's nothing there" (Raphael & Au, 2005, p. 210). In this case, the student was encouraged to talk with a peer to see if the peer could help. As the authors put it: "Armed with QAR language, students can communicate about what they are doing and request help they need to answer or ask questions effectively" (Raphael & Au, 2005, p. 210). By contrast, looking up the name of a particular Revolutionary War general, a setting where a battle occurred, or the date for a specific event involve *In the Book* strategies when this knowledge is unknown to a reader. *In the Book* strategies such as rereading, skimming, and scanning texts may also provide students with information. When they fail, however, students should have other options available to them. They should be taught to appreciate the different sources of information that can help them understand what they read.

Figure 8-3 shows two additional facets of the QAR framework: *Think & Search* (*In the Book* category) and *Author & Me* (*In My Head* category). *Think and Search* and *Author & Me* strategies may be slightly more advanced than the previous strategies. They tend to require more integration of information. For example, *Think & Search*, another *In the Book* strategy, involves finding answers that are in the text. But just as the strategy's name suggests, readers have to exert additional energy—that is, use more effective searching skills—to be successful. The answer may be across sentences, paragraphs, or book chapters. *Right There* answers, on the other hand, are usually in the same sentence. We could say that *Think & Search* targets a macrolevel of discourse, whereas *Right There* has more of a microlevel (sentence-level) focus.

Consider the questions posed in Box 8-5. Both answers are *in the text*, but finding the correct answer requires different *In the Book* savvy.

Readers of this text can appreciate the difference between these two *In the Book* strategies. In addition to the connected discourse demands in the *Think & Search* component, SLPs might be able to contribute information about the different linguistic levels of the reading comprehension questions. For example, the first question asks for a specific detail, whereas the second question requires more abstract, inferential thinking. Indeed, although the answer to question 2 is *In the Book*, its full meaning, coupled with its embeddedness in connected discourse, may contribute to its level of difficulty. Speech-language pathologists might also share information with teachers about any syntactic differences that

---

BOX 8-5   *QAR Framework*: **Examples of In the Book Questions**

Questions
1. Which river did George Washington cross in the winter of 1776?
2. What did George Washington do in the winter of 1776 to show that he was a capable of winning the war for independence?

In-the-Book Answers
Right There
Washington knew it was his last chance to prove his leadership of the army so he decided to cross the Delaware River in the winter of 1776 to attack the British.

Think & Search
The winter of the first year of the war for independence was extremely cold. George Washington's troops had lost many battles and Washington's leadership was being questioned by Congress. So General Washington thought hard about his next move. He knew his career was in jeopardy and that the war might be lost. He decided to take a big risk. In the dark of night on a cold December evening in 1776, General Washington gave the order to get the ships and troops ready. They were going to cross the Delaware River and attack the British in Trenton, New Jersey.

might also affect comprehension (e.g., the complement/that construction of sentence 2 may contribute to its difficulty). According to Raphael and Au (2005), the *Think & Search* strategy may be a powerful one to teach students because of its relevance to curricular activities in social studies and science and other school subjects. Students are asked frequently to answer end-of-the-chapter questions and integrate information across texts and materials.

Finally, *Author & Me* questions are part of *In My Head* strategies, as shown in Figure 8-3. They involve using background knowledge and past experiences to comprehend text. But *Author & Me* questions take readers a bit beyond *On My Own* approaches. In *On My Own* approaches, readers use their own experiences and knowledge to figure out what might happen, what a character might do in a specific situation, or what list of books an author might present in his summary of a favorite writer's accomplishments. When one has prior knowledge of a topic, his or her "guesses" (or inferences) before reading a text have a greater probability of being accurate or of matching an author's words or intentions. *Author & Me* strategies bring background knowledge and text together by asking readers to think about how what they already know fits with the text. Our students who used background knowledge to predict what might be in the text by considering the title, "Christopher Columbus: How History Was Invented," made some connections to the topic by using past experiences that were based on what they had read and what they had been taught. On further reading of this particular text about Columbus *(Author & Me)*, they had to rethink their perceptions. Of course, readers also have the option of rejecting an author's claims or point of view. Using the George Washington example presented in Box 8-5, we could ask students to engage in *In My Head* strategies by asking them, for example, what they think "leadership" means or who are leaders they admire. They could expand on this exercise by listing "leadership qualities" and relate their prior knowledge about leaders and leadership to what they think the text might say about Washington's leadership qualities. Then they could read the text to determine what was actually written about our first president.

Both *In the Book* and *In My Head* strategies are important rungs on the comprehension ladder. According to Raphael and Au (2005), children as young as second grade have been successful at learning to appreciate and use both *Right There* and *Think & Search* strategies, and fourth graders can usually distinguish all four QAR components (*Right There, Think & Search, On My Own,* and *Author & Me*). They also point out that reading groups can provide opportunities for dialogues among children. For example, for one child an answer may be *On my Own* because she already knew about a particular topic; for another child the answer was *Right There* because he had to get the information from the book.

Clearly, additional research is required in the LLD arena, but the value of strategic teaching and strategic language intervention cannot be underestimated. As put by Raphael and Au (2005): "The QAR framework can be a starting point for conversations that lead teachers to think deeply about reading comprehension instruction to promote sustained changes in practice" (p. 216). Frameworks such as QAR and others that offer guidelines for both spoken and written language provide ways for teachers and specialists such as

SLPs to open up a dialogue. The conversation might be about how to improve literacy instruction and how to "stay on the same page" for students in academic trouble. "Staying on the same page" does not mean doing the same things but doing complementary things, as emphasized throughout this text. Speech-language pathologists can tease out the language skills needed to engage children in these strategies, such as the semantic-syntactic requirements of questions or the cohesive devices needed to keep text together. Teachers can implement *In the Book* and *In My Head* strategies across curricular areas or cycles of reading (before reading, during reading, and after reading). Speech-language pathologists can help students acquire both macro and micro discourse skills needed to participate in *Think & Search* strategies. Teachers can apply *Think & Search* strategies to questions students have to answer at the end of chapters in their texts.

Speech-language pathologists might also take on leadership roles by introducing the strategies (QAR and others) to teachers in in-class demonstration lessons. Teachers can then follow up by modeling strategies and teaching their students to use the strategies across curricular and high-stakes testing situations. Indeed, there are many opportunities for developing shared responsibilities in the education of students. Raphael and Au (2005) encourage the creation of a shared language among teachers and specialists. They outline the benefits of having a coherence in literacy policies that lead to "sustained whole-school reform aimed at higher standards for literacy learning and teaching" (p. 218). There are many challenges facing us as we embark on the journey to help all students acquire higher standards of literacy. But there are voices of reason coming from many sources that keep the bigger picture in mind and offer alternatives to intervention and instruction practices that are too far removed from the real world of students.

School's Back in Session: An Integration of Literacies

As SLPs, teachers, and other specialists work toward creating joint and complementary responsibilities in literacy, students become the fortunate recipients of a more integrated and language-based education. In addition, when our interventions and instruction are authentic and occur within the context of difficulty, the likelihood of success for our students increases (Palincsar & Duke, 2004). By contrast, when our interventions take more abstract and indirect paths, such as implementing those that fall under the umbrella term of "central auditory processing" and similar therapies (e.g., oral-motor training), our focus on the linguistic demands of the curriculum becomes obscured. Knowing what we now know about both spoken and written linguistic demands of the curriculum brings home the need to work toward the integration of fundamental and subject-specific literacies.

Palincsar and her colleagues (e.g., Palincsar et al., 2000; Palincsar & Duke, 2004; Palincsar & Magnusson, 2001) reiterate concepts discussed by many of the researchers in language, reading comprehension, and writing. Palincsar and Duke (2004) emphasize the benefits of exposing students to texts that connect primary reading instruction to content-area material. Their preliminary research findings suggest that when informational texts are combined with material that is meaningful to advancing students' subject-matter knowledge, students' success rate for acquiring both primary and content-based literacy improves. Further, combining informational (expository) texts with narrative texts provides a potentially better outcome for students than when narrative text is the sole focus of instruction or intervention. Their research also suggests that when activities have an authentic component to them—that is, when there is an actual purpose for what they are reading or writing in the real world—children perform better and are more engaged in learning. (See Palincsar and Duke's [2004] review of research from the Center for the Improvement of Early Reading Achievement [CIERA]).

For SLPs, who do not teach or reinforce curricular content directly, *using content-area materials* in their language intervention sessions has the potential to help students "see" how the linguistic skills and strategies that are part of their language intervention sessions connect to learning in the classroom. Language intervention has more authenticity when it relates to students' textbooks and class requirements. In addition, the depth of speech-language pathologists' background in language, including knowledge of both the assessment and intervention of connected discourse, creates collaborative opportunities between SLPs and teachers who can discuss their views about the "best ways" to help students master a variety of text genres. Palincsar and Duke (2004) remind teachers and other specialists who work with students who have reading and academic difficulties that they need to stay focused on what is relevant. They should expose children to the genres of texts that they want them to read and write (and talk about). Many researchers and practitioners agree with Palincsar and colleagues that we need to consider the role of text and the mastery of a variety of text genres in learning. There is also discussion in the literature about introducing informational/expository text to students as early as the first grade (e.g., Duke, 2000; Hall et al., 2005). Palincsar and colleagues (2004), among others, add that while it is important to expose children to a variety of genres, additional research is needed to determine the long-term effects of both content-based literacy and text-based intervention and instruction for students with and without LLD.

Science Revisited

As outlined in the previous chapter, science has its own way of expressing itself to learners. By understanding its specialized literacy requirements, speech-language pathologists take a first and important step toward creating curriculum-relevant language intervention. Many of the guidelines and other activities presented throughout this text can also be applied to science. In this section, we will take a closer look at how some of the suggestions can work together to combine primary and content-specific literacy. Although some of the activities described are directed toward teachers, we will comment on the language-based activities that have a more direct connection to intervention and offer opportunities for collaboration among SLPs, teachers, and literacy specialists. We will start with some of the suggestions from Palincsar and colleagues (2004), whose research was mentioned in the previous section. As part of a series of projects for CIERA, they studied second and third graders' science instruction as it related to students' evolving literacy skills. These researchers offer us some astute observations about text-savvy teachers and also provide suggestions for practice that are based on their research findings.

Creating Authenticity: A Pragmatic Notion. An example of authentic reading and writing of an informational text in science would be to have students research and write a brochure about pond life for visitors who will attend a lecture at the local nature center. Creating a brochure for the local nature center (and similar assignments) is an activity that may have more meaning for children since they live in the area and are familiar with the center (Palincsar and colleagues, 2004). Palincsar and colleagues (2004) provide another example of having students write an instructional (procedural) piece for a future class about how to care for tadpoles because many of their class tadpoles had died. Many of the examples they provide include writing expository pieces related to science for "real" audiences that go beyond the teacher—a point made earlier in the previous chapter. Palincsar and colleagues (2004) talk about having children write for groups at a distance (pen pals in other countries), write for local audiences (other classes in their schools), and write for their own class and different classmates within the class. For example, students could be supported to write pieces about the weather or a current event in science. These pieces might be used within a classroom or they could have a wider audience. Students could also write invitations to other classes in their school, inviting them to attend their latest science project exhibition. The invitations could have summaries describing the projects to encourage students to attend.

According to Palincsar and Duke (2004), preliminary data suggest that more authentic activities such as the ones described result in a higher growth in students' abilities to read and write expository text, particularly as it relates to informational and procedural texts in science. They added that "tailoring instructional activities to specific texts—in particular to the purposes and real-world instantiations of these texts—seemed to support children's development" (Palincsar & Duke, 2004, p. 191; from Purcell-Gates & Duke, 2001). For SLPs, the concept of creating "real" and more authentic communication situations—that is, those that make sense pragmatically—should be part of the fabric of language intervention. As SLPs' roles have expanded in literacy and in-class participation, they have taken a more active role in helping students "get to the point" where they can participate in Palincsar's and others' authentic classroom activities. For example, SLPs can expose students to narrative and expository text differences, they can facilitate the use of syntactic structures that will provide the raw material for connected discourse, and they can engage their children in meta-vocabulary activities using graphic webs to help students with word relationships, naming, and word-finding strategies, among other content-form-use interactions.

> The concept of creating authentic communication situations—those that make pragmatic sense—should be part of any language intervention.

Language intervention goals that answer the following question help us create relevant targets: What language skills do my students need to participate in the brochure-writing activity, and others the teacher might be using to develop science literacy in the early elementary grades? For students with LLD who are beyond Grades 3 or 4, where the curriculum moves faster, is denser, and is driven by textbooks, SLPs should continue to work toward helping their students develop the language and literacy skills needed to access the curriculum. But they might also focus on higher levels of text (such as dealing with the specific language of science), as well as incorporating and modifying some of the ideas proposed by Palincsar and Duke (2004) that have a language pragmatic framework.

Using Accessible Text to Create Content Knowledge. Studying kindergarten to fifth-grade classrooms, Palincsar and Magnusson (2001, 2002; see also Palincsar & Duke, 2004) observed children using science notebooks. The science notebooks are adaptations of more traditional, informational-expository heavy, textbooks. They are written in first person and have more of a "think aloud" format. The "character" who is the author for the notebook is a fictional scientist called Lesley Park. She generates questions, plans, interpretations, and conclusions about various science problems. For example, she might ask, Will something heavy and something light always get to the bottom of the hill in the same amount of time? Then, in a series of discussions, Lesley tells her readers about an experiment she creates to answer the question. Palincsar and colleagues point out that these texts promote interaction between students and the text (recall *Author & Me* strategies) because students are encouraged to predict what will happen and bring their own experiences into play. They note that because texts such as the science notebooks are written to encourage the readers to actively use observations familiar to them, to ask questions, and to form their own conclusions before finding the answers in the text, students become more comfortable with scientific reasoning and critical thinking (Palincsar & Duke, 2004). And although traditional texts also support children's learning about topics, the notebooks help them develop strategies (such as inquiry and prediction) that have a positive effect across content areas. Results suggest that the conversations around the science notebooks were richer and brought the text's content to life. Talking about the use of "narrative-like" characters and first-person experiences to enhance science content knowledge, the authors stated the following:

> This type of conversation was far less likely to occur during the reading of the traditional text in which the phenomenon and its explanation were presented for the students and then illustrated in additional contexts. [Further] science instruction supported the teaching of significant general literacy skills such as text preview, identifying text features and their typical purposes, reading across texts (intertextuality), and vocabulary learning (technical terms associated with scientific inquiry). (Palincsar & Duke, 2004, p. 194)

Palincsar and Duke (2004) offer readers much to think about. Although they were not talking about students with LLD (or struggling readers) specifically, we can see the applicability of their work for these populations. Indeed, if efforts to integrate content area and reading instruction have the dual benefit of advancing both fundamental and derived literacy, it becomes easier to appreciate the benefits of creating spoken and written language intervention programs that use subject-relevant and subject-specific materials.

Speech-language pathologists can do much to help students with LLD manage the more "accessible science-related texts" described by Palincsar and colleagues. Helping students develop macro and micro aspects of narrative text

8

is part of the SLP's intervention repertoire. Using stories that have a scientific bent to them—such as science notebooks where a character goes through the actions, plans her experiments, and so on—has the added benefit of helping students use language to think scientifically. We could also create a correlate for social studies (as in the previous chapter). Speech-language pathologists can also help their students acquire the oral language skills that are needed to "talk around" a text. For example, can they form and respond to inferential questions? Do they have the lexical savvy to engage in conversations with Lesley Park, our fictional scientist? Do they know what the words *heavy, light, always,* and *amount* mean when Lesley asks herself the question, Will something heavy and something light always get to the bottom of the hill in the same amount of time? Do they comprehend the "linguistic glue" words that often accompany scientific experiments, such as *cause, effect, as a result,* and *conclusion*?

Again, helping students acquire the language needed to participate in and complete a task, along with the strategies needed to comprehend a variety of texts for a variety of purposes, is a complex business. As Singer and Bashir (2004) reminded us earlier, it is important to know where and when specific techniques, tools, and strategies work and for what desired outcome. Unlike students without LLD, students with LLD often need explicit, repeated, and clear direction.

Understanding the Text Itself: Matching Text Activities to Content-Area Subjects. The current literature in both language intervention and literacy fields has addressed the issue of "connectedness" for those professionals whose services reside literally or figuratively "outside" of classrooms. We have emphasized curriculum-relevant therapy in this text (inspired by Ehren, 2000), and literacy professionals and curricular specialists have emphasized the need to integrate basic and derived literacy. Likewise, educators who teach across content areas have emphasized the primacy of language in the learning content, including mathematics (e.g., Abedi & Lord, 2001). Palincsar and Duke (2004) mirrored this thinking in the studies that were highlighted earlier. Much of their research recognizes the importance of the "conversations" that surround text. They recognize that students have to manage the complexities of expository text eventually but propose many innovative ways to help them "get there."

Palincsar's group also reported some interesting findings about expository text instruction. Their data suggested that teaching children about the components of expository text in general—for example, that expository text has the following features—may be helpful, but when taught "in isolation," it loses some of its meaning. In other words, it may be more effective to teach students to read and write exposition for a specific purpose or as it relates to mastering a specific subject. For example, a SLP might work with a middle school or high school student who needs help comprehending and writing expository text. Her intervention might include using graphic organizers (such as the one shown in Figure 8-4) as scaffolds. Included in her instructions could be some variation of the following: "We are going to practice with this special kind of problem-solution graph. Remember when we worked on the compare-contrast graph for history?" (Hopefully, the student does not have a blank stare on his face at this point.)

Science Report Diagram

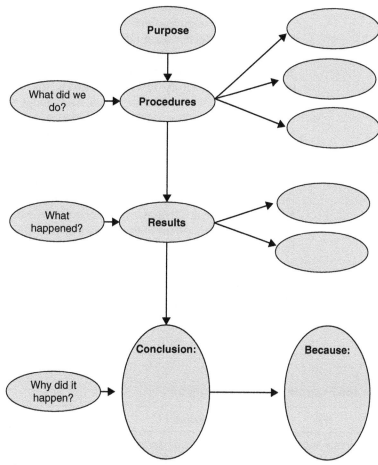

Figure 8-4 ■ A graphic representing the organization of a science report. *(Adapted from Westby, C. E., & Clauser, P. S. [2005]. The right stuff for writing: Assessing and facilitating written language. In H. W. Catts & A. G. Kamhi [Eds.], Language and reading disabilities [2nd ed., p. 302]. Boston: Allyn & Bacon. Modified by Beck, A., & Knoll, C. [2006, May]. Curriculum-based and collaborative language intervention. Paper prepared for the Department of Communicative Disorders at California State University at Long Beach, Long Beach, CA.)*

"This new graph will help you to organize your science report. We'll paste it in your notebook after we finish today as a reminder of how science experiments follow certain steps." Figure 8-4 presents a graphic organizer for science from Westby and Clauser (2005) as modified by Beck and Knoll (2006). It relates specifically to activities and requirements that are part of science.

Thus working on expository text as part of a core of activities that connect to class activities may have more relevance for the student and, as a result, have a bit more "staying power."

The idea of creating intervention goals and objectives that lead to more "staying power" or "generalizability" is an important one. If science is a subject that requires an understanding of how to build an "argument" (e.g., Pappas, 2006; Yore et al., 2004)—for example, finding support theories or statements—then exposure to expository texts that include the components of an argument is another potential way to link textual knowledge with science knowledge. Both macro (overall structure) and micro (sentence and word) aspects of argumentative text can be targeted in language intervention. Westby and Clauser (2005) provide an excellent summary in this area. They say that this aspect of writing (and comprehension) is particularly difficult for students with LLD. Many of the concepts related to forming an argument are abstract (Westby & Clauser, 2005). One also has to have the linguistic and metalinguistic ability to form effective arguments—a skill that some adults have yet to acquire. Westby and Clauser (2005) note that an argument is made up of the following three parts:

1. A claim (an assertion)
2. A warrant (a principle by which one gets the data to make the claim)
3. Data (the "proof' that substantiates the claim)

Table 8-1 shows Westby's and Clauser's (2005) outline of the components of an argument for the following claim: *The rain forests should not be cut down to make room for ranches and farms.*

Table 8-1
Outline for Argument Comprehension

Claim	Warrant	Data
The rain forests should not be cut down to make room for ranches and farms.	1. Loss of the rain forest will alter weather patterns around the world.	1a. Worldwide rainfall will decrease, creating more deserts. 1b. It will contribute to global warming, causing icecaps to melt.
	2. Cutting the rain forest will result in loss of valuable resources.	2a. Rare plans that can be used to develop medicines against cancer and AIDS will be lost. 2b. Unique animals will be destroyed.
	3. There is no need for additional ranch land and farmland.	3a. Present farmland could provide better yields if crops are rotated. 3b. People are eating less beef and more chicken; chickens don't require the large amounts of land required by cattle.

From Westby, C. E., & Clauser, P. S. (2005). The right stuff for writing: Assessing and facilitating written language. In H. W. Catts & A. G. Kamhi (Eds.), *Language and reading disabilities* (2nd ed., p. 296). Boston: Allyn & Bacon.

Clearly, the complexity of the language and the required organization of the discourse needed to make a complete, effective, and sophisticated argument is evidenced in Table 8-1. Quoting the work of Golder and Coirier (1994), Westby and Clauser (2005) remind practitioners that the development of argument is a long and gradual one. A continuum that outlines the degree to which an argument is made is presented by Golder and Coirier (1994), as summarized by Westby and Clauser (2005, pp. 297–298) in Box 8-6, with the Kobe Bryant examples provided by the author of this text.

BOX 8-6	*Development of an Argument*

Preargumentative Text

0 = No claim is made.

  Example: Kobe Bryant plays for the Los Angeles Lakers.

1 = A claim is made.

  Example: Kobe helps the Lakers win many games.

Minimally Argumentative Text

2 = A claim is made with a supportive statement that is self-related.

  Example: Kobe Bryant should be more of a team player. Then I would be happier because the Clipper fans wouldn't tease me so much.

3 = A claim is made and supported by a non–self-related argument.

  Example: Kobe Bryant should be more of a team player. His selfishness caused the Lakers to lose in the playoffs to the Phoenix Suns.

Elaborated Argumentative Text

4 = A claim is made and supported by a general argument plus one or more statements of clarification.

  Example: Kobe Bryant has been the driving force of the Los Angeles Lakers. But his attempts to try to do it all have caused the Lakers to lose the chance to win two NBA titles in a row. But the team is really weak so that he doesn't have the support he needs to bring another championship to Los Angeles.

5 = A claim is made, supported by a general argument, plus some level of speaker endorsement.

  Example: Many people think that Kobe Bryant is one of the premiere players in the game of basketball. Still in his twenties, his record of accomplishments demonstrates that this is an accurate statement. (Statistics can be added here to strengthen the argument.) Others disagree, saying that he had Shaq (Shaquille O'Neill) to back him up. As a loyal Laker fan, I think it is easy to criticize Kobe Bryant, who brought the Lakers further than they might have gone in 2006.

Data from Golder, C., & Coirier, P. (1994). Augmentative text writing: Development trends. *Discourse Processes, 18,* 187–210. Summarized by Westby, C. E., & Clauser, P. S. (2005). The right stuff for writing: Assessing and facilitating written language. In H. W. Catts & A. G. Kamhi (Eds.), *Language and reading disabilities* (2nd ed., pp. 297–298). Boston: Allyn & Bacon.

As with all continua, the Golder and Coirier (1994) rendition of the road to argumentative text can provide us with some understanding of students' efforts to speak, comprehend, or write this text. Although a later acquisition, covering ages 11 to 16 when argumentative text abilities become stronger, children can certainly be exposed to this type of exposition in the early grades. Temple and colleagues (1993) provide some wonderful examples of first and second graders' argumentative text writing with topics such as "Why should students be allowed to come to school only when they want to?" and "Write to your parents to persuade them to let you do something you really want to do." Modifying the content by using familiar topics that students know something about is a way to introduce the components of argument. Moving from sports topics such as Kobe and the Lakers to topics covered in science such as global warming and others is another avenue to pursue in our quest to relate text to the subject-area content. (The reader is directed to Westby and Clauser [2005] for detailed coverage of the subject.)

Other examples of science-based ideas for helping students manage the language and organizational structure of science come from Bittel and Hernandez (2006), Hansen (2006), and Straits (2005), among others, who tie together language knowledge and science content. Bittel and Hernandez's (2006) science "flipbook" is a variation of Westby and Clauser's (2005) graphic organizer for science and Singer and Bashir's (2004) vertical story sequence graph shown in Figure 8-2. The flipbooks function like a photo album with pages that are stacked in a vertical arrangement. Flipbooks have different sections for each part of an experiment. The sections include areas such as purpose, what we want to find out, steps taken, and so on that help students summarize what happened in the experiments using the flipbook framework. Students "flip" to each section where they may have a sentence starter or a visual image or any other kind of supportive scaffold to help them record steps and appropriate data (Beck & Knoll, 2006). For example, the SLP might provide a sentence starter in one of the flipbook sections such as the following: "The purpose of this experiment was to…" or "We discovered three things: (1)…" More or less language can be supplied in each "flipped" section depending on a student's needs. The flipbooks help students keep a written record of their experiments, help them review the language needed to summarize these experiments, and help them practice with the underlying structure of expository text, particularly as it relates to describing the planning and completing of science experiments. The flipbook sections form an outline that provides a concrete representation of the "steps" involved in the scientific method.

Hansen's (2006) "process grids," originally developed for English-language learners, help students organize information in a three-column format similar to Ogle's (1986) K-W-L sheets. For example, in an earth science unit covering different types of rock formations, the column headings used would include the following: Type of Rock and Its Illustration (drawn by the student); How & Where It's Formed; and Examples of the Rock Types. In brief, many ideas are currently available that bring language and curricular content together. Speech-language pathologists and teachers should be natural partners in sharing responsibility for the language and the specific content that coexist in the suggested techniques and tools.

History Repeating Itself: An "In-Class" Example

The ideas proposed by Palincsar and others encourage school-based practitioners to think along the lines of the following three connected concepts:

1. Work toward creating authentic tasks.
2. Create intervention and instructional goals and objectives that integrate "generic" literacy skills and content-specific literacy.
3. Understand the requirements of the text itself.

VanSledright (2002a, 2002b, 2004) and many curriculum planners and researchers have made similar points about social studies and mathematics. Others have brought these concepts into discussions about learning how to write academic discourse (e.g., Bashir & Singer, 2006; Brock & Raphael, 2003).

In an article with a clever title—"Should Social Studies Textbooks Become History?"—Villano (2005) presents a summary of some of the techniques she used and the steps she took to reach her fifth graders who could not manage the concepts and language of their textbooks. She notes that fifth grade is particularly dense in terms of the amount and level of content reading required. As put by Villano (2005): "As students are being pushed to read and understand more content, many students struggle with not only *what* the text is about but also *how* to read it" (p. 122). Lack of experience with expository reading, says Villano (2005), creates learning roadblocks for students who do not know how to deal with these texts. In addition to lacking familiarity with the text's overall structure, her students were also confused by the unfamiliar sentence structures and transition words used in the texts. Again, the reality of tough content coupled with tough text helps us to appreciate how teachers (handling the *what* aspect) and SLPs (handling the *how* aspect) can split the professional difference, so to speak, when working with students with LLD. Although not using the LLD categorization specifically, Villano (2005) added that some of her students were one- to two-plus years below expected reading levels. This below-reading situation created the dual-literacies challenge we have been discussing.

Villano's (2005) model classroom brought information processing concepts to life. It also helped students "move" from contextualized to more decontextualized activities and from more oral styles of language to more literate styles of language. That is, students progressed from handling new content in easier and more accessible texts (such as narratives) to handling that content in more abstract, unfamiliar texts (such as expository texts). Villano's (2005) plan involved the orchestration of a number of activities before students actually opened their textbooks to read about a topic. The "horizon" for Villano (2005) was getting her students to a place where they could read and comprehend the content of the fifth-grade textbook. And although the textbook *guided* her curriculum, it did not *become* the curriculum (Villano, 2005, p. 128).

The activities Villano (2005) created had a logical sequence to them, including building background knowledge by using illustrated picture books with simpler text and encouraging discussions about the various characters or key figures

8

who were part of the unit's content (such as George Washington and James Madison). Villano (2005) also introduced students to a number of genres such as historical poetry in addition to narrative and expository text to, as she put it, expand their horizons about a topic. Using nonfiction read-alouds, choral reading, and note-taking, among other integrated oral-to-written and written-to-oral oral activities, Villano (2005) built a familiarity with both content and structure that students brought with them when they finally opened their texts. Some examples of what occurred in a history unit about the "Early Years of the United States Government" are as follows:

- Reading aloud from the picture book *A More Perfect Union: The Story of the Constitution* (Maestro & Maestro, 1987). Key words and phrases are emphasized and the illustrations are used to familiarize the students with key characters and places. (This book was chosen for its beginning-middle-end story grammar text and its illustrations that complemented the spoken and written word.)
- Introducing a K-W-L sheet (Ogle, 1986) to students before a second reading of the *Perfect Union* book. Students write (or talk about) three or four facts or ideas they remember from the previous reading.
- Engaging students in discussions about the illustrations that might move them from literal (Who is he?) to inferential (What important piece of paper do you think John Adams is signing?) comprehension.
- Reading a poem, "The Challenge—June 11, 1776" (Katz, 1998), which is written from the point of view of Thomas Jefferson (Villano, 2005). Students are asked to predict what the poem might be about. They listen to the poem and discuss the colonists' point of view (as per the Samantha Stevens story from Chapter 7, p. 196). They also listen to, read, and write poems that express British citizens' and colonists' feelings and opinions about the Revolutionary War.

Villano (2005) provides additional examples of activities that prepared her fifth graders for the content that would be in their textbooks. She makes a number of important points about using these supplementary materials and activities. She says, for example, that although it is time consuming to pull together these units, it is worth the effort. She reiterates her earlier statement by saying that it is unreasonable to expect children, especially struggling readers, to absorb complex content from textbooks alone. This is a statement that reflects the challenges facing clinicians and teachers who work with students with LLD. At the very least, "it is helpful to remember that when learning complex content, young students typically need several reiterations of ideas as well as opportunities for discussion in order to clarify and elaborate their initial understandings" (Villano, 2005, p. 129). Villano (2005) adds that "historical genres offer the perfect venue for preparing students for further learning on similar topics" (p. 129). In other words, students can learn about scaffolding techniques, clarifying, and elaborating on topics through a study of history. These are strategies that can be helpful across subject areas and that complement subject-specific strategies.

In her summary remarks, Villano (2005) recognizes that these supportive activities and materials are not substitutes for textbooks. Students must learn to deal with complex text and new content, sooner rather than later. Further, the activities and materials chosen to introduce students to key figures in history,

SLPs should focus on creating language intervention programs that have a strong connection to the challenges facing students in classrooms.

such as narrative texts or illustrated picture books, should be used with an eye toward how they help us help students reach the ultimate goal—reading and writing expository text and comprehending new and less familiar content. Again, we want to create intervention and instructional programs that have a "directness" to the challenges facing students. Villano (2005) believes that a balance can be struck between using textbooks and supportive approaches to deliver the curriculum to students. For school SLPs, being part of this balance is critical. Getting to the core of language that lies beneath many of the classroom and curricular requirements places SLPs in a unique and well-qualified position.

Teasing Out the Language: Macro and Micro Components Come Together in a Backdrop Drawn from Classroom Content

School-based SLPs have many opportunities to bring oral language, metalinguistic language, and written language requirements together. As we have seen in Villano's (2005) class description, a good portion of her alternative methods included group discussions of the pictures, poems, stories, and so on. This section highlights additional intervention ideas that combine spoken and written language and curricular content. Some of the activities that follow are more micro focused such as the "sentence chunking" and the verb categorization examples; others are a combination of macro and micro components such as the "stoplight organization" and "out-of-order text" examples. The first section reminds practitioners to keep the metacognitive and metalinguistic aspects of intervention in the forefront of intervention at school-age levels.

The "Big" Strategies: Keeping Students Thinking About What They Are Doing and Why

Reciprocal Teaching Strategies. From the original work of Palincsar and Brown (1984), these strategies including summarizing, seeking clarification, questioning, and making predictions to help students develop improved comprehension and awareness of how to monitor comprehension. Myers (2006) adapted some of these techniques for children as young as kindergarten to complement the decoding activities that are often the focus of reading activities in the early grades. Using puppets to represent the Princess (who told or read stories), Quincy Questioner (who asked "easy" questions to see who is listening), and Clara Clarifier (who doesn't always understand everything or who asks questions that may or may not be found in the story), children learned that reading is more that sounding out words and developed a better awareness of how to comprehend what one reads. The puppet format appears to have promise for younger readers and offers some interesting possibilities for elementary school–age students with LLD. We would drop the puppet idea for older students but incorporate the reciprocal teaching components and modeling of the strategies to improve comprehension of text. And as discussed previously, we should help our students continue to use a TWA approach to reading—*think* before reading, think *while* reading, and think *after* reading (Mason, 2004; Mason et al., 2006; see p. 222, this chapter).

While trying to keep the "bigger picture' in mind, Ogle's (1986) K-W-L (what I *know*, what I *want* to know, and what I *learned*) technique might stay in the foreground of language intervention activities at school-age levels. A slight modification of the K-W-L technique is to have the student complete the K (what I *know*) and W (what I *want* to know) columns using information from his or her science, social studies, or math curriculum. One could choose the subject that is proving to be the most difficult for the student. The L column (what I *learned*) could be modified (or a column could be added) to include "what I *learned* about *language*" (LL). For example, consider the Grade 6 science information summarized as follows:

K	W	LL
All living things are made of cells.	What are the parts of cells?	How to organize a descriptive and enumerative paragraph.
Cells are the basic units of structure and function of living things.	What is a nucleus?	That the word *unit* means "part."

The K-W-L sheet could also be modified to include a two-tiered sheet listing the same K-W-L columns. Students can fill in the content information from their textbooks on the "top floor" and the language K-W-L components on the "bottom floor." It would look like the following:

_____ K _____W_____ L _____

The Science

_____

The Language

_____

Stoplight Organization. Suggested by Mason (2004) and as summarized by Charlton and Christie (2006), this activity moves a bit more to the sentence level but has a strong self-monitoring component. It is an interesting idea that may need modification for students with LLD if and when they are ready for this type of analysis. Mason (2004) uses the image (or concept) of green, yellow, and red stoplights to help students appreciate the main idea (green), supporting facts (yellow), and details (red) of a text, as follows:

- Green means GO. The author is telling the reader what the paragraph is going to be about. It is a main (or big) idea.
- Yellow means SLOW DOWN. The author is telling the reader reasons why the green statement is true (or is believed to be true by the author).
- Red means STOP. The author is going to provide little pieces of information that say more about the yellow statement.

In stoplight organization, Mason (2004) uses green to help students see the main idea, yellow to indicate the supporting facts, and red to highlight the text's details.

These are called *details.* The reader may want to spend a little time digesting all of these facts. For example, the text that follows would be color-coded in the following way:

Green: **General Benedict Arnold was a hero in many Revolutionary War battles but he was about to become a traitor to the cause.**

Yellow: *While he was in charge of Fort Arnold, which is now West Point, he made a deal with the British to provide them with the details of George Washington's upcoming battle plans.*

Red: There were several events that led up to Arnold's decision to side with the British after being such a capable and well-respected leader of the Continental Army

(The text would continue.)

The bold, italicized, and underlined print used to demonstrate the changes in color that might appear on the page can also represent a modification of Mason's original idea. In addition, one might consider adaptations to this idea that may be more focused for students with LLD. For example, one might focus on color-coding or bolding the main ideas only. (Sometimes a main idea appears in different order; for example, it can be the second or even the last sentence.) The aim of the stoplight organization technique is to help students become more aware of text structure and, ultimately, to improve their comprehension and written language abilities. By reading the text, students gain exposure to expository structure; by color-coding text ideas on their own as they progress, they develop an awareness of the way ideas can be organized. And beyond the use of colors or font changes to signal main ideas, explanations, and details, the purpose would be to help students internalize the elements of text and form a mental representation of text as suggested by Lahey and others (e.g., Lahey & Bloom, 1994).

"Hard-Core" Linguistic Knowledge: Helping Students Become More Knowledgeable about the Ways Language Works

Charlton and Christie (2006) summarized a number of additional techniques that appeared in the literature from a variety of sources, including speech and language, English as a second language (ESL), literacy, curriculum, and educational journals. Speaking to SLPs, they saw ways that SLPs' particular and unique training becomes an important link to the curriculum. The ideas that Charlton and Christie (2006) presented are discussed in the following sections.

Sentence-Chunking Strategies: From Simple to Complex. The idea of understanding the "who did what to whom" in a sentence involves understanding the relations among actors, action, and objects. In social studies and science, the "doers" or agents of an action are not necessarily humans or individuals. In history, agents and receivers may be represented by groups, states, or nations. These groups, states, or nations can also cause things to happen. Extracting the semantic, underlying relations among words in a sentence (and in a connected text) can be a difficult task for students with and without LLD.

Adapted from Schleppegrell and Achugar (2005) and Medina (2005), Figures 8-5 and 8-6 provide examples of graphic organizers that can be used before, during, or after reading the content of a social studies unit. They can also be used to help students prepare a summary or written report. The SLP can decide how much language she or he will write in the sections for the student. These types of scaffolds can be modified to match the content of other subjects. The idea is to help students comprehend the "who did what to whom" and acquire the metalinguistic ability to talk about the relations. These activities have the potential to help students acquire the syntactic proficiency needed to navigate through the complexity of their textbooks. (See the section on "Literate Language Revisited" later in this chapter.)

According to Charlton and Christie (2006), SLPs can help students manage history text, but they have to be aware of the way that text changes, rising in complexity with each grade level. Indeed, history text (and the texts of other subjects) becomes more abstract, syntactically heavy, and rich in its use of cohesive markers, time words, and metaphorical language, especially from Grade 4 onward. Consequently, students have to learn how language works—how grammar functions—to create complex meanings (Medina, 2005). A series of questions can follow the graphing of information using the sentence organizers to reinforce the idea that phrases and words have specific functions

Simple Sentence Chunking

Agent	Actor	Receiver of Action
A conquistador named Hernando Cortés	attacked	the Aztec Indians in Mexico.
Cortés and his soldiers	defeated	the Aztec.
They (the conquistadors)	took	their (the Aztecs) gold, silver, and jewels
He (Cortés)	tore down	the city of Tenochtitlán.
The Spanish	built	Mexico City as the capital of New Spain.

Figure 8-5 ■ Sentence-chunking chart. *(Redrawn from Schleppegrell, M., & Achugar, M. [2003]. Learning language and learning history: A functional linguistic approach. TESOL Journal, 12[2], p. 21-27. Reproduced with permission of Teachers of English to Speakers of Other Languages in the format Textbook via the Copyright Clearance Center. Modified by Medina, K. [2005]. Building academic literacy through history. Paper presented at the meeting for the California History Social Science project. Funded by the University of California at Irvine, Irvine, CA; and Charlton, S., & Christie, J. [2006, May]. Language intervention for elementary history. Paper prepared for the Department of Communicative Disorders at California State University at Long Beach, Long Beach, CA.)*

The Text
One of the patriots who did the most to change public opinion in the colonies was Thomas Paine. In January 1776, Paine published a pamphlet called *Common Sense*. In it he attacked George III as a bully and questioned the idea of one person having all the authority to rule.
(From Harcourt Brace & Co. *Social Studies: Early United States:* Grade 5 (2000), p. 285.)

Put the Puzzle Pieces In the Box: Find the Meanings

TIME MARKERS	CHARACTERS (Focus: DOERS)	WHAT'S DONE	WHAT HAPPENED? OUTCOME	OTHER INFO. NAMES/PLACES DESCRIPTIONS +
	One of the patriots Thomas Paine	*did something*	*change public opinion*	*colonies*
January 1776	Paine	*published*	*pamphlet*	Common Sense
	He	*attacked*	*George III*	*bully*
		questioned	*idea*	*one person having all the authority to rule*

Left Overs?   *Tricky Words?*   *Easy and Confusing?*

Figure 8-6 ■ A graphic organizer used to facilitate comprehension of history text. *(Data from Medina, K. [2005]. Building academic literacy through history. Paper presented at the meeting for the California History Social Science project. Funded by the University of California at Irvine, Irvine, CA; and Charlton, S., & Christie, J. [2006, May]. Language intervention for elementary history. Paper prepared for the Department of Communicative Disorders at California State University at Long Beach, Long Beach, CA.)*

8

(Schleppegrell & Achugar, 2005). For example, Figure 8-5 could include the accompanying questions:

1. Who are the main participants in these events? (Cortes, Spanish conquistadors, the Aztec Indians.)
2. Are they people? If so, are they individuals or groups? (There are people and two cities; the conquistadors are a group, the Aztecs are a group, etc.)
3. Are they agents or receivers of the action? (The conquistadors are agents, the Aztecs are receivers of the action; Mexico City receives the action, etc.)
4. What participants are only agents? Why? (The conquistadors are the agents. They are the only ones doing all of the "bad things.")

5. Who are the only receivers of the action? Why? (The Aztecs are the receivers of the action. They are the ones getting conquered. The two cities are receivers.)

Speech-language pathologists reviewing the sentence organizers shown in Figures 8-5 and 8-6 will appreciate the complex interactions among semantic, syntactic, and discourse knowledge. Lexical and syntactic knowledge certainly interface with one's facility with connected text and with each other. For example, after students learn something about the concept of actor–action–receiver of action and the subject-verb-object form of sentences, do they understand the meanings of words such as *group, individual, participants,* and so on? Taking the actor-action-object/subject-verb-object structure of our sentence discussion further, we might ask whether students understand the differences between active and passive sentences. In a passive sentence such as "The Aztecs were conquered by the Spanish conquistadors," the "actor" (or doer) of the action appears at the end of the sentence (in the object position), and the "receiver of the action" appears at the beginning of the sentence (in the subject position). These syntactic changes, common in literate forms of communication, can be confusing for students.

Further practice with sentence-meaning relationships is shown in Figure 8-6. Using the graphic organizer, students outline the key elements of the sentence and write their responses in the appropriate boxes. The boxes are designated with the following categories: Time Markers, Characters (the "doers" or "actors"), What's Done (or spoken about), What Happened or Outcome, and Other (added) Information (other names, places mentioned, descriptions, etc.). The focus is on semantics—finding the meaning—but students are exposed to textbook language at the same time. They discuss "leftover" and tricky words and make judgments about the easy and confusing parts of the text with their clinician. Clearly, balancing the two extremes of "watering down" and "overloading" the language remains a challenge for clinicians whose goal it is to find authentic and relevant ways to help their students acquire the skills needed to move successfully through the pages of history.

Putting "Out-of-Order Text" in Order. Charlton and Christie (2006) combined lexical and sentence comprehension work in a metalinguistic activity using sentences from the curriculum that can be confusing to students with LLD. Villano's (2005) fifth graders might also have some trouble with the following sentence:

> The Boston Tea Party was the colonists' response to an unfair tax instituted the prior year by the British Parliament.

Understanding "who did what to whom" in the "Boston Tea Party" sentence is no easy task for many students. One reason is that more abstract concepts are being expressed in the sentence. In addition, the British Parliament and the colonists are "doers" or agents of some action, whereas the colonists serve a dual function of also being the receivers of an action—the unfair tax. In addition to completing a semantic analysis (such as talking about who did what to whom), understanding the way time markers work is also important. Phrases such as "the prior year" signal the actual order of events, but the meaning may be missed by students. Clearly, the use of complex syntactic structures, in this case a passive/multiclause sentence,* contributes to possible comprehension difficulties.

Charlton and Christie (2006) suggest working on key words and their meanings along with "breaking up" sentences to show students how these smaller linguistic units influence our understanding of the order of events. With the purpose of helping students develop a keener understanding of syntactic-semantic relationships, they expose students to sentences in which the word order does not follow the order of events. (Recall the discussion of comprehension strategies in Chapter 3, p. 66–70.) An example of Charlton and Christie's (2006) "out-of-order text" activity is presented in an adapted form in the following sections.

Step 1. Key words chosen by the clinician are written and read with the students. Students can be encouraged to use these words in sentences to describe events in their own lives, among other topics:

Before	After	While
Prior	Following	Meanwhile

Step 2. The sentence is presented in written form and read by the student or the clinician. Student and clinician discuss the "main ideas" or "main words" expressed in the sentence and how the word "prior" (or phrase "prior year") connects to them. (Color coding can be used as per the "Benedict Arnold" passage presented earlier to make connections more or less explicit.)

The Boston Tea Party PRIOR TO unfair tax
Unfair tax PRIOR TO Boston Tea Party
Question: How does the word *prior* relate to these pieces of the sentences? (Discussion of the meanings of *prior* and *before*)

Step 3. The phrases are written on separate cards by the student (or clinician). They are moved around (as per above) and the correct order of events is discussed.

Unfair tax PRIOR TO Boston Tea Party
(The unfair tax by the British came *before* the Boston Tea Party.)

Step 4. Does it make sense? Why? (Something would have to make you mad before you did something about it.)

Order of events:
- British tax (that makes colonists mad) is enacted.
- They do something.
- Dump tea in the harbor. Called Boston Tea Party.

Step 4 can also be a place to start after key words are highlighted. In this arrangement, the students are given the actual order and work through the syntax to observe and analyze how this sequence and the relations are expressed.

8

---

*An object relative clause sentence with "that was" implied; the final clause defines the unfair tax.

Several variations on the theme are possible using science and math content as a backdrop. Various time markers (before, after, etc.) and other smaller linguistic units (if...then, between, by contrast, etc.) can be chosen to demonstrate how syntax and meaning connect. Additional syntactic-semantic ideas will be included later in this chapter.

Attending to Tricky Words and Phrases and Putting Them Back Together Again. Following from the previously mentioned sentence-word combinations, additional suggestions encourage practitioners to help students analyze and talk about language. Researchers and practitioners across disciplines say that helping students become more aware of key words, time markers, cohesive ties in discourse, and verb categories can facilitate comprehension (Burns, 2004; Medina, 2005; Schleppegrell & Achugar, 2005). For example, words can be written under math symbols (e.g., + or −) that signal "plus," "minus," "more than," and "less than" to compile a group of synonyms. Students can practice with these words in familiar and meaningful events first and then apply meanings to specific math problems from textbooks. As per the Boston Tea Party sentence in the previous example, conjunctions can be highlighted to help students attend to them more carefully when completing assignments on their own. Building on sentence structure work (through activities surrounding Figures 8-5 and 8-6 and the section that follows), students can go back and analyze the verb categories in a paragraph more specifically. This activity becomes a guide to discussing what the author's main points might be. The added "meta" practice can be useful for vocabulary building not only for comprehension but also for developing a richer language repertoire for writing. Schleppegrell and Achugar (2005) found that talking in terms of *action verbs* (signaling a sequence of events), *thinking/feeling verbs* (presenting an author's bias), *saying verbs* (signaling a conversation, a quote, or a reporting of something), and *relating verbs* (signaling description) can be facilitative to comprehension. For example, students can look through a social studies text and chart the verb categories:

Various interdisciplinary researchers note that helping students become more aware of key words, time markers, cohesive ties in discourse, and verb categories can facilitate comprehension.

Action Verbs (Events)	Thinking/Feeling Verbs (Comments/ Opinions)	Saying Verbs (Reporting)	Relating Verbs (Description)
fought	*believed*	*said*	*was*
returned		*screamed*	*had been*
ordered			
surprised			

In some cases, the verbs chosen by an author may dominate a passage. This suggests that a piece is emphasizing a summary of events, but texts are often mixed. Social studies textbooks frequently present detailed descriptions of events. Clearly, although useful, this type of activity should serve a purpose and be considered as part of a broader focus on processing and comprehension. Indeed, bringing individual words and phrases back to connected discourse is recommended. Medina (2005) suggests having students circle time markers in text (especially in history text) to remind them when an event occurred, which is difficult for many students (and adults). How many of us can remember which year George Washington was elected the nation's first president? (It was 1789.) Likewise, Medina (2005) indicates that students should also circle nouns or nominal phrases and draw an arrow to the pronoun or referent it refers to. For example, consider the following:

> *Benjamin Franklin* went to France to get help for the war in the colonies, which was not going well. *He* spent many years in France before *he* was successful. *This famous inventor, statesman, and patriot* was also an amazing *diplomat.*

The italicized words refer to the same person, Ben Franklin. As the text continues, adding the names of Thomas Jefferson and John Adams, who also came to France, makes the text more confusing because the reader has to keep track of "who" is being discussed and the roles they took in procuring France's help in the war. Students with LLD frequently have difficulty with cohesive ties, especially when they are embedded in complex text and less familiar content.

Literate Language Revisited: Integrating Form, Content, and Use with a Strong "Meta Twist"

Back to Textbooks. Consider the following excerpts from Grade 4 and Grade 6 science texts:

"Class: Please open your textbooks..."
Grade 4 Science: Topic—Energy and Change of State:

> As the particles in the solid gain energy, they move farther apart. If they gain enough energy, the particles move far enough apart so that they can slide past each other. The matter begins to melt. **Melting** is the change of state from a solid to a liquid. (Pictures of ice in a glass pot on a stove and numbers for each paragraph to signal the steps in the process serve as supports for comprehension of the content. Selected words are in bold to highlight key concepts.) (*Science Discovery Works*, Grade 4, p. B40.)

Grade 6 Science: Topic—Structure of Matter and Particles in Motion:

> The moving specks of dust offer evidence of the structure and nature of matter. Matter is composed of very tiny particles that are constantly in motion. The particles that make up matter are much smaller than the tiniest speck of dust. These particles are so small, in fact, that they can't be seen, even with the best microscope your school owns. Air is made up of such particles, moving through space. As the particles of air move about, they collide with each other and with everything in your room, including the specks of dust. The movements of dust specks are caused by the particles of air bouncing the specks of dust around! (*Science Discovery Works*, Grade 6, p. C19.)
> (An illustration of a slide projector in a darkened room showing illuminated specks of dust provides some supportive context.)

These examples are familiar to readers of this text. They remind us, yet again, to consider the level of language that is assumed to be intact by the time children reach these grades. Westby (2005) points out that "by middle elementary school children must be capable of producing a variety of independent and dependent clause structures…linked by coordinating and subordinating conjunctions" (p. 309). They must also deal with passive constructions such as those shown earlier and others that change the order of "who did what to whom." Examples of complex syntactic forms are seen in the science book excerpts. Elaborated noun phrases, relative clause sentences, various embedded phrases and clauses, and passive forms are evidenced in the passages. We also see the nominalization of the verb "melting" in the form of a gerund.

An analysis of many of the texts that students must use includes the use of complex literate-syntactic forms to express ideas. And although the study of syntax became a bit obscured as pragmatics, connected discourse, and other aspects of language study came to the forefront of interest, syntactic proficiency has been seen in more recent years as part of a framework that connects to literate language—the language of teachers and textbooks. Eisenberg (2006), Nippold (1998), Scott (2005), Westby and Clauser (2005), and Westby (2006), to name only a few, have contributed much to our understanding of the role of complex syntax in language and literacy learning and academic success. They recognize, as do other researchers (e.g., Tyree et al., 1994), the reality that textbooks are often designed for the above-average reader, a point that Villano (2005) made when discussing the challenges facing her fifth graders who were trying to learn history. And the above-average reader has a tremendous advantage over struggling or limited readers because good readers have an understanding of and proficiency with literate language forms, along with other linguistic and metalinguistic abilities such as being a fast and fluent decoder of words and having a strong lexical inventory.

Grammar Still Counts? In her elegant discussion entitled "Grammar: How Can I Say That Better?" Eisenberg (2006) asks us to take a hard look at the state of the art of that piece of language intervention that focuses on helping students acquire grammatical skills. She provides useful information about expectations and efficacy and offers research-based suggestions for ways to translate what is known into daily practice. One of the first steps in understanding "where we might go" therapeutically with students is determining what the grammatical targets might be. Those of us in the business of helping children acquire language, that is, SLPs, must be versed in what the later-developing grammatical structures look like. (Can we identify the subject and object relative clause sentences in the science excerpts?) Using examples from the work of Nippold (1998) and Weaver (1996), Eisenberg provides us with a summary that is reproduced in Box 8-7. The majority of these grammatical structures are acquired after age 5 and are often part of the literate repertoire that children develop not only from talking and listening to language but also from reading and writing their language, a point made throughout this text.

According to Eisenberg (2006), many different techniques for syntactic development have been widely used in speech and language intervention sessions. Imitation, modeling, and expansions are among those that are familiar to clinicians. Gillam and Ukrainetz (2006) summarized some of the more efficacious techniques in Box 6-4 (p. 155, this text). Reminding us of the significant differences between preschool and school-age language, Eisenberg (2006) notes that

BOX 8-7   *Later-Developing Grammatical Structures*

Noun-Phrase Expansion
- Adjective phrase with two or more adjectives (the *three main* parts)
- Adjective phrase with adverbs (the *extremely* cold conditions)
- Post-noun modifying prepositional phrase (the details *of the plan*)
- Post-noun modifying relative clause (Thomas Edison, *who invented the light bulb*)
- Post-noun modifying nonfinite clause (the best way *to study*)
- Post-noun modifying appositive (Gonaïves, *the country's third-largest city*)
- Post-noun elaboration (Other countries *such as Italy and France*)

Verb-Form Expansion
- Perfect aspect (The enemy *had reached* the outskirts of the town.)
- Passive voice (The evidence *was found* after a long search.)
- Combination of modals and auxiliaries (The company *could have been spending less.*)

Predicate Expansion
- Combination of two-object noun phrases (The architect showed *the town council the plans for the new building.*)
- Combination of object-noun phrase and prepositional object (The assistant leaked *the scandal to the public.*)
- Combination of object-noun phrase and locative (The attorney placed *the confidential papers in a locked cabinet.*)

Conjunctions
- Coordinating conjunction (She had missed breakfast, *but it was still too early for lunch.*)
- Subordinating conjunction (The storm destroyed many homes *even though its intensity had lessened.*)
- Correlative conjunction (Elevated blood sugar increases the risk of heart disease *not only in people with diabetes but also in those with high-normal readings.*)

Complement Clauses (Nominal Constructions)
- Infinitive clause (The general decided *to invade* before dawn.)
- Tensed verb clause (The woman realized *that she had seen the stranger before.*)
- *Wh* clause (They didn't know *when the attack would start.*)
- Participial clause (The bank recently began *charging* for money machine withdrawal.)

Adverbial Constructions
- Adverbs (I can't, *unfortunately*, get you more paper.)
- Adverbial clause with a subordinating conjunction (The space capsule crashed *when its parachutes failed to open.*)
- Adverbial clause with an infinitive verb form (He saved up his money *[in order] to buy a new computer.*)

Continued

8

BOX 8-7   *Later-Developing Grammatical Structures—cont'd*

Other Complex Sentence Constructions
- Subject complement clause (*Patients taking the new medications* had not been told the risks.)
- Subject relative clause (*The students who had taken the review course* scored higher on the exam.)
- Preposed subordinate clause (*As the dust cloud drew closer,* the man could see that there were four horsemen riding toward him.)
- Cleft construction (*It was yesterday that* she came home from the hospital.)
- Extraposition construction (*It would be sensible* to leave early.)
- Sentences with three or more clauses (*Because the state has underfinanced its public schools, some schools have been forced to cut programs.*)

From Eisenberg, S. L. (2006). Grammar: How can I say that better? In T. A. Ukrainetz (Ed.), *Contextualized language intervention* (pp. 150–151). Eau Claire, WI: Thinking Publications. Data from Nippold, M. A. (1998). *Later language development: Ages nine through nineteen.* Austin, TX: Pro-Ed; and Weaver, C. (1996). *Teaching grammar in context.* Portsmouth, NH: Boyton/Cook Publishers.

syntactic work for older students includes the use of some similar techniques used at preschool levels, such as modeling and expansions. These techniques, however, must go well beyond the conversational formats that predominate in preschool intervention. Further, school-age intervention should be targeted with connected discourse in mind and include and be interactive with written language. It should also occur within meaningful and authentic activities (Eisenberg, 2006). She goes on to say that there may be times when we may "pull out" specific linguistic forms and present mini-lessons that engage students in focused practice with particular targets, but we should bring these lessons back to reality as quickly as possible. Again, the notion of keeping our interventions direct and relevant is reflected in Eisenberg's (2006) suggestions.

As seen in the activities presented in the previous section, connecting syntactic awareness activities to social studies, science, and other school subjects is one way to keep grammatical intervention more relevant to students. In addition, says Eisenberg (2006), clinicians should choose instructional procedures with care. Research suggests that integrative activities, that is, those that combine activities in meaningful contexts, have the most promise of success. For example, modeling with production and sentence formation procedures that include combining sentences, paraphrasing, and expanding sentences are intervention options. On the other hand, Eisenberg (2006) says that some techniques should be "retired," such as having students memorize parts of speech out of context. She adds that while students should have knowledge of grammatical categories such as word classes (nouns, verbs, etc.) and subjects and predicates, "these concepts can be incorporated into comments about grammar during meaningful activities" (Eisenberg, 2006, p. 164). The focus on meaning and how forms help readers and writers "get there" for some purpose is the critical point. Figures 8-5 and 8-6 provided examples of ways to connect sentence activities to the curricular content that children have to learn. But Eisenberg (2006) suggests exercising caution when using (or overusing) these types of sentence analysis activities because they appear to be less effective than other techniques, especially when they are delivered "in isolation"—separate from classroom materials or activities. Thus the suggestions discussed in the following sections are best viewed with Eisenberg's (2006) cautionary comments in mind.

Helping Students Appreciate Literate Forms. Westby and Clauser (2005) also talk about using a number of different techniques to help students gain an appreciation for and a competence with complex syntactic forms. Referencing the work of Killgallon and Killgallon (2000), they say that exposing students to the structures through modeling and reading to them (with the target structures in mind) is one way to begin. This introductory section should be followed by a number of systematic activities that include identifying the structures, combining sentences, unscrambling sentences, expanding sentences, and, eventually, producing novel sentences. Like Eisenberg (2006), Westby and Clauser (2005) emphasize the importance of bringing students' newly learned syntactic knowledge to connected discourse and those discourses that they are reading or participating in at school. In an earlier rendition, Wallach and Miller (1988) talked about having students see "the whole" before manipulating a sentence into its parts.

Identifying/Becoming Familiar with Target Forms. This aspect of intervention can be delivered in a number of ways. Killgallon and Killgallon (2000) provided definitions and examples of structures to students. Eisenberg (2006), as per her previously discussed remarks, prefers having the student use the structures in meaningful situations and suggests a balance between the two ideas (defining forms vs. exposure and use of forms). In the adaptation presented next, students read or are read to while following along with the print. For example, consider the following sentences:

> Topic of interest **(sports)**: Derek Jeter *who is the captain of the Yankee team* hit a home run last night.
> Curriculum topic **(science)**: The formation of bubbles *that is forming in the pot* means the liquid is beginning to boil.*

The key form (or aspect of the form to be targeted and learned) is italicized or color-coded. Specific instructions can be provided in a mini-lesson to highlight the form, in this case, a relative clause sentence. Clinicians can add comments such as the following: "The first sentence, 'Derek Jeter…,' is called a relative clause sentence. It has an extra description that tells us more about a person or thing or event. Let's practice reading a few sentences like these from the sports page (or the science text, social studies text, literature). Then we will practice building sentences together and on our own" (adapted from Eisenberg, 2006, p. 164). Again, the instructions may vary depending on the individual abilities and needs of students.

8

*Modified from *Science Discovery Works*, Grade 4, p. B40.

Sentence Combining. This activity, which has been shown to be effective clinically and educationally (see Eisenberg, 2006), gets students involved in creating sentences with a good deal of scaffolding initially. Westby and Clauser (2005) used sentences from the book *Harry Potter and the Chamber of Secrets.* Students are given the following two sentences (Westby & Clauser, 2005, p. 313):

1. The red envelope ^ burst into flames and curled into ashes.
2. It was the red envelope which had dropped from Ron's hand.

Their task is to combine them into one sentence. They are told to use the underlined section of sentence 2, inserting it where the ^ is shown in sentence 1. The result is the following complex relative sentence: "The red envelope, which had dropped from Ron's hand, burst into flames and curled into ashes."

In a previous discussion of syntax (and semantic connections), Wallach and Miller (1988) also stated that students should be exposed to the complex sentences in stories and other connected text genres before (or in conjunction with) syntactically oriented activities that isolate sentences. They also reminded their readers, as we did in Chapter 3 of this text (pp. 66–70), to consider the comprehension strategies used by students. For example, Charlton and Christie's (2006) "Boston Tea Party/Unfair Tax" sequence asks us to pay attention to the way students attempt to comprehend what they hear and read. Do students follow the word order? Do they attend to the smaller linguistic units that change meaning? Are they confused when the word order and meaning are not matched?

A variation of the sentence-combining activity presented earlier involves a combination of (a) exposure to the model form and (b) putting sentence pieces (i.e., clauses) together (adapted from the original work by Wallach & Miller, 1988). Students read (or follow along with the clinician as he or she reads) the following sentence:

3. The general who was one of Washington's most respected field commanders was about to commit treason.

Students are asked to decide which of the following four ideas forms the relative clause sentence:

1. The man will commit treason.
2. The man is a general.
3. The man was one of Washington's most respected field commanders.
4. Benedict Arnold decided to fight for the British.

Note that the fourth choice represents an inference from the given information. This is not necessarily an incorrect choice from a discourse standpoint, but it is not the focus of this activity. This type of activity, which requires predicting what the next sentence could be or what might logically "fit" in the discourse (inferential processing), is an important aspect of intervention for school-age students. Clinicians should always be cautious about doing too many things at once and making their instruction explicit. At some point, clinicians and students should discuss given and inferential information differences such as the *In the Book* and *In My Head* strategies.

The four choices can vary depending on the clinician's purpose. For example, one could substitute different nouns (e.g., the officer) for the phrase "the man." Ultimately, the repetition of "man" for the referent can be modified to create a session on cohesion and appropriate word substitutions. But if syntactic manipulation is the major goal, adding too many possibilities should be exercised with caution.

A variety of sentence forms can be used in all the activities presented. Sentences can be modified to help students focus on different aspects of structure. Clauses can be manipulated to vary the syntactic complexity—for example, embedded sentences are generally more difficult to comprehend than nonembedded sentences. Sentence 3 on the previous page is a relative clause sentence. The clause is embedded, and it modifies the subject. Other variations include clauses that appear at the end of the sentence and word-order variations that may affect comprehension. For example, the following sentence is also a relative clause sentence, but the modifying clause is at the end of the sentence: "Washington respected Benedict Arnold who was a great field commander and a soon-to-be traitor." In the next sentence, we see the addition of another noun (a key figure) and a somewhat confusing word order: "Washington who John Adams was talking to was concerned about his field general, Benedict Arnold." There are certainly many possible variations to the syntactic theme. It might be an understatement to say that SLPs and language arts teachers would be well served to be versed in syntactic development and disorders.

Smaller Linguistic Units: Sentence Completions and More. Westby and Clauser (2005), referencing the work of May (1994) and Strong (1986), as well as presenting their own ideas, provide examples of ways to improve students' comprehension and use of connective words. Appendix D contains an extensive list of clausal connective words, their definitions, and words with similar meanings compiled by Westby and Clauser (2005). The appendix is a useful resource for speech-language and other professionals who are interested in helping students with these constructions. In a brief summary, Westby (2006) lists the meanings expressed by cue words used to form complex sentences:

Time:	after, as long as, before, until, when
Place:	where, wherever
Condition:	even though, if, unless, whether
Cause:	as, because, since
Purpose:	so that, in order that
Concession:	though, although
Comparison:	than
Manner:	as, as if, as though

In their chapter, Westby and Clauser (2005) provide examples of conversational, sentence-combining, and connected text formats. Consider the following examples from Westby and Clauser (2005, p. 309).

- Student 1: What will you be doing while I _____? *(Student adds action word.)*
- Student 2: While you're (action word), I'll_____. *(Student adds alternative activity.)*
- Student 1: What will you be doing while I wash the dishes?
- Student 2: While you're washing the dishes, I'll play tennis.

The scaffolded conversational format may be a reasonable starting point. Clinicians should move to, or integrate, written and curricular materials for school-age students as early as possible. Using or creating stories (or expository text excerpts) that emphasize a particular conjunction is another technique presented by Westby and Clauser (2005). For example:

> It was the job of Ray and Pete to take care of the yard work at their house. They made up a list of jobs. While Ray did the top half of the list, Pete did the bottom half. (May, 1994, p. 232; as reported by Westby & Clauser, 2005, p. 309)

Students can continue the story in spoken or written form, using *while* at key points as directed by the clinician. Students can also read (with the clinician) a story that is written with "and" as the only connector in the piece. Students work toward substituting another word for "and," for example, "while," "when," "after," and so on. Questions can also follow the reading of narrative or expository pieces with target connectors. *Cloze* procedures (providing blanks at selected places for students to write in the connector) can be added as a variation on this theme. Reading from the curriculum is also recommended to familiarize students with these smaller linguistic units. For example, consider the use of *as*, *if*, and *so that* in the following excerpt:

> *As* the particles in the solid gain energy, they move farther apart. *If* they gain enough energy, the particles move far enough apart *so that* they can slide past each other. The matter begins to melt. (From *Science Discovery Works*, Grade 4, p. B40)

Returning to sentence-combining activities, Westby and Clauser (2006) introduce simple sentences with target constructions indicated as key words that will join the simple sentences to make a complex sentence. The curriculum-based examples are modifications of the Westby and Clauser (2005) idea, as follows:

(General idea for sentence combining)
I like driving.
It is very exciting. (BECAUSE)

> Result: *I like driving because it is very exciting.*

(Curriculum-based sentence-combining example)
The Civil War was a bitter and long-term conflict.
The North and South had very different views regarding states' rights and the issue of slavery. (BECAUSE)

> Result: *The Civil War was a bitter and long-term conflict because the North and South had very different views regarding states' rights and the issue of slavery.*

Eisenberg (2006) provided another example of sentence combining using content from the *New York Times* (Eisenberg, 2006, p. 173, quoting Steinhauer, 2005). The example shows the creation of a that-complement structure:

Some experts say SOMETHING.
The problem stems from preschool itself. (THAT)

> Result: *Some experts say that the problem stems from preschool itself.*

Practicing with Other Semantic-Syntactic Combinations and Navigating through Word-Order Confusions. In their original work (adapted here), Wallach and Miller (1988) also talked about how conjunctions/connector words such as "if," "because," "before," and "after" make comprehension difficult for younger children and for students with LLD. Wallach and Miller (1988) also outlined activities for advancing students' syntactic knowledge. They discussed the ways conjunctions and clausal connectors were used, as well as the ways clauses can be ordered in sentences (main first/subordinate second vs. subordinate first/main second). They suggested using sentences such as the one that follows to help students become more aware of form-meaning (syntactic-semantic) connections. A prototype of an "if" sentence follows:

If the hot sun comes out, the snowman will melt.

(Subordinate clause first)
(Cause-effect follows the order of events)
The snowman will melt if the hot sun comes out.

(Main clause first)
(Cause-effect is the opposite of the clause order)

In a variation of the sentence-combining activities mentioned previously, the clauses would be written on cards:

THE HOT SUN COMES OUT   THE SNOWMAN MELTS
(IF)

Students decide where the "if' (or other conjunction) would go. Then they write the complete sentence. Discussions follow about why choices were made, and so on. To expand on the task, students are asked to create an original sentence. Next, they find sentences in their textbooks that replicate the "if" structure. Making up a sentence that might come before or after the target sentence works toward helping sentences make predictions and connect individual sentences to connected discourse. Differences between "because," "and so," and other connectors can follow.

Along similar lines, we might consider the complexity of "before" and "after" sentences. These structures are often confusing for students with LLD, especially when they are embedded in more decontextualized situations (such as classroom instructions) and unfamiliar text. Helping students acquire some syntactic savvy and flexibility can make a difference to comprehension and is a skill that should prove useful in school.

Wallach and Miller (1988) used before-after sentences that were ordered (the word order matches the order of events) and nonordered (the word order violates the order of events; it is in reverse order) to help students acquire better syntactic proficiency for instructional language, reading comprehension, and writing. Starting with familiar sequences, they moved students to more abstract, and curriculum-based materials. Examples of these sentence types are provided in Box 8-8.

8

BOX 8-8	*Examples of Before-After Sentences*

The Familiar Event Sequences
Before Sentences
- The boy brushed his teeth before he went to bed. (Ordered)
- Before he went to bed the boy brushed his teeth. (Nonordered)

After Sentences
- After he put on his bathing suit the boy jumped into the pool. (Ordered)
- The boy jumped into the pool after he put on his bathing suit. (Nonordered)

The Curricular-Related/Instructional Sequences
Before Sentences
- Jayne counted the money she had saved up before she went to the ski shop. She had a total of six 5-dollar bills, twenty quarters, and four 1-dollar bills. If the ski poles cost $100, how much more does she need to buy the poles? (Also an *if* structure) (Math problem: ordered *before* structure)
- Before you answer the questions at the bottom of the page, read the whole paragraph and tell me what the author's trying to tell us. (Instruction: Nonordered *before* structure)

After Sentences
- After President Abraham Lincoln appointed him to the position, Ulysses S. Grant became Commanding General of all the Union forces during the Civil War between the States. (History: Ordered *after* structure)
- Pick up the big yellow circle after you touch the big white square. (Decontextualized instruction/test item: Nonordered *after* structure)

High-context activities surrounding syntactic awareness work would include using pictures to represent spoken or written sequences. Again, using vocabulary and content from students' textbooks is always recommended along with (or shortly after) using more familiar scenarios. Oral and written work should be combined. Sentences can be presented in ordered (spoken matches real-world sequence) and nonordered (spoken order is the reverse of the real-world order) forms. A number of "meta-level" activities surround the construction and use of these complex sentences, as in the following examples:

- *Picture cues (ordered):* Students are presented with two pictures. (The number can vary with the complexity of sentences or short passages.) The pictures are ordered initially so that the events follow their real-world sequence, for example:

BOY BRUSHING TEETH   BOY GETTING INTO BED (BEFORE-AFTER)
PICTURE OF LINCOLN   PICTURE OF U. S. GRANT* (BEFORE-AFTER)

Students produce a spoken or written sentence to "match" the picture. As per the sentence-combining activities, the before-after conjunction is presented as part of a "warm-up" or mini-lesson (from Eisenberg, 2006).

■ *Picture cues (nonordered):* Pictures can also be "out of order" in terms of their representation of events, for example,

BOY GETTING INTO BED   BOY BRUSHING HIS TEETH
                                   (BEFORE-AFTER)
PICTURE OF U. S. GRANT   PICTURE OF LINCOLN
                                   (BEFORE-AFTER)

Students work on before-after words and choose a structure that works with the pictures. (Clinicians should remember that "sequence" is a relative term. It can mean many things and is not a static [always in order] occurrence.)

■ *Choosing sentences:* Students are given two sentences with one set of pictures. For example, the BOY BRUSHING TEETH and BOY GETTING INTO BED picture sequence could have the following two sentences beneath the pictures:
1. *After* the boy brushed his teeth, he went to bed.
2. *Before* the boy went to bed, he brushed his teeth.
(The curricular pictures would appear with similar picture choices.)

Students (or clinicians) read the sentences. The clinician may use stress and prosody to help students attend to critical pieces of the sentence. Color-coding or italicizing the key words, phrases, or clauses (similar to the stop-light and other activities) may be used with the goal of eliminating these extra cues as quickly as possible. The supportive cues in print are provided initially to help students acquire more effective processing (and writing) strategies. Different variations can be practiced and the sentence-to-picture matches discussed. Caution should be exercised since judgments such as the one just presented (the synonymous after-before "brushing teeth" example) and the example that follows are later language acquisitions and have a strong metalinguistic focus to them (Nippold, 1998; van Kleeck, 1994).

A variation of the sentence-to-picture matches presented in the previous section involves having students make sentence-to-sentence matches. In this activity, students are given a written sentence (in this case, a passive sentence) that is semantically constrained/nonreversible. This means that there are limited possibilities about "who can do what to whom." In the sentence that follows,

8

---

*Recall Villano's (2005) use of pictures of historical events to help her students become familiar with key characters and events in history.

"Wolf Blitzer" can discuss "the crisis" but "the crisis" cannot discuss "Wolf Blitzer." The nouns are semantically constrained; one noun cannot be substituted for another in the sentence and still make sense (see Chapter 3, pp. 59, 77, this text). On the other hand, if the sentence had two nouns, for example, "Wolf Blitzer" and "Charles Gibson," it would be nonconstrained and reversible. Passive sentences are more literate forms that appear more often in written text and formal situations such as lectures. Consider the following nonreversible passive sentence:

> The crisis in the Middle East was discussed by Wolf Blitzer of CNN. (Target Sentence)

(In a passive sentence, the actor occurs last and the receiver/object appears first. The active version appears in the choices that are presented next.)

Students are given three written sentences (which can be read to them) and are asked to decide which one means the same thing as the target sentence:

1. Wolf Blitzer of CNN discussed the crisis in the Middle East. (Answer)
2. The Middle East discussed the crisis with Wolf Blitzer of CNN.
3. He said the Middle East crisis was becoming a tremendously dangerous situation.*

Judgments become more difficult when the passive sentences are reversible, as in the following:

> Charles Gibson of ABC was congratulated by Wolf Blitzer of CNN for his great reporting. (Target Sentence)
> 1. Charles Gibson of ABC congratulated Wolf Blitzer of CNN for his great reporting.
> 2. Wolf Blitzer of CNN was congratulated by Charles Gibson of ABC for his great reporting.
> 3. Wolf Blitzer of CNN congratulated Charles Gibson of ABC for his great reporting. (Answer)

Any number of variations are possible, and additional support may be provided as needed. For example, we might color-code the doer of the actions as a clue. We might provide presentence cueing by presenting short stories before working on the target sentences. We might consider engaging the students in *In My Head* activities and explore the background knowledge they bring to the syntactic judgment tasks. Do the students know who Wolf Blitzer is? Have they heard of CNN? Do they know anything about the Middle East crisis? Do they know what "congratulate" means? And so on.

In sum, there are many twists and turns on the road to acquiring advanced syntactic ability, as well as the ability to pull it apart, put it back together, and make judgments about it. In a sense, the examples presented may reflect the proverbial "tip-of-the-iceberg phenomenon." They are prototypes of what is possible and they remind us to keep the micro aspects of language in our intervention goals and objects. At the same time, however, Eisenberg (2006)

---

*An inference or possible next sentence, which can be another activity for another purpose.

notes that grammatical intervention needs to reside "within meaningful reading, writing, and speaking activities that provide repeated opportunities [for students] to learn and use grammatical forms to express meaning and to participate in discourse" (p. 187).

The Discourse Is Terminated Temporarily

We have continued our journey through the maze of basic and derived literacy. With each path taken, there is even more to say about what we can do to help students with LLD. So many of the things that come naturally to students without LLD are a greater challenge for the students we serve. And, in actuality, how many things really come naturally for students once they leave preschool? Armed with intact language, children without LLD do have an advantage because they can use their language and evolving metalinguistic skills to tackle content-specific reading and writing. But as we have seen in the examples from science and social studies, these subjects make many demands on the cognitive and linguistic systems of the best of us. So, we will continue to explore, question, and reflect on the information covered thus far in the next chapter. Chapter 9 will pull some of the pieces together with additional examples of both macro and micro language components, beginning with a look at expectations across the grades from within the prism of selected state standards and benchmarks.

8

Part IV

Toward a Summary

PART OUTLINE

9 Back into the Field
   Starting to Pull the Missing Pieces Together

10 The End Becomes a New Beginning
   Coming Full Circle

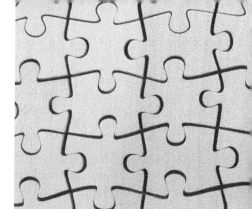

To address children's language needs, the SLP must maintain a long-term functional view of language and learning... A functional view recognizes language as a means of sharing ideas with others and accomplishing a wide range of goals... Consequently, language must be thought of as more than the mastery of syntactic structures or pragmatic functions.
(Norris, 1997, p. 50)

9 Back into the Field

Starting to Pull the Missing Pieces Together

SUMMARY STATEMENT ▰▰▰▰▰▰

Chapter 9 begins to pull some of the pieces of language intervention goals and objectives together by continuing to explore the contexts in which professionals have to practice—school settings that are encumbered by their standards, benchmarks, and high-stakes testing. We will continue to weave macro and micro aspects of text together while continuing to ask the following question: Why did I make these choices for my students? The chapter delves a bit further into "word-level" considerations but keeps these aspects of language under the umbrella of connected text and curricular concerns. Through a presentation of different activities, school scenarios, and diagnostic conclusions in this chapter and in Chapter 10, readers are encouraged to form discussion groups with colleagues both within and across their disciplines. This chapter restates the idea that although we have come a very long way, we still have much to tackle on the road less traveled. The era of evidenced-based practice (EBP) may be upon us, but the roadmap for "getting there" is, at this writing, a work in progress. The current chapter suggests that practitioners who work with children and adolescents in the front lines of schools are a critical piece of EBP endeavor. Indeed, while we push for strong collaboration among the different professionals who

---

work directly with children, so, too, must collaboration occur among researchers, clinicians, and teachers (Kamhi, 2006; Nail-Chiwetalu & Ratner, 2006).

KEY QUESTIONS ■■■■■■■■■

1. How do state standards and benchmarks inform language intervention at school-age levels?
2. What should practitioners know about skills such as "vocabulary knowledge and use," and how do these word-level abilities influence

and interact with literacy learning and academic success?

3. What do the language intervention activities and tools we choose say about our knowledge of the theoretical foundations that ground them and the functionality and relevance of their use?
4. Can we maintain our view of the "bigger picture" when we work on micro pieces of language such as word knowledge and syntactic structure?

INTRODUCTORY THOUGHTS

It is difficult to believe that Norris (1997) wrote the words that appear at the beginning of this chapter a decade ago. The article that accompanied her words, "Functional Language Intervention in the Classroom: Avoiding the Tutoring Trap," was among a number of contributions in the 1990s that encouraged speech-language pathologists (SLPs) to look beyond their "speech rooms," tests, and intervention approaches that isolated language from its contexts—the classroom and the curriculum. Fortunately, the writings of the past two decades in particular have helped us reevaluate the creation of goals and objectives that live outside of the classroom and that "pull apart" the components of language without putting them together again. Norris's (1997) contribution, among others, offered us many suggestions that integrate language intervention and classroom goals.

As this text suggests, we have come a long way from viewing syntactic forms or pragmatic functions as separate and distinct pieces of language that should be taught "away from" classroom and curricular contexts and still have relevance for school-age students with language learning disabilities (LLD). Syntactic and pragmatic dimensions of language often remain in the forefront of intervention goals, but they are painted on a much broader canvas than they were two decades ago. Indeed, the particular pragmatics of school versus the pragmatics of other communicative situations are now recognized and understood. And as Norris's (1997) words suggest, maintaining a long-term functional view of language is also critical in the intervention process. As a way to revisit our goal of creating curriculum-relevant and strategic intervention programs, we will engage readers in a three-pronged discussion covering the following topics in this chapter:

■ Ways that state standards and benchmarks inform intervention
■ Word knowledge and decoding as important micro aspects of intervention

- Intervention activities and tools that beg the question, What's the point of this activity?

State Standards and Benchmarks: An Example of Keeping Language Functional and Relevant

Ehren (e.g., Ehren, 2004) has talked a great deal about the evolving role of SLPs in schools. She has also talked about how professionals' understanding of state standards and benchmarks helps set a direction for language intervention. For SLPs specifically, knowing one's state standards and understanding their language underpinnings is one way to keep language intervention focused and relevant. But, again, as emphasized throughout this text, SLPs should avoid replicating the work of classroom and content-area teachers. Rather, they should be asking the following questions, as pointed out by Ehren (2004):

- What are the attitudes, knowledge, skills, and strategies my students need to meet the standard?
- What are the teacher's instructional demands (Ehren, 2006a)?
- What is the "language reason" a student "can't" meet a standard? What language abilities are assumed to be intact and already acquired that relate to the standard?

Consider the examples of state standards from the California State Department of Education for Science (www.cde.ca.gov/be/st/ss/scgrade4.asp) presented in Box 9-1. After reviewing these standards, then what?

Even a fast read of the abbreviated excerpts from the California Grade 4 Science Content Standards brings home, yet again, the complexity of content required at this relatively early grade level. Students are expected to demonstrate an understanding of the relationships among events and the animate and inanimate beings and objects that inhabit the earth. They are also expected to absorb new, abstract, and multilayered (and multisyllabic) terminology. Indeed, the level of background knowledge and linguistic savvy needed to "crack the standards" seems almost overwhelming (for both clinicians and the students they serve). But, again, SLPs' knowledge of the standards helps them to frame language intervention goals within a context of expectations for a particular grade. Working collaboratively with classroom and content-area teachers is a natural step in the process. Teachers' perceptions about their students' academic vulnerability (as per the standards) provides data that should join with their SLP's evaluation of the language knowledge and skills required. Results from the SLP's language assessments (which may include both formal and informal and in- and out-of-classroom curricular components) contribute information that identifies language gaps that are influencing—or blocking—a student's ability to meet all or some of the standards. Assessments should also shed light on students' strengths.

As we look across the science standards listed, we can see that there are several clues in the standards that speak to their language underpinnings. By perusing the standards, we not only gain an understanding of the language demanded to "get" the concepts expressed but we also acquire an appreciation for what teachers and students have to accomplish by the end of fourth grade. In terms of language, we might ask the following questions: Does the student know enough about basic cause-effect relationships? Does he or she

9

| BOX 9-1 | *Grade 4 Science Content Standards* |

Students are required to meet science content standards across a variety of topics, including physical sciences, life sciences, and earth sciences.

Life Sciences
Standard 3
3.0. Living organisms depend on one another and on their environment for survival. As a basis for understanding this concept:
  a. *Students know* ecosystems can be characterized by their living and nonliving components.
  b. *Students know* that in any particular environment, some kinds of plants and animals survive well, some survive less well, and some cannot survive at all.
  c. *Students know* that many plants depend on animals for pollination and seed dispersal, and animals depend on plants for food and shelter.
  d. *Students know* that most microorganisms do not cause disease and that many are beneficial.

Earth Sciences
Standard 5
5.0. Waves, wind, water, and ice shape and reshape Earth's land surface. As a basis for understanding this concept:
  a. *Students know* that some changes in the Earth are due to slow processes, such as erosion, and some changes are due to rapid processes, such as landslides, volcanic eruptions, and earthquakes.
  b. *Students know* that natural processes, including freezing and thawing and the growth of roots, cause rocks to break down into smaller pieces.

From California State Board of Education. (1998, October). *Grade four science content standards.* Sacramento, CA: California State Board of Education. Retrieved January 9, 2007, from www.cde.ca.gov/be/st/ss/scgrade4.asp.

have sufficient lexical knowledge and naming ability to connect the dots among causal (and other) relationships expected for this grade level?

Specific to the standards presented, we might consider the significance of phrases such as "are characterized by" and "depend on," among others mentioned in this text (e.g., the smaller linguistic units/connector phrases, etc.). Although students may not have to use these specific words in their explanations, the concepts behind the words should be part of their language learning repertoires. Likewise, can the student organize (in writing and otherwise) a compare-contrast text (beyond science requirements)? We can appreciate the need for students to understand ways of comparing and contrasting "living" and "nonliving" things and "slow" and "rapid" processes by reading the standards. Does the student with LLD have enough "surrounding vocabulary"—that is, those words that "accompany" content-area lexicons? For example, a comparison of living and nonliving things would include the comprehension and use of words and phrases such as "alike," "different," "these have some similar traits," "these do not belong because...," and so on. (Recall the connector words listed in Appendix D.)

In addition, SLPs can consider students' morphophonemic abilities as they connect to reading (including decoding and comprehension), writing, and developing strategies for learning new words. We see words such as "ecosystems," "nonliving," and "microorganisms," among others, that consist of root words plus their prefixes and suffixes. Do students have an understanding of and a strategic approach for breaking up words? Do they know what the separate morphological pieces mean (such as "micro" and "organism")? Do they understand that morphological skills can "carry over" to other word attack and comprehension-heavy situations? Do they have strategies for finding the meanings of unfamiliar words (DeKemel, 2003d; see upcoming section on "Words")? Although other questions might be posed for science as noted in this text, these aforementioned examples that relate more specifically to state standards provide us with additional food for thought. Again, the integration of derivation and fundamental literacies should be a goal for professionals who work both within and outside of classrooms.

A Continuing Exploration of Standards

Consider the complexity of concepts covered as early as Grade 4 in social studies, as represented in excerpts from the California State Standards (www.cde.ca.gov/be/st/ss/hstmain.asp) (Box 9-2) and ask, What language skills are required?

What the Social Studies Standards Say. Again, it is a worthwhile endeavor to look through one's state standards. As with the science standards, professionals who work outside of classrooms—such as SLPs—may not be as familiar with the standards as teachers must be to meet the standards for their grades and specialized content areas. But clearly, speech-language pathologists and teachers can form strong partnerships when they engage in dialogues about the standards. As noted previously, SLPs can contribute information about the language knowledge required to meet the standards and offer suggestions for those students in trouble. Indeed, the language skills that underpin the standards are striking, not to mention the information load outlined in the curricular content. We see the terms *describe, explain, identify, discuss,* and others that give us a sense of how students must demonstrate their newly acquired knowledge—if they have it or if they "get it." Acquiring proficiency with semantic relations and associations among words, sentences, and connected text is necessary because these elements form a foundation for success. Understanding and using those genres that code cause-effect, problem-solution, and enumeration, among other expository structures, are also among the language skills that weave their way through the social studies standards. It may not be an overstatement to say that we can see why social studies presents many students with challenges as noted here and throughout this text.

BOX 9-2	*Grades 4 and 5 History–Social Science Content Standards*

Grade 4

Students learn the story of their home state, unique in American history in terms of its vast and varied geography, its many waves of immigrants beginning with pre-Columbian societies, its continuous diversity, economic energy, and rapid growth. In addition to the specific treatment of milestones in California history, students examine the state in the context of the rest of the nation with an emphasis on the U.S. Constitution and the relationship between state and federal government.

4.2. Students describe the social, political, cultural, and economic life and interactions among peoples of California from pre-Columbian societies to the Spanish mission Mexican rancho periods.

1. Discuss the major nations of California Indians, including their geographic distribution, economics, legends, and religious beliefs; describe how they depended on, adapted to, and modified the environment by cultivation of land and use of sea resources.

2. Identify the early land and sea routes to, and European settlements in, California with a focus on the routes of the North Pacific (e.g., by Captain James Cook, Vitus Bering, Juan Cabrillo), noting especially the role of mountains, deserts, ocean currents, and wind patterns.

3. Describe the Spanish exploration and colonization of California, including...(continues).

4. Describe the mapping of, geographic basis of, and economic factors in the placement and function of the Spanish missions...(continues).

(Additional objectives are listed under standard 4.2.)

Grade 5

Students in grade five study the development of the nation up to 1850, with an emphasis on the people who were already here, when and from where others arrived, and why they came. Students learn about the colonial government founded on Judeo-Christian principles, the ideas of the Enlightenment, and the English traditions of self-government. They recognize that ours is a nation that has a constitution that derives its power from the people, that has gone through a revolution, that once sanctioned slavery, that experienced conflict over land with the original inhabitants, and that experiences a westward movement.

5.5. Students explain the causes of the American Revolution.

1. Understand how political, religious, and economic ideas and interests brought about the Revolutionary resistance to imperial policy, the Stamp Act, the Townshend Acts, and taxes on tea, Coercive Acts.

2. Know the significance of the first and second Continental Congress and the Committees of Correspondence.

BOX 9-2 *Grades 4 and 5 History–Social Science Content Standards—cont'd*

> 3. Understand the people and events associated with the drafting and signing of the Declaration of Independence and the document's significance, including the key political concepts it embodies, the origins of those concepts, and its role in severing ties with Great Britain.*

From California State Board of Education. (1998, October). *History–social science content standards.* Sacramento, CA: California State Board of Education. Retrieved January 9, 2007, from http://www.cde.ca.gov/be/st/ss/hstmain.asp.
Grade 5 information from http:www.cde.ca.gov/be/st/ss/hstgrade5.asp.
*A final objective relates to understanding the course and consequences of the American Revolution.

BOX 9-3 *Grades 5 and 7 English/Language Arts Content Standards*

> **From Grade 5**
> **2.0. Reading Comprehension (Focus on Information Materials)**
> Students read and understand grade-level appropriate material. They describe and connect essential ideas, arguments, and perspectives of the text by using their knowledge of text structure, organization, and purpose. The selections in *Recommended Readings in Literature, Kindergarten through Grade Eight* illustrate the quality and complexity of the materials to be read by students. In addition, by grade eight students read one million words annually on their own, including good representation of grade-level appropriate narrative and expository text (e.g., classic and contemporary literature, magazines, newspapers, online information). In grade five, students make progress toward this goal.
>
> **Structural Features of Informational Materials**
> 2.1. Understand how text features (e.g., format, graphics, sequence, diagrams, illustrations, charts, maps) make information accessible and usable.
> 2.2. Analyze text that is organized in sequential or chronological order.

9

Continued

English/Language Arts Content. When we consider the state standards for Grades 7 or 8 in the English/Language Arts Content, we note that they include more in-depth knowledge of fiction (including plot-theme-character), nonfiction, poetry, and text structure and organization. Students are expected to come very far by the end of their elementary–middle school careers. For example, consider the California state standards that are listed in Box 9-3.

BOX 9-3   *Grades 5 and 7 English/Language Arts Content Standards—cont'd*

Comprehension and Analysis of Grade-Level Appropriate Text
2.3. Discern main ideas and concepts presented in texts, identifying and assessing evidence that supports those ideas.
2.4. Draw inferences, conclusions, or generalizations about text and support them with textual evidence and prior knowledge.

Expository Critique
2.5. Distinguish facts, supported inferences, and opinions in text.

Grade 7
2.0. Reading Comprehension (Focus on Informational Materials)
The statement reads the same as the above 2.0 for grade seven with the exception of the last sentence that notes: In grade seven, students make substantial progress toward this goal.
   Foundational skills are recognized for the standards. Among the foundational skills listed are the following:
■ Make inferences
■ Make predictions
■ Develop strategies for reading: visualizing and connecting
■ Recognize compare-contrast organization
■ Develop strategies for reading informational texts: skimming, scanning, and understanding graphics
■ Draw conclusions and make judgments
■ Analyze text that uses main idea organizational pattern
■ Analyze text that uses the chronological order/sequence order organizational pattern

Structural Features of Informational Materials
2.1. Understand and analyze the differences in structure and purpose between various categories of informational materials (e.g., textbooks, newspapers, instructional manuals, signs).
   Foundational skills: Understand and analyze an instructional manual; identify main idea and supporting detail.
2.2. Locate information by using a variety of consumer, workplace, and public documents.
   Foundational skills: Understand functional reading materials including product information, public notices, and workplace documents.
2.3. Analyze text that uses the cause-effect organizational pattern.

Comprehension and Analysis of Grade-Appropriate Text
2.4. Identify and trace the development of an author's argument, point of view, or perspective in text.
   Foundational skills: Identify overgeneralizations.
2.5. Understand and explain the use of a simple mechanical device by following technical directions.

BOX 9-3 | *Grades 5 and 7 English/Language Arts Content Standards—cont'd*

Expository Critique
2.6. Assess the adequacy, accuracy, and appropriateness of author's evidence to support claims and assertions, noting instances of bias and stereotyping.
Foundational skills: Recognize fact and opinion; identify and distinguish between statements of fact and fiction; identify author's purpose.

From California State Board of Education. (1997, December). *English–language arts content standards.* Sacramento, CA: California State Board of Education. Retrieved January 9, 2007, from www.cde.ca.gov/be/st/ss/engmain.asp.

Looking at specific areas in the English standards, for example, across fiction and nonfiction, one would observe the Grade 7 standards and the foundational skills that form a cluster needed for mastery of the standards (McDougal, 2002), as outlined in the following box:

Grade 7 English/Language Arts Content Standards

Reading Domain
Fiction
Some of the standards that relate to fiction would include (among others in both the Writing and Language Conventions Domains) the following:

- Standard 1.3. Clarify word meanings through the use of definition, example, restatement, or contrast.
- Standard 3.2. Identify events that advance the plot and determine how each event explains past or present action(s) or foreshadows future action(s).
- Standard 3.3. Analyze characterization as delineated through a character's thoughts, words, speech patterns, and actions; the narrator's description; and the thoughts, words, and actions of other characters.
- Standard 3.4. Identify and analyze recurring themes across works (e.g., the value of bravery, loyalty, and friendship; the effects of loneliness).

Nonfiction
Standards that relate to nonfiction would include the following:

- Standard 1.2. Uses knowledge of Greek, Latin, and Anglo-Saxon roots and affixes to understand content-area vocabulary.
- Standard 1.3. (Overlaps with above. Clarify word meanings through the use of definition, example, restatement, or contrast.)

Continued

Grade 7 English/Language Arts Content Standards—cont'd

- Standard 2.3. Analyze text that uses the cause-and-effect organizational pattern.
- Standard 2.6. Assess the adequacy, accuracy, and appropriateness of the author's evidence to support claims and assertions, noting instances of bias and stereotyping.
- Standard 3.1. Articulate the expressed purposes and characteristics of different forms of prose (e.g., short story, novel, novella, essay).

From California State Board of Education. (1997, December). *Grade seven English–language arts content standards.* Sacramento, CA: California State Board of Education. Retrieved January 9, 2007, from www.cde.ca.gov/be/st/ss/enggrade7.asp.

Among the foundational skills for the standards that cluster around fiction as a subarea of English/Language Arts are the following:
- Using contextual clues to determine word meaning
- Making inferences
- Recognizing cause-effect relationships
- Analyzing settings
- Determining central conflict in a plot
- Identifying major and minor characters
- Identifying character traits and motives
  The foundational skills in the nonfiction cluster include the following:
- Using contextual clues to determine word meaning
- Analyzing text organization in chronological order
- Clarifying an understanding of texts by creating outlines, logical notes, summaries, or reports
- Identifying the author's purpose
- Identifying and distinguishing between statements of fact and statements of opinion

Looking Across State Standards

As we look across grade-level and subject-area standards, we gain a better understanding of the role that SLPs can play in unraveling the language abilities that underlie and interact with the requirements of standards. Clearly, aspects of syntactic, semantic, and pragmatic components come into play in systemic harmony (ideally, of course) in spoken and written connected text to form a backbone for mastery of the standards. SLPs, in concert with teachers and content area specialists, determine which standards (or areas) are most problematic and develop literacy-focused priorities to help students with LLD manage the curriculum requirements as defined by the standards. According to Ehren (2004), who looked across state standards in Grade 8 reading, there are many common language underpinnings that cut across standards within a grade and across grades. For example, many Grade 8 standards require students to "summarize the literal gist of a selection," "identify main ideas," "synthesize a group of main ideas into a big idea," and "paraphrase text." Among the language underpinnings according to Ehren (2004) that relate to these and other standards in reading would be the following:

■ *For summarizing gists/identifying main ideas/synthesizing ideas:* understanding the notion of concept hierarchy (big ideas, smaller ideas, even smaller ideas, etc.); and being able to place ideas in the correct hierarchy in relation to one another

■ *For paraphrasing text:* being aware that there is more than one way to express a thought; knowing synonyms for words; having facility with a variety of syntactic patterns; identifying key ideas in a unit of syntax; and manipulating syntax without changing meaning (as per Ehren, 2004; Chapter 3, this text)

Along with the language skills and abilities that students are taught, they must learn to *use* what they know to match the demands of the situation.

Thus although we may not be able to know everything about every standard for all grades and subjects, it is clear that having knowledge about one's state standards, perhaps starting with English/Language Arts, is an important component in the development and delivery of language intervention services at school-age levels. The listing of foundational skills under the California state standards can also be helpful to consider but, again, students with LLD may require additional language exposure and practice to acquire these skills, which are viewed as "prerequisites" for the standards. Clearly, SLPs must stay in a posture of discovery that takes them through the many "layers" of ability needed to get to the core of a student's language challenges. We are reminded of another image of "layered language"—the basic versus metalinguistic layer—that was discussed in our introductory chapter (see Chapter 1, p. 8–10). Metalinguistic proficiency, the ability to talk about, manipulate, analyze, synthesize, and judge language, forms another cluster of abilities that cuts across standards and curricular requirements throughout the grades.

A Word about Words: Another Thought about Keeping Language Intervention Functional and Relevant

Acquiring a working knowledge of state standards helps us to appreciate the horizon of skills required at each grade level and the way the curricular requirements are expressed. "Vocabulary" is another area that is predominant in the intervention goals and objectives of SLPs. We frequently talk about students with LLD as having limited lexical knowledge. Learning new words, including learning their basic and figurative meanings, as well as their content-specific meanings, among other skills, is a challenge for students with and without LLD. The science and social studies standards, for example, remind us that students have to absorb and use many new and unfamiliar words in spoken, read, and written contexts in school. It is staggering to think of the idea as noted in the California standards that "by grade eight, students read one million words annually on their own" (www.cde.ca.gov/be/ss/ela.grade8.asp). It is clear that the standards assume that students have and will acquire many vocabulary-related skills. For example, students in Grade 4 have to differentiate different rock formations by finding words to describe their properties and formations. Grade 7 students are required to clarify word meanings through the use of definitions, examples, restatement, or contrast. We have touched on this aspect of semantics in various sections of this text, but it is important to reconsider this aspect of language intervention with the caveat of keeping the bigger picture and the curriculum in mind when choosing to work on "vocabulary." The areas of evolving lexical knowledge, word naming, and word retrieval have been studied by many researchers whose work has helped bridge the gap between many theoretical constructs and daily practice (e.g., Blachowicz, 1994; DeKemel, 2003d; German, 1991, 1992, 2000; Kail & Leonard, 1986; Nelson & Van Meter, 2006).

Aspects of Word Learning for Consideration

Wallach and Miller (1988) used a classic quote at the beginning of their chapter that included a discussion of vocabulary and naming abilities. The chapter presented ways to combine spoken and written activities similar to some of the suggestions we will provide in this chapter. The quote from Bashir (1987) went like this: "It is not only a matter of asking what a word means, it's a matter of asking *what else* the word means." Bashir's (1987) eloquent words asked SLPs and teachers to think about the broad-based and complex nature of lexical knowledge and use. Clearly, as students move through the grades, knowing the literal meanings of words will take them only so far. Students have to appreciate many things about words, including the different ways that idioms, similes, metaphors, and other nonliteral forms manifest themselves in speech and in print (Milosky, 1994; Nippold et al., 2001; Owens, 2001; van Kleeck, 1994). Being "word savvy" is an important skill that will influence and interact with academic success. Having a rich and elaborated repertoire of words at one's disposal and having strategies for learning and retaining new words are lifelong pursuits.

> As students advance through grades, they must appreciate the ways that nonliteral forms manifest themselves in speech and writing.

In addition to developing a basic lexicon for their spoken language repertoires, students have to learn how to read and write both common and curriculum-specific words. They also have to develop proficiency in using those "literate" forms and text-related words that are required in particular situations, for example, expressing persuasive arguments that call for more formal, stylistic modifications in speech and on paper (Nippold et al., 2005). Students also need to acquire the self-monitoring skills that will help them use effective strategies for learning new words and finding the meanings of unfamiliar words. The increased language flexibility and creativity that develops in the school years, some of which is manifested in students' abilities to go beyond the "literalness" of word and text meaning, is a critical transition that we hope to help our students achieve.

Volumes have been written about "vocabulary," an area of semantics that has been studied widely, offering varying opinions about how vocabulary knowledge connects to cognitive ability, how to teach vocabulary, and how deficits in vocabulary relate to literacy, among other topics (DeKemel, 2003d). Clinicians and educators have always been concerned about and focused on this area using information about vocabulary acquisition and growth from many sources. Owens (2001), for example, provides an excellent summary of the research on the semantic and lexical development; DeKemel (2003d) applies some of this research to students with LLD. On the reading side, literacy researchers and reading specialists have long studied the effects of vocabulary and related decoding abilities on comprehension (e.g., Kamhi & Catts, 2005; Tabors et al., 2001; Torgeson et al., 2005).

Marion Blank's "space excerpt" on p. 56 in Chapter 3 provided us with an example of the way that lexical knowledge interacts with text comprehension. Our history, science, and math examples have also shown how "smaller linguistic units" (i.e., individual words) influence comprehension. And as readers of this text well know, much has been written about the links between vocabulary ability and traditional measures of intelligence, although the vocabulary-intelligence correlation is certainly fraught with controversy (e.g., Baddeley et al., 1998; Nelson et al., 2006; Stahl, 1986; Sternberg, 1987). Although there are no easy answers in theory and practice, we do know that having a "way with words" is critical to surviving and thriving in the clinics and classrooms of America. In her classic article describing vocabulary approaches in school, some of which are still popular today, Blachowicz (1986) provided readers with a typical scenario characteristic of the fast-moving sequence that occurs in many middle and high school situations, as follows:

Monday: Learn new words.
Tuesday: Look them up and write a dictionary definition.
Wednesday: Write a sentence.
Thursday: Study words.
Friday: Take a test.

More recently, DeKemel (2003d) explored the complex and multilayered nature of semantic knowledge, which she notes is sometimes defined under the general heading of "vocabulary." And "vocabulary" is often thought of as learning new words and their definitions. Recognizing that learning to define words is an aspect of semantic knowledge predominant in academic learning, DeKemel (2003d) encourages clinicians and teachers to think beyond "definitional activities" and consider a number of elements that encompass "vocabulary knowledge" (Box 9-4). For example, one of the elements of vocabulary knowledge that may be familiar to SLPs is *concept formation*. *Concept formation* relates to a student's underlying idea of what a word could mean based on his or her perceptions, experiences, and world knowledge. So when a student sees the word "war" or "compromise" in a fifth-grade social studies text, does he or she have any concept of what the word could mean from past experience? Does the student have "wars" with his little brother (or play games that involve "war"), or does she have to "compromise" with younger siblings? Clearly, words such as "dog" are easier to attach perceptual features to or to visualize (form a concept for) than more abstract words such as "compromise."

DeKemel (2003d) outlines additional elements of vocabulary that relate to school success. She reminds practitioners to think about helping students acquire lexical proficiency across a variety of areas, including *content words* (such as nouns, verbs, and adjectives), *antonyms* (understanding opposites), *synonyms* (understanding meaning equivalences), and words with *multiple*

9

BOX 9-4	*Elements of Vocabulary Knowledge*

- Concept formation (underlying idea of a word's meaning based on perceptions, experiences, and world knowledge)
- Content words (nouns, verbs, adjectives)
- Antonyms (opposites)
- Synonyms (meaning equivalences)
- Multiple meanings (words that change based on context)
- Superordinate and subordinate categories (relationships; e.g., superordinate category *American League*, with subordinate category *New York Yankees*)
- Semantic features (characteristics; e.g., for a baseball team: nine players, first baseman, manager, etc.)
- Selective restrictions (items that cannot be used together; e.g., hot snow, male mother)

Data from DeKemel, K. (2003). Building a power lexicon: Vocabulary acquisition in language-learning disabled students. In K. DeKemel (Ed.), *Intervention in language arts: A practical guide for speech-language pathologists* (pp. 79–94). Philadelphia: Butterworth-Heinemann.

meanings (words that change based on context). For example, the word "bat" has multiple meanings that change across contexts, such as when one is referring to a baseball game or a Halloween story. According to DeKemel (2003d), students must also learn about *superordinate* and *subordinate* categories. Thus "American League" could function as a *superordinate* category with Yankees, Angels, White Sox, and so on serving as examples of *subordinate* words in the category. Each team name could be delineated further with the names of individual players. Using "National League" as a *superordinate* category, we would find Mets, Dodgers, Cubs, and so on as *subordinate* words in the category. Complex semantic networks also allow us to see different superordinate-subordinate relationships. For example, the Yankees and Mets both fall under the umbrella of "New York" teams, the Dodgers and Angels represent "California" or "Los Angeles–area" teams, and the White Sox and Cubs represent Chicago teams. Other elements of semantic knowledge that relate to word knowledge include learning about *semantic features* (e.g., a baseball team has a number of features, such as nine players, with the positions of pitcher, catcher, first baseman, etc.; each team has a manager and coaches; each team represents a city or state; etc.) and *selective restrictions* (e.g., Kobe Bryant cannot be listed under "baseball players," and we cannot use "male mother" or "hot snow" as noted by DeKemel, 2003d, p. 80).

DeKemel (2003d), Ehren (2003), and Nelson and Van Meter (2006), among other researcher-practitioners, recognize the importance of mastering these aforementioned aspects of word knowledge. But they remind us to keep the "relevance" of our choices in the forefront of our clinical and educational decisions when working on these facets of "vocabulary." This has been a recurring theme of this text and is emphasized in current research. For example, Ehren (2003, 2004) has reminded us time and again that many school-related activities require underlying lexical ability. Ehren's (2004) example of "paraphrasing" as a reading comprehension strategy comes to mind (as noted on p. 279 in this chapter and on p. 54 in Chapter 3). One of the language underpinnings of paraphrasing is the understanding that you can substitute words for one another (using *synonyms*) and maintain the meaning of a sentence or text. Likewise, organizing an expository report, such as comparing and contrasting the contributions of American presidents in social studies and fast and slow processes in science, may also be facilitated by an understanding of superordinate and subordinate relations among words. This understanding of superordinate-subordinate categorizations may facilitate organizing one's ideas into major and minor points and is reminiscent of the often-used notion of "finding the main idea." Again, we can see how lexical knowledge weaves its way through other aspects of linguistic proficiency, but we also recognize that "vocabulary work" should be embarked on within an eye toward its connection to the curriculum and larger pieces of text. In a similar sense, decoding abilities should be seen as part of the picture toward comprehending what one reads with accuracy and fluency.

Although readers may agree with the previous points, we could also ask: Is it ever appropriate to teach words out of context? We might only think back to the SATs or GREs to know that words are often tested and taught "in isolation." Recall Blachowicz's (1986) scenario of a school week noted earlier. Thus learning about words—their definitions and roots—and learning how to use words in sentences are useful classroom skills. DeKemel (2003d) recognizes this reality but points out that there is still much controversy surrounding the "best way" to teach vocabulary to students with and without LLD. Research suggests that providing students with both a definitional and contextual component and many exposures to new vocabulary, plus encouraging students to talk about, think about, and use words in different situations, are effective vocabulary teaching methods. In agreement with multidimensional approaches, DeKemel (2003d) also encourages us to keep the bigger picture of connected text in mind when we are including "vocabulary intervention" into therapy sessions. She makes a point about the whole being bigger than its parts when she talks about sentence comprehension. She wrote the following:

> Sentences represent a meaning greater than the sum of the individual words that make up that sentence; listeners and readers tend to focus on whole-sentence meaning, and to do that, they must readily understand relationships between and across the words in a sentence. (DeKemel, 2003d, p. 80)

Nippold and colleagues (2005) make some very interesting observations about words and word knowledge (and various aspects of syntax, semantics, and pragmatics) in their study of persuasive writing in children, adolescents, and adults. They remind us of the oral-to-literate transition when they write that "effective persuasive writing...requires the use of literate vocabulary, words that have a low frequency of occurrence in the language in general but do occur in formal written contexts" (Nippold et al., 2005, p. 127; see also

Nippold, 1998). One of the things that students do as they get older—advancing from sixth to twelfth grades—is make better use of later-developing connectors such as *therefore, on the other hand, meanwhile, similarly, conversely, rather,* and so on to frame their arguments. In addition to these connector words, some of which were mentioned in other sections of this text, Nippold and colleagues (2005) say that other types of *literate vocabulary* improve during adolescence and interact with one's ability to write (or express) persuasive language. Two categories of words are mentioned by these researchers: (1) word learning that focuses on abstract concepts; and (2) the use of metalinguistic and metacognitive verbs ("metaverbs"). We know from our discussions of curricular content that words mastered by middle school (and earlier) involve abstract concepts. Nippold and colleagues (2005) use the examples of abstract words such as *diversion, federalism,* and *implication.* We saw history words such as *emancipation, tyranny,* and *freedom,* among others, in this text. Metaverbs are those that refer to acts of speaking (*assert, concede, predict, argue,* etc.) and thinking (*hypothesize, remember, doubt, assume,* etc.) (Nippold et al., 2005, p. 127). According to Nippold and colleagues, metaverbs such as *say, think,* and *know* may be in the repertoires of younger school-age children whereas less common verbs such as *predict, conclude,* and *interpret* evolve later.

> **Metaverbs** refer to acts of speaking (e.g., *assert, concede, predict, argue*) and thinking (e.g., *hypothesize, remember, doubt, assume*).

Nippold and colleagues (2005) contributed information about the acquisition of various aspects of language in relation to the writing of persuasive text. But they also brought word-level/semantic knowledge back to connected text. In terms of word-level/semantic abilities, Nippold and colleagues (2005) found that connector words, abstract nouns, and metaverb usage increased from childhood to adulthood. For example, younger students (below sixth grade) tended to use *also, so,* and *then* when making points, whereas adolescents (above sixth grade) were more likely to use *on the other hand, consequently,* and similar connectors. Use of a variety of abstract nouns increased with the greatest frequency when compared with the overall use of both connectors (which remained difficult) and the more advanced metaverbs. Although readers are encouraged to go to the original article for a detailed discussion of the acquisitions across semantic, syntactic, and pragmatic areas, the important point here is that persuasive writing has the potential to encourage the use of certain categories of words such as metaverbs, which may be more "common" or which may fit more "naturally" into this type of text as Nippold and colleagues (2005) suggest. In other words, our genre choice may have the added benefit of encouraging the use of vocabulary for a purpose and within a context. We will come back to some of the implications of their study later in this chapter in the section entitled "Why Am I Doing This? A Meta Exploration of Selected Intervention Activities."

Although not a specific aspect of this discussion, it should be noted that syntactic and pragmatic advances found by Nippold and colleagues (2005) included gradual increases in essay length, mean length of utterance, and uses of complex syntactic forms such as relative clauses. Older writers, not surprisingly, had a more refined pragmatic sense in that they added many reasons for their points of view to make them clear to the reader, and they tended to acknowledge the opinions of others in their essays. Again, the interaction of macro (type of discourse) and micro (word-level choices) aspects of language is demonstrated in Nippold and colleagues (2005) and many other current works (e.g., Nelson & Van Meter, 2006; Gillam & Gorman, 2004).

Word Finding, Word Retrieval, and More: The LLD Connection

A 12-year-old student with LLD was taking a science exam. One of the "true-false" items is as follows:

TRUE or FALSE: The backbone is made of vertebrae.

The student wrote FALSE for this item. When asked to read the sentence, the student read: "The backbone is made of vegetables." Following the logic of his read rendition, one could see why he indicated that the answer was false. The student's misstep and others like it ask us to ask a number of questions that speak to the connections (and disconnections) among word knowledge, word retrieval, and word recognition (decoding). For example, is the word "vertebrae" in his spoken language repertoire? Does the word have meaning for him? Can he define or explain what it means or make a connection to other words he knows? Can he use the word (produce it) in an oral presentation? Or is "vertebrae" an unknown word to him? If it is more or less "unknown" or unfamiliar to him, how much meaning would it hold in this sentence even if his decoding skills were more precise? And, looking at his decoding skills, we note that he attempts to "find the word" with a first phoneme "stab," at the beginning of each syllable, using the "v," "t," and "b," which leads him to the lexical entry of "vegetables"—a familiar word that is part of his spoken repertoire.

Referring back to some of the ideas discussed in Chapter 5, we know that it is not uncommon to substitute a familiar-sounding (or looking) word for an unfamiliar one in both spoken and written language. Indeed, listeners and readers search for patterns and familiarity to make sense out of what they are hearing and seeing. For the student who misread the word "vertebrae," both semantic and phonological aspects of word knowledge and retrieval were targeted in his language intervention program (and embedded in and interactive with connected discourse skills). That is, his intervention included expanding his understanding of words (conceptual and semantic features), facilitating his word naming and retrieval abilities (phonological renditions), and improving his word recognition (decoding) skills. Moreover, he needed to develop *strategies* for learning new words, expanding their connections to other words and alternative meanings, and connecting new lexical entries to print.

Nelson and Van Meter (2006) support this last statement. They remind clinicians and teachers that they cannot teach students every word they need to know. And while SLPs can help students use and understand selected connector words and other key words that pull text together, their goals should also be geared, as mentioned, toward strategic outcomes for students. As expressed beautifully by Nelson and Van Meter (2006):

It is important to remember that there are far too many words to teach, either explicitly or implicitly. Students need to become better and more independent word learners. They need to know how to recognize when they don't know a

9

word or when they need a word. For reading, students need to know how to figure out the word from context or morphological analysis. For writing, they need to know how to reflect on their own knowledge to seek words that will express the desired meanings. Finally, students need to know how to use tools, such as thesauri and dictionaries, to further comprehension and expression goals. (p. 100)

German's landmark work (e.g., German, 1986, 1994), among the work of many other researcher-clinicians (e.g., Kail & Leonard, 1986; Lahey & Edwards, 1996), have taught us much about word-finding and word-retrieval deficits in students with LLD. Some of readers of this text who are considered part of the "baby boomer" generation may identify with how it feels to have word-retrieval problems when they are challenged by the common phenomenon of "losing words" and trying to find them. To say the least, it is a frustrating experience to "know" what you want to say and then to stop seemingly "dead in one's tracks" when the name of a person, place, or thing escapes you. The word may "resurface" after a time (such as 2:00 AM), but it is a daunting experience when the "lost word phenomenon" happens, especially if it starts to happen with increasing frequency. (See German [2001] for a fascinating discussion.)

But clearly, the boomers have some advantages that students with LLD may not have. As readers and writers of language, baby boomers have the benefit of print, which can help them retain old words as well as learn new ones. Boomers may also have the background (conceptual) knowledge, comprehension, and elaborated meanings for words that are "in their heads." Although they "lose" the phonological representation (the actual name of something), there is always the potential to "get it back." Boomers (hopefully) also have various strategies for finding both old (lost) and new words. For example, they may use a prompt such as going through the alphabet to find a lost word. They might visualize what something looks like or visualize a situation to retrieve a word. They might wait for someone else in the room to produce the name of a guest. To disambiguate less familiar or rarely used words, boomers (and younger proficient readers) might use the context of an article to figure out a word's meaning or they might use a dictionary to search for a closely matched meaning.

The boomers may try any number of strategies, making judgments about which ones work best and why, to retrieve words. For students with LLD, word-knowledge and word-retrieval problems are certainly just as daunting as, and maybe even more daunting than, they are for the baby boomers. Coupled with background knowledge and written language gaps, students with LLD often have a steep slope to climb to enhance their "vocabularies." Additionally, many students with LLD lack or have limited strategies for finding, learning, and retrieving new words.

What complicates the area of "vocabulary" study—its acquisition, instruction, or intervention—as discussed by DeKemel (2003d) and mentioned earlier, are professionals' perceptions of what "vocabulary" means and their different views about how students should be taught vocabulary. In addition, professionals may use the expressions "word finding" or "word retrieval" differently to describe problems that students may have acquiring, absorbing, and using words. "Word recognition," a skill that intersects with spoken language abilities, enters the mix because it refers to the "ability to construct meaning while attending to the printed word" (Gillam & Gorman, 2004, p. 63). As we saw in the "vertebrae" sentence, word knowledge (both semantic and phonological aspects) and decoding were both issues for this particular student. For others, the core of the problem may be different. For example, a student could have words in his or her vocabulary that he or she cannot read or spell (Nelson & Van Meter, 2006). Nonetheless, in the reality of a language learning disabled world, we are advised to exercise caution when viewing problems such as word finding or word recognition (decoding) in a "vacuum." Gillam and Gorman (2004), among others, suggest staying focused on a dynamic view of systems where complex interactions among word, text, and other processing units, including orthographic, phonological, and morphological units, exist and influence one another.

As DeKemel (2003d) pointed out, word learning is facilitated by a *conceptual and experiential base,* and an experiential repertoire, if words are to have any real meaning and if words are going to become part of one's written language inventory. The act of naming, on the other hand, involves the expressive representation of concepts. In essence, names are phonological summaries of semantic information. Children can have a concept (and be able to show you nonverbally that they have it) but not know (or remember) the name for the concept (Rubin & Liberman, 1983; Nelson & Van Meter, 2006). Thus naming difficulties can be related to lack of background knowledge (the semantic base), limited verbal exposure to and practice with the word itself (the phonological structure), or a combination of both. Word learning involves a long and complex process so that individuals may have a partial knowledge of words or, in the case of some students with LLD, they may have a restricted or concrete idea about what a word means (German, 1994). For example, a student may know the meaning of the word "seal" (as an animal) but fail to understand the meaning of the phrase, "he sealed the deal" (German, 1994).

Consider the following examples from Rubin and Liberman's (1983) now-classic study, which considered oral naming errors in relation to word decoding errors in reading:

Target Words (Picture Shown to Child)	Response
Wheelchair	"The thing you sit on when you're sick"
Helicopter	"Airplane"
Escalator	"Elevator"
Scissors	"Sister"

According to Rubin and Liberman (1983), the responses for "wheelchair" and "helicopter" are semantically oriented. Note the circumlocution for "wheelchair" and the substitution of a semantically associated word for "helicopter." The circumlocution may be indicative of some background knowledge and experience with wheelchairs. The airplane response for "helicopter" is certainly in the semantic ballpark, but we would want to know more about the responder's knowledge of helicopters before drawing any conclusions about his or her naming abilities. The responses for "escalator" and "scissors" are especially interesting. "Elevator" and "sister" are phonologically close to the target words. The elevator/escalator pair represents semantic and phonological closeness whereas the sister/scissors pair appears to have phonological closeness alone. Rubin and Liberman (1983) say that phonological stabs such as "sister" for "scissors" (discounting the idea that the student thinks the scissors are his sister) may be considered sophisticated because they show that the child/student is going for structure. As we have noted, students may substitute words they already know for words they cannot pronounce or remember. (Recall our discussion of so-called "auditory processing" errors in Chapter 5.) Thus we might look at "stabs" at words in both spoken and written domains with a careful eye toward what they may say about a student's strategic approach to words and his or her prior knowledge of words.

Indeed, both phonological and semantic approximations for both spoken and written words warrant careful consideration. Although current research suggests that many good readers appear to have more accurate phonological representations of words than poorer and problematic readers (Troia, 2004), there is much to learn about language learning disabled/reading subgroups, as noted in Chapter 2 (Catts & Kamhi, 2005c). Poor readers tend to have difficulty retaining and accessing the phonological representation of words, which may lie in both conceptual/semantic and phonological components. Some poor readers may have "good" semantic skills but still have difficulty with accessing the phonological representation of words (Catts & Kamhi, 2005c). Early on, Rubin and Liberman (1983) suggested looking at decoding problems in connection with potential naming difficulties. Indeed, when we think about it, it becomes clear that decoding, particularly *fast and efficient* decoding, involves coming up with the phonological representation—the pronunciation—of the printed word. (See also Lahey & Edwards [1996] on naming and naming latency in children with language disorders.)

German (1992, 1994) reiterated a number of concepts already mentioned. Her research in word finding and word retrieval led her to the proposal of three major subgroups of children. Recognizing that research is ongoing, she observed the following:

- *Subgroup 1: Retrieval Difficulties.* This group has word-finding difficulties with apparently intact understanding of spoken words. The problem is focused on the production, rather than the comprehension, of target words.
- *Subgroup 2: Comprehension Difficulties.* These students have difficulty comprehending words and using words that are unfamiliar to them or are absent from their lexicons. Their knowledge of target words may be minimal, concrete, or nonexistent.
- *Subgroup 3: Comprehension and Retrieval Difficulties.* The students in this subgroup, as the label suggests, have underlying difficulties learning the meanings of words and they also have problems retrieving the targets. These students usually have difficulty retrieving "known" words, as well as adding new words to their lexical repertoires.

Along with many of her colleagues, German (1994; and personal communication, 2007) reminds practitioners to exercise caution when evaluating the nature and severity of word-finding difficulties. Consistent with informational processing models, German (1994) notes that vocabulary knowledge and its acquisition, along with the word-finding difficulties that may accompany LLD, are influenced by several variables. The *situation or context*, the *nature of the target word*, and the *presence or absence of facilitating cues* are factors that come together to influence one's perceptions or conclusions about what word-finding difficulties look like. For instance, in constrained situations that are common in standardized test scenarios, the student is often asked to name pictures (nouns, verbs, or categories), complete sentences, or provide descriptions of something. According to German (1994), these tasks call for the retrieval of a specific target word. On the other hand, spontaneous situations or discourse-related activities may call for a different level of productivity, lexical savvy, and word-finding ability, as we have seen in various discussions throughout this text (see, for example, Geddes & Fukumoto, 2005, and Chapter 7 in this text; see German, 1991). Discourse abilities are certainly influenced by one's lexical choices, one's repertoire of available words, and one's ability to find words quickly and seemingly effortlessly. Likewise, the type of text in which words are embedded (e.g., Chapter 7) may influence and interact with the type and severity of word-finding problems that may occur (Blank, 2002; Geddes & Fukumoto, 2005; German, 1991).

> The situation or context, the nature of the target word, and the presence or absence of facilitating cues all influence a person's perceptions or conclusions about word-finding difficulties.

Following from constrained versus spontaneous and discourse-related activities, practitioners should also consider the influence that word classes and retrieval cues might have (or not have) on word-finding abilities. For example, it is suggested that nouns may be the easiest to retrieve, followed by verbs, followed by superordinate categories (German, 2000). Similarly, different prompts may or may not enhance a student's retrieval ability. For example, one should consider the facilitative influence of a variety of prompts, including the following: *phonetic prompts* ("/ko/" to prompt comb), *semantic prompts* ("It's not a pear; it's an _____"); and *multiple choice prompts* ("It's either apple, dog, green, or big"). And it is important to remember that a prompt that "works" for one student may not work for another (German, 1987, 1994, 2000, 2001).

Other researchers and practitioners would mirror German's thinking, especially her words of caution about drawing conclusions from limited samples of word-finding abilities. As with many labels and characterizations of students, some writers also suggest that in daily practice we sometimes use the expression "retrieval problem" too quickly to describe word-finding difficulties (e.g., Kail & Leonard, 1986; Levelt et al., 1999; West et al., 1993). From the earlier days of research in this area, Leonard (1986) asked clinicians to consider the possibility that the inability or difficulty some children have in coming up with labels on fast naming and similar tasks is a bigger problem than accessing a word *they already have*. Many naming problems, said Leonard, have more to do with semantic elaboration problems. In other words, many language learning disabled children have not had enough exposure to and practice with the words they supposedly cannot "retrieve." This idea centers around the notion that the more words one has, the richer the associations one can make among words—and thus the faster one can find words to meet the needs of various communicative situations (Kail & Leonard, 1968; Nelson & Van Meter, 2006). Coupled with the research of West and colleagues (1993) and the more recent language-to-reading research (e.g., Catts & Kamhi, 2005a), we might think about the challenge of learning new words for students with LLD, *especially those who are nonreaders or poor readers*. For example, West and colleagues (1993)

9

suggest that nonreaders or poor readers are at a particular disadvantage for learning new words because many rare, moderate-frequency, and low-frequency words appear in print rather than in speech. They point out that children's books contain 50% more rare words than prime-time television and adult conversations, and much of the new vocabulary of the middle grades (not to mention complex syntax) is gleaned from books.

Regardless of the differences that exist among professionals, most researchers agree that semantic elaboration problems and information processing glitches can contribute to word-finding difficulties (Nelson & Van Meter, 2006). And, regardless of one's "take" on the subject, most clinicians and teachers would also agree that lexical and semantic-related deficits are frequently seen in students with LLD. Moreover, these difficulties cut across curricular areas. DeKemel (2003d) reminds us that there are many ways that these deficits manifest themselves. Students who may have shown delayed expressive and receptive vocabulary acquisition in the preschool years may now have difficulty learning new vocabulary in their school years. They may show limited variety and flexibility in word use and diversity. For example, they may use circumlocutions, repeat words in connected discourse, and use less elaborated vocabulary. Students with LLD may also lack a "meta" set or curiosity toward words or they may lack strategies for looking up words or finding words that they fail to understand (see DeKemel, 2003d, p. 87). Thus practitioners are challenged once again to understand students' language learning problems and to find ways to help them overcome their problems. Standardized tools are certainly helpful in this area (see, for example, German, 1990, 1991, 2000), but as our cautionary words suggested earlier, we should also observe lexical performance across contexts, text genres, and curricular content in spoken and written modes.

Intervention Directions: The Text's Themes Continue to Reverberate

Reiterating the themes that permeate this text, DeKemel (2003d) wrote the following:

> Our goal [in semantic intervention] should be not to just add words to the child's lexicon (like adding pennies to a piggy bank); rather our goal should be to teach the child multiple strategies for processing new vocabulary that he or she encounters in context (e.g., in written texts, spoken dialogue, classroom discourse)...The child who has truly mastered meaning-based strategies will be successful at adding new words and concepts throughout life. (p. 87)

Following up on her statement, DeKemel (2003d) provides readers with a number of suggestions that relate to semantic/lexical aspects of language intervention. She indicates that we should keep the following in mind (DeKemel, 2003, p. 88):

■ Have a *metalinguistic* focus in our approach to word learning and its acquisition. She reminds us that the "second layer" of language learning is critical in this endeavor. Help students become aware of how they might learn new words and help them to understand the advantages of having a rich and elaborated vocabulary.

■ Keep *connected discourse* in mind when working on vocabulary building. Expose students to many literary genres, including narratives, poetry, and various types of expository text, which will introduce students to new vocabulary that can be highlighted, discussed, and analyzed.

■ Teach students how to *use context* to deduce word meanings. But, also, work with *other tools* to help them discover word meanings, such as using dictionaries, thesauri, and online aids.

■ *Connect new or elaborated meanings* to students' existing words in addition to adding new words to students' repertoires. Encourage the student to use his/her background knowledge to figure out the meanings of unfamiliar words.

Providing a detailed, integrated, and practical view of semantic/lexical acquisition, DeKemel (2003d) presents a model that demonstrates how goals and objectives can be written in individualized education plans (IEPs), as seen in Box 9-5.

Showing how the "pieces can be pulled together," DeKemel (2003d) encourages practitioners to use curricular vocabulary and take into account the "discovery strategies" needed to acquire new words and build on words already known.

Nelson and Van Meter (2006) also discuss aspects of *meta awareness* as it relates to word comprehension and word decoding. They encourage students to use self-talk strategies as part of a series of activities that are aimed toward helping students connect word forms and word meanings. They propose a series of questions followed by strategies (sometimes additional questions) that cut across curricular materials that appear most often in print. For example, a general question is, What can I ask myself when I don't know how to read a word? Follow-up questions (strategies suggested by Nelson & Van Meter, 2006) are as follows:

■ Do I know this word? (This question is related to oral language/naming ability.)
■ What are the parts I recognize?
■ Does it look like a word I already know?

BOX 9-5

Goals and Objectives for Semantic and Lexical Acquisition

Goal

To improve lexical and semantic language abilities (i.e., vocabulary, word meanings, and word relationships) to levels commensurate with chronological age and grade-level expectancies.

Objectives

1. Student will *identify, describe,* and *use* curricular vocabulary encountered in story books, nonfiction books, textbooks, etc. (target = approximately 10 to 15 new vocabulary items or concepts per story or thematic unit, for a total of approximately 30 to 45 new vocabulary items or concepts per 6-week grading period). Progress will be measured using the following rating scale: 0 = student has no idea what the word or concept means; cannot identify, describe, define, or use the item expressively in context; 1 = student has limited idea of what the word or concept means; may be able to identify, describe, define it (with prompting or cueing), but still cannot use the word or concept spontaneously and expressively in context (e.g., when retelling or discussing a story); 2 = student has a fully developed understanding

Continued

BOX 9-5

Goals and Objectives for Semantic and Lexical Acquisition—cont'd

Objectives—cont'd

of what the word or concept means (able to identify, describe, define it), beginning to be able to use it expressively in a limited fashion (with prompting or cueing); 3 = student has a fully developed understanding of what the word or concept means; can identify, describe, define, and use the word or concept correctly and spontaneously in context, when retelling or discussing the story.

2. Student will demonstrate *context-based strategies* for acquiring new vocabulary words or meanings such as the following:
    a. Using picture clues to infer word meanings
    b. Using whole-sentence meaning (i.e., the rest of the sentence) to infer the meaning of individual words within the sentence (e.g., "Skip that word for now and read the rest of the sentence, and then we'll go back and figure out what that word means.")
    c. Using previously read material and background word or world knowledge to infer or predict the meaning of new words (e.g., "This book, *Heidi*, is about a girl who lived in the *Swiss Alps*. Look at the picture, and tell me what you think *alps* are. That's right, alps are a type of mountain. What do you already know about mountains?")
    d. Using phoneme or grapheme cues to infer meaning of a new word (e.g., from the story *Heidi*: "That word begins with the letter *H*, and it tells you the *name* of the girl in this book. What girl's names do you know that start with *H* that make sense here?" or, "That word begins with the letters *c-h* and refers to the *type of food* that Heidi's grandfather made from goat's milk. What type of dairy product do you eat that comes from milk and starts with ch?" Rating scale: 0 = no mastery of skill; 1 = limited mastery of skill; 2 = complete mastery of skill.

3. Student will demonstrate *dictionary skills and formal strategies* for acquiring new vocabulary including the following:
    a. Ability to locate words in a dictionary using guide words and alphabetization skills
    b. Ability to use phonetic pronunciation key in a dictionary to pronounce words correctly
    c. Ability to identify usage and parts of speech using abbreviations in a dictionary entry
    d. Ability to read and understand definitions in a dictionary
    e. Ability to read and understand sample sentences in a dictionary entry
    f. Ability to subsequently define words without looking at the dictionary entry
    g. Ability to subsequently use words correctly in self-generated sentences without looking at the dictionary entry
    h. Ability to generalize new words and meanings to spontaneous classroom discourse

From DeKemel, K. (2003). Building a power lexicon: Vocabulary acquisition in language-learning disabled students. In DeKemel, K. (Ed.), *Intervention in language arts: A practical guide for speech-language pathologists* (p. 92). Philadelphia: Butterworth-Heinemann.

A more specific question is, What can I do to say this word? Follow-up strategies include the following:

- Look at the word parts or syllables.
- Say each syllable.
- Practice saying each syllable and see if the word makes sense.

A final question is, What can I do to figure out the meaning of this word? Strategies that can be used include the following:

- Read the whole sentence and see if that helps me to learn about the word.
- Look at parts of the word and see if those pieces remind me of a word I already know.
- Read across sentences to determine whether the word still makes sense and fits with the other sentences.
- Ask someone if my word meaning is correct.
- Practice using the new word when writing or talking.

In addition to discussing the importance of self-monitoring and word awareness strategies, Nelson and Van Meter (2006) provide many examples of both academically focused and pragmatically relevant activities for "finding words." Examples of scaffolds in the form of semantic maps and other tools, some of which will be covered later, are outlined by Nelson and Van Meter (2006), who emphasize the importance of establishing contexts that create opportunities to learn and to be exposed to new words many times. They support many of DeKemel's (2003d) points about embedding vocabulary into meaningful, authentic, and purposeful activities so that students see the value of what they are doing in their intervention experiences (and other instructional endeavors) and take ownership over the things they have been taught. In addition, they say that intervention should also encourage "the natural and joyful processes of learning new words" (Nelson & Van Meter, 2006, p. 109).

Nelson and Van Meter (2006) add that there are three factors that contribute to making vocabulary intervention successful:

1. Students must "see" the need and purpose for learning new and interesting words.
2. Students need to be engaged in meaningful interactions across a variety of adult-peer and peer-peer interactions with interesting and motivating topics that encourage and enhance word learning. (For example, an Angels-Yankees topic might be of interest to a baseball fan, as seen in Chapter 7.)
3. Once the student has participated in some positive experiences enhancing new and known words, intervention can then target the specific areas of need and focus on helping the student acquire strategies for comprehending and using a variety of words for a variety of purposes.

Reminiscent of many of our previous discussions (e.g., Ehren, 2000; Norris, 1997), Nelson and Van Meter (2006) also ask practitioners to keep in mind the differences between instruction and intervention (see Ehren's model in Chapter 4, Figure 4-3, p. 90). Although there are times when instruction and intervention streams may not seem very distinct, vocabulary *intervention* often involves different lexical targets and more specific and pointed scaffolding for students with LLD. That is, these students need "more explicit, intensive, individualized scaffolding and repeated opportunities to encode words in their mental lexicons on multiple levels (semantically, phonologically, orthographically) in order to develop deep associations and automaticity" (Nelson & Van Meter, 2006, p. 101).

Blachowicz (1986, 1994) and her colleagues (e.g., Blachowicz & Fisher, 2004) also see vocabulary instruction (and intervention) from within a strong information processing framework. Nelson and Van Meter's (2006) use of the words "association" and "automaticity" in the previous quote speak to this framework. Blachowicz (1994) noted that if we consider the development of vocabulary (and its remediation and intervention) within a more generalized constructive comprehension framework, we approach the issue of vocabulary learning, in part at least, as a connection between "old" and "new" information. In other words, says Blachowicz (1994), students should be actively involved in the process of "figuring out" what new or unknown words mean, using clues from an author or speaker, trying to match a new word to one already known, and knowing what one needs to know to tackle tough words. She also notes that learning words is not an "all or nothing proposition" (Blachowicz, 1994, p. 319). Word meaning and use also develop and change on a continuum that moves from unknown to very familiar. In the "middle" of the two extremes as per other continua (see, for example, pp. 35–37) are words that we may know slightly or have heard or seen but are not quite sure of their meanings. We might also have restricted or limited meanings attached to certain words, as is the case for some students with LLD. According to Blachowicz (1994), it is important for clinicians and teachers to recognize that word knowledge is a slow and gradual process involving abilities that change over time; we not only learn new words but also learn new meanings for old words, and we get better at dealing with words in increasingly more abstract, refined, and "meta" ways.

Similar to DeKemel (2003d) and Nelson and Van Meter (2006), Blachowicz (1994) and, more recently, Blachowicz and Fisher (2004) suggest the following guidelines for vocabulary instruction in content classes. Speech-language pathologists may find the guidelines useful and create adaptations for students with LLD accordingly, as follows:

- Establish what students already know about the words they must use and comprehend. This aspect of instruction includes the activation of one's prior knowledge. Where is the student "coming from," and how can the student begin to connect what he or she knows to the new and unfamiliar word?
- Highlight the new by encouraging students to brainstorm about possible meanings. In this case, Blachowicz (1986) suggests avoiding "giving" the students the correct meaning too soon. Helping students look for cues they may have failed to notice is part of the process of learning new words "on their own."
- Generate as many connections as possible between "known" words and "new" ones. Students should be encouraged and guided through a series of questions that lead them to generating possible connections, which they must verify, clarify, and so on. Blachowicz (1994) suggests including known words in every introduction to new words so there is always a framework of knowledge to "fall back on."
- Practice gathering information that can help solve the problem (of getting the meaning of an unknown or unfamiliar word). Contextual reading, says

---

Word meaning and use develop and change on a continuum that moves from unknown to very familiar.

Blachowicz (1994) is one way, among others, to start to verify if "word meaning guesses" (hypotheses) can be verified.

■ Facilitate self-monitoring and consolidation. As per Nelson and Van Meter's (2006) suggestions, students check their connections (and disconnections), consider what they need to do to get to the word meaning, and discuss next steps with their teachers or clinicians.

Word Savvy Summary: A Curriculum Connection Worth Repeating

Learning, retaining, and retrieving new words is a challenge for students with and without LLD. The question of when a student really "has" a word—or any other aspect of linguistic content or form—will never be an easy one to answer. It may be that a student takes ownership of a vocabulary item when he or she relates it to an appropriate word already known (Thelen, 1986). It may be that the student uses the word appropriately in different contexts across different genres and language systems (speaking and writing). It may be that the student develops multiple and more elaborated meanings for words that exist in his or her lexicon. But there is a consensus building that the important question for clinicians and teachers, as mentioned earlier, is not necessarily to ask, "How can I get this word into the student's head?" but rather to ask, "What is it that the student already knows about that [word or concept] that I can use as an anchor point, as a way of accessing this new concept?" (Thelen, 1986, p. 606).

As we have seen throughout this text and in many of the readings that have been referenced, the curriculum requires in-depth mastery of many content-specific and unfamiliar words. The assumption is also made that students come to the curriculum with word attack strategies and a repertoire of words and word-learning strategies that form a foundation for academic learning. Fortunately, as discussed in earlier chapters of this text, language is coming to the forefront of many discussions in educational settings. Curricular specialists are also writing about the level of language required for science, social studies, and other subjects, including the ability to comprehend, retain, and use a variety of new and complex terms. Many researchers and practitioners who are not speech-language professionals have begun to discuss in more explicit terms the idea that the mastery of content-area subjects cannot be seen separately from the mastery of language (e.g., VanSledright, 2004, see Chapters 7 and 8).

In earlier writings covering the connection between language and school success and highlighting word learning and related areas, Stephens and Montgomery (1985) wrote that "categorizing words, supplying synonyms and antonyms, formulating complex sentences, offering multiple definitions, recognizing ambiguity, and explaining nonliteral aspects of language are only a few of the linguistic and metalinguistic demands made by upper-grade curricula" (p. 43). Thus we see the weaving together of words, sentences, and discourse skills in our language intervention programs. As clinicians, we should keep one eye focused on the immediate needs of our students and the other eye focused on the horizon of a curriculum that becomes more complex as students move through the grades.

9

As we have often said, the choices we make should also be couched within a *meta* framework that begs the question, *Why am I doing this?* Underlying the "why" are other questions that include how our choices connect to the curriculum, how they focus on the language underpinnings of the curriculum (not teaching the curriculum itself), and where the theoretical and evidence-based data for our approaches "come from." Importantly, our choices should also consider the ways that they will help our students become more active and independent learners. In the next section, we will present examples of activities that may be part of language intervention programs for vocabulary development, as well as other aspects of language. We will be asking "why questions" for these activities and exploring the pros and cons of our choices as another way to begin to pull the pieces of language together.

Why Am I Doing This? A Meta Exploration of Selected Intervention Activities

The activities outlined in this section are presented for the purpose of reviewing some of the key concepts covered in this text. The activities are snapshots taken from the larger canvas of language intervention across time. They appear out of context and thus, as the cliché phrase suggests, *it goes without saying* that caution should be exercised when applying any of the ideas to practice. The supportive tools and the activities that accompany the examples are based on currently available research and are inspired by the works of those referenced in addition to this author's. The out-of-context/summary format of this section was chosen to encourage discussion among the professionals who share responsibility for the education of students with LLD. Professionals are encouraged to discuss their ideas about the activities, including ways that they might modify and adapt activities for their students. In addition, professionals serving students with LLD who are the front lines of service delivery in school settings should take an active role in contributing intervention data to the growing body of evidence-based "best practices."

Activity 1

Figure 9-1 is an example of an exclusive brainstorming activity inspired by Blachowicz (1986, 1994). Students are presented with a preselected list of words and phrases. They are asked to read each word, receiving help if decoding is difficult for them. The next step is to eliminate words and phrases that "do not belong" to the topic. Students are then led through a discussion about why they have chosen to delete and include words or phrases for a topic chosen from curricular content.

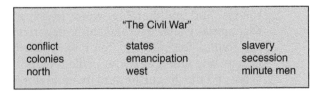

	"The Civil War"	
conflict	states	slavery
colonies	emancipation	secession
north	west	minute men

Figure 9-1 ■ Activity 1: brainstorming. *(Data from Blachowicz, C. L. Z. [1986]. Making connections: Alternatives to the vocabulary notebook.* Journal of Reading, 29, 643–649; *and Blachowicz, C. L. Z. [1994]. Problem-solving strategies for academic success. In G. P. Wallach & K. G. Butler [Eds.],* Language learning disabilities in school-age children and adolescents: Some principles and applications *[pp. 304–322]. Boston: Allyn & Bacon.)*

The Whys. The prototype brainstorming activity is a blend of text, word knowledge, and meta awareness. We also see an activity that works toward connecting "old" (known) and "new" (unfamiliar) information. This activity helps us understand a little more about "where" a student might be in terms of this group of vocabulary items. (For example, he may be familiar with the word "conflict" as in "having a conflict with a younger sibling," a concept mentioned earlier in this chapter.) Students with word-recognition/decoding difficulties have the opportunity to practice with both the form and content of these words in this type of activity. The pragmatic function—judging the appropriate use (and exclusion) of words for a topic—adds to the "contextualization" of word learning. The activity could continue with the construction of spoken and written pieces that embed the words in connected text. The scaffolding that is provided by the clinician in the form of who writes what and how much, and the kinds of supports used (e.g., visual maps, sentence-completion frames, etc.), will vary from student to student. Strategies for finding the meanings of unknown works can be incorporated into the session or later sessions. Words from various subject areas, including literature, can be selected.

Remember: SLPs should be helping students develop linguistically based strategies that they can use across content areas. It is not the goal of SLPs to teach or reinforce the history/social studies content. The curricular content as reflected in this activity and others serves as a backdrop for language intervention goals like those of Ehren (2000) and others.

Activity 2

A rating checklist is presented to students (Figure 9-2). A list of words is preselected as per the previous activity. Students read each word (with or without

How much do you know about these words?			
	Can define	Have seen/heard but not sure	Don't know (?)
algae	X		
diatom			X
protozoan			X
ethanol		X	
fermentation		X	
fungi	X		
multicellular		X	

Figure 9-2 ■ Activity 2: self-evaluation vocabulary knowledge checklist. (*Data from Blachowicz, C. L. Z. [1994]. Problem-solving strategies for academic success. In G. P. Wallach & K. G. Butler [Eds.],* Language learning disabilities in school-age children and adolescents: Some principles and applications *[p. 319]. Boston: Allyn & Bacon.*)

appropriate and needed support). They are guided through the list to make a determination of their knowledge of words from various topics.

The Whys. The word knowledge rating scale is a supportive tool that speaks to developing vocabulary-related activities that help students appreciate the idea (from Blachowicz, 1994) that learning words and their meanings is not an "all or nothing" event. Blachowicz (1994) says word-consciousness activities can include a number of questions to help students become more aware of what they know, as well as what they need to know, as per Ogle's K-W-L activities mentioned elsewhere (e.g., see Chapters 7 and 8, pp. 174–246, this text). Questions such as the following might be included in vocabulary activities to bring students' knowledge (or lack thereof) to the surface:

■ Which are the hardest words (for you)?
■ Which words do you think most of us (the class or the group) probably don't know?
■ Which are the easiest ones?
■ Which are the history words?
■ Which are the science words?

Word recognition, vocabulary growth, and metalinguistic awareness come together in this type of activity.

Remember: SLPs may choose to use curricular materials or they may opt to focus on heightening students' meta awareness of the "tricky" or "connector" words and phrases that surround curricular content words (e.g., words such as "prewar," "postwar," "cause," "effect," "dependent," "similar," "different," etc.).

Activity 3

In this activity, students use key vocabulary words presented to construct a spoken story (or expository piece) before they read it. A "predict-o-gram," shown in Figure 9-3, is used to help students make some educated guesses, that is, inferences, about the way words will be used in the story to express the

PREDICT HOW THE AUTHOR WILL USE THESE WORDS IN THE STORY TO TELL ABOUT:		
The Setting A fishing boat Coast of New 　England	**The Characters** captain fishing crew family	**The Goal or Problem** unexpected storm radar damage
The Actions calling stranded	**The Resolution** back-up systems	**Other things** weather reports taking risks motivation

Figure 9-3 ■ Activity 3: predict-o-gram. *(Redrawn from Blachowicz, C. L. Z. [1986]. Making connections: Alternatives to the vocabulary notebook.* Journal of Reading, 29, *648.)*

story's key elements. For example, the clinician/teacher asks the following questions (Blachowicz, 1986):

- "From the words you know and the ones we have just read, what might the story (or chapter) be about?"
- "What other words might we add to the predict-o-gram?"
- "Do these words (or phrases) 'fit' the whole idea of the story (or chapter)?"
- "Do we have to look up any words we're not sure of?"

Predictions are verified after reading (or listening to) the story.

The Whys. Similar to the ideas outlined in the previous activities, word learning can be an active process that connects known and unknown (or less familiar) information. Exposure to and practice with selected vocabulary, when embedded in connected discourse, has the added benefit of helping students learn to appreciate how words are used to express meanings in various genres. We could choose to start modeling and practicing with meta awareness techniques such as these using information that is familiar to students. For example, the brainstorming, rating scales, and predict-o-grams could cover sports, shopping, or other topics that may be student favorites before transitioning to curricular words and concepts. The visual aids may also serve as scaffolds for organizing written reports and other in-class assignments. The predict-o-gram presented represents a narrative genre. A different visual scaffold would be created for expository text (see, for example, Figure 9-4 and the comparison-contrast figures in Chapter 6, pp. 165 & 167).

Remember: Language intervention should be aimed at helping students "take ownership" of word-finding, prediction, and organizational strategies (Ehren, 2000, 2006a). As students listen to and read stories and selections from

Directions: Use the information from the graphic organizer to complete this writing frame. Write the position first, then reasons to support that position. Conclude with a restatement of the position.

I think that _____

_____

I believe this because _____

_____

To support my opinion, _____

_____

Another reason would be _____

_____

All these reasons should persuade you _____

_____

Figure 9-4 ■ Activity 4: persuasive writing game. (*Redrawn from Hutson-Nechkash, P. [2004]. "Help me write!" [p. 230]. Eau Claire, WI: Thinking Publications.*)

Language intervention should help students take ownership of word-finding, prediction, and organizational strategies (Ehren, 2000, 2006a).

their textbooks, they should take with them a "meta-approach" to refining their predictions and preconceptions about the words and texts facing them (Blachowicz, 1994). Any of the figures presented are merely tools to help us help students develop mental models for processing and organizing linguistic information across spoken and written domains (Lahey & Bloom, 1994).

Activity 4

Students are presented with the following persuasive writing frame presented in Figure 9-4. The sentences within the frame provide an outline for reports and oral presentations of opinion-related topics. The frames help students to offer their opinions and then think about facts that would support those opinions. They are also taught to present arguments in an organized way and to persuade a listener or reader about something. Clinicians may start by guiding students through discussions and written renditions using more familiar topics. They move students toward the handling of more complex curricular topics. For example, a more familiar topic might be persuading the principal to allow students to have a particular event. A more difficult topic might be a discussion of the dangers of global warming. After students fill in the frame (or the clinician does it for the limited writers), they read the piece aloud and ask whether it makes sense with questions to lead the editing portion of the activity (e.g., "Do you have a sentence for each item in the graphic organizer? Do we need to add another sentence?"). Students are encouraged to get feedback (help) from their clinician, their teacher, or a peer.

The Whys. The inclusion of various activities that encourage persuasive writing, as with other genres of expository text, exposes students to the language of their textbooks and the curriculum. Students throughout their school careers will be required to write and discuss various pros and cons of issues. The frames, plus a discussion of what is written, reinforce the "meta" set required to edit one's writing. Reminiscent of the work of Nippold and colleagues (2005), persuasive writing also encourages the use of a whole set of vocabulary that matches the particular purpose and context of persuasive arguments. Recall that Nippold and colleagues (2005) talked about how persuasive text encourages the use of metaverbs such as "think" and "know." These are two verbs that might be more familiar to students. Less familiar verbs such as "predict," "conclude," and "interpret"—verbs that might also be very helpful in science—can be embedded in and learned through practice with persuasive pieces. Learning to present arguments in an organized way, a long developmental process noted by Westby and Clauser (2005), combines many skills, including linguistic, cognitive (reasoning), and pragmatic skills that connect a speaker-writer and his or her audience.

Learning to present organized arguments combines linguistic, cognitive (reasoning), and pragmatic skills.

Remember: Many activities might precede or accompany the writing of an expository persuasive piece. The writing frame presented in Figure 9-4 can be modified to include as little or as much scaffolding as needed. Additional verbs or vocabulary might be added to the framework (e.g., words and phrases such as *therefore, by contrast, on the other hand, similarly, conversely,* etc.), and curricular content might be used. Hutson-Nechkash (2004) provides many more ways to scaffold students' writing.

Activity 5

This activity may be used to facilitate word knowledge and the building of semantic networks among words. An 11-word, 5-line poem, an adaptation of the cinquain form, is the framework of choice, as seen in Figure 9-5. In addition to practicing with the vocabulary used in the poems, students become familiar with grammatical terms such as *noun, adjective,* and *verb* in a more functional way rather than just listing words on worksheets and putting them into their appropriate categories (Eisenberg, 2006).

The clinician guides the student through each line of the poem offering examples, using sentence-closure techniques, and other scaffolds, such as reading stories with targeted words, to help students complete the task. The level of written work required will vary based on students' abilities.

The Whys. The poetic-based activity heightens students' awareness of grammatical categories while at the same time providing them with a wordplay activity within the context of a poetry genre. The need to provide a synonym for the title word at the end of the cinquain has the potential to help students acquire a more elaborated word bank. Finding additional applications for the poetry's word choices could form a next step. For example, the poem's words could serve as a foundation for creating a narrative about a fire. Similarly, the cinquain's words may be used in an expository piece on fire prevention. And, finally, exposing students to printed text helps those who have word-recognition difficulties.

Remember: SLPs can work with teachers and other professionals so that activities such as this one become embedded into classroom routines. Vocabulary choices can also be shared—or negotiated—between teachers and SLPs. Using the words across genres and contexts and helping students answer the question "Why am I doing this?" are factors that will influence both intervention

---

Line 1: One word, the title (a noun)

Line 2: Two words, each describing the title (adjectives)

Line 3: Three words, each expressing an action (verbs)

Line 4: Four words, expressing a feeling (start with an adjective)

Line 5: One word, a synonym for the title (a noun)

Flame
Hot, bright
Burning, raging, spreading
Warm on my face
Fire

Figure 9-5 ■ Activity 5: meaningful grammar-word practice using poetry. (*Redrawn from Eisenberg, S. L. [2006]. Grammar: How can I say that better? In T. A. Ukrainetz [Ed.],* Contextualized language intervention *[p. 176]. Eau Claire, WI: Thinking Publications.)*

and instructional outcomes. As with any intervention activity, tool, and technique, keeping the ultimate purpose and direction of one's choices in mind is key.

Activity 6

Consider the following assignment given to a student:

> Alexander the Great was an effective and important leader. He quickly won the love and respect of his people, but did not keep it throughout his time as their ruler. Discuss what he did to win the devotion of his people and explain what caused his popularity to decline. (Singer & Bashir, 2004, p. 251)

As an initial step in the EmPOWER strategy (Singer & Bashir, 2004), students are taught to Evaluate the assignment. They are prompted (by the **E** in Evaluate) to ask the question, What is this assignment asking me to do? As shown in Figure 9-6, first the student finds and *circles the action words*. These are the words that tell the student to take some action. Next, the student underlines the key words that will tell him or her what to do. These are the words that give more information about the actions to be taken.

The Whys. Just a glance at the assignment makes it clear to the reader how "dense" school text can be. As a consequence, as noted by Singer and Bashir (2004), students need to be guided through the maze of complicated text. They need—to use one of our introductory metaphors in a slightly different way—to see the "trees" away from the "forest." The approach described here is only one piece of the EmPOWER strategy (see Chapter 8, p. 226, and the original from Singer & Bashir, 2004; also see Bashir & Singer, 2006). EmPOWER helps students to develop a method for approaching writing assignments. The circle-and-underline strategy also highlights key vocabulary words and reinforces learning their meanings. For students who have limited reading skills, the assignment can be read to them, and they can follow along with the appropriate level of scaffolding.

Remember: Students with LLD may need additional support and more intensive levels of scaffolding to get them to Singer and Bashir's level of analysis and segmentation. Clinicians have to ask themselves more questions. Does the student

---

Assignment after a student completes the first step of E (Evaluate):

Alexander the Great was an effective and important leader. He quickly won the love and respect of his people, but did not keep it throughout his time as their ruler. Discuss what he did to win the devotion of his people and explain what caused his popularity to decline.

Figure 9-6 ■ Activity 6: sample assignment with the Evaluation component from the EmPOWER strategy. (*Redrawn from Singer, B. D, & Bashir, A. S. [2004]. EmPOWER: A strategy for teaching students with language learning disabilities how to write expository text. In E. R. Silliman & L. C. Wilkinson [Eds.],* Language and literacy learning in schools *[p. 251]. New York: Guilford Press.*)

know what action words are? Does he or she have an understanding of "verb" categories? Does the student know the meanings of the action verbs circled? If students understand action words and verb categories, how do we help them avoid misusing the strategy by circling *all the verbs* in the instructions? Additional strategy work may be required to teach students how to focus on those action words that tell them specifically what to do to compete the writing assignment (Singer & Bashir, 2004).

Activity 7

Students are presented with a written sentence that is a semantically constrained (nonreversible) passive (see p. 68, this text, Chapter 3, and Chapter 8, pp. 263–264). The subject (doer) and object (done to) change places in passive sentences, with the subject appearing at or toward the end of the sentence, whereas the object appears at the beginning. In the case of semantically constrained/nonreversible passives, only one noun can logically "act on" the other noun. In the sentence that follows, "Sam" can discuss Iran, but Iran (per se) cannot discuss "Sam." Passive forms occur more frequently in literate-style communicative situations. The discourse of most textbooks involves literate-heavy language structures including passives, such as the following:

> The Iran crisis was discussed by Sam Donaldson of NBC.*

Students are given three written sentences (which they read or which can be read to them as they follow along). Students are asked to decide which one means the same thing as the target sentence. Discussions follow about their choices:

1. The Iran crisis was discussed by Charles Gibson of ABC.
2. Sam Donaldson of NBC discussed the Iran crisis. (or NBC's Sam Donaldson discussed the Iran crisis.)
3. He said the crisis was a tremendously dangerous situation.

The Whys. Students must use and process complex sentences shifting to the management of literate style forms in both reading and writing. Likewise, students' ability to understand the different ways that meanings can be expressed relates to their ability to paraphrase what they have read and what their teacher's lectures convey in the classroom. The ability to use a variety of complex syntactic forms to complete any number of class assignments places syntactic intervention where it is most needed. The use of curricular content, as always, adds to the relevance of working on sentences "out of context." The activity can be modified and expanded on (and individual sentences put into a broader context) by discussing the idea that one of the sentences (in this case, sentence 3) could follow the target sentence if we were writing a paragraph about the newscast. The meta focus, once again, contributes to students' awareness of the ways language can be manipulated for different purposes.

---

*The original sentence from Wallach and Miller (1988) is still a topic for current events at this writing, with the exception that Sam has since retired (or semi-retired).

Remember: Judgments may become more difficult when the sentence forms used are reversible. For example, in a sentence such as "The president congratulated the reporters," the reporters can congratulate the president, and the president can congratulate the reporters (Wallach & Miller, 1988). Consequently, the "who did what to whom" is less predictable. In addition, the amount of scaffolding needed must be adjusted accordingly. For example, we might color-code the doer of the actions as a clue. We might provide presentence cueing by presenting short stories before working on the target sentences. We might encourage a discussion of the sentence's topic to tap background knowledge. What do the students already know about the crisis? Do they know the reporters named? Do they watch the news at all? On a particular station? Or do they get their current affair facts from the Internet? Do they know the meaning of the word "crisis" and others that appear in the sentence selections?

Activity 8

A sentence appears on the board or paper or on a series of cards with selected vocabulary words or phrases on each card, such as the following example:

> The 16th President issued the Emancipation Proclamation which freed the slaves during the Civil War.*

Students read the sentence (or have it read to them). They are then guided through a paraphrasing activity. They *cross out words* as directed and put others in their place while maintaining the sentence's meaning. Again, depending on the needs of students, there can be more or less scaffolding provided at this point. Some students may need to have word/phrase choice substitutions made available for them that "match" the crossed-out slots. The result should look something like the following:

> Abraham Lincoln wrote (or came out with) an important paper (or a historical document) which gave the slaves freedom in 1863.*

Students write the substituted words above the original words that have been crossed out. Thus the name "Abraham Lincoln" would appear above the original phrase "The 16th President," "wrote" would appear above the word "issued," and "an important paper" would appear above the words, "the Emancipation Proclamation," and so on. Again, the amount and type of paraphrasing required is controlled by clinicians and teachers and based on the existing knowledge and skills of their students.

The Whys. Similar to the passive sentence activity described in activity 7, this activity by Ehren (2003, 2006a) helps students acquire the skills needed for paraphrasing. As she has noted many times, paraphrasing is an important reading comprehension strategy (e.g., Ehren, 2005b). It will be a useful tool for students to have as they progress through the grades and as curricular content becomes more difficult. The activity, using the curriculum as a backdrop yet again, adds to a student's familiarity with tough concepts, unfamiliar vocabulary, and highly structured materials. Paraphrasing activities have the added benefit of helping students with LLD build stronger semantic networks among words, an issue that was discussed earlier in this chapter.

Paraphrasing helps students with LLD to build stronger semantic networks among words.

---

*From Ehren (2003 [presentation]).

Remember: Students with LLD may not have a lexical repertoire that is as broad as one may need to be successful with the paraphrasing tasks. But with enough scaffolding, for example, providing students with word choices they might use for their substitutions, the processing and retrieval load demanded by the activity may be lessened. Of course, as with any activity presented, there may be many steps that precede its use.

Activity 9

Students participate in a sentence-building activity inspired by the works of Athley (1977), which was originally reported by Wallach and Miller and modified here. They are given various semantically-based propositions and are required to form complete sentences from the core ideas. The following propositions appear on the board or on cards:

Getting darker	Rain coming down
Jim tall	John short
Lion growled	Bob terror
Sally dreamed	Famous doctor

Students read the phrases. A general brainstorming activity starts the session. In a situation with a limited amount of scaffolding, students talk about ways that the two thoughts could be combined. Next, students are directed to use a word (a conjunction) that joins the two ideas. For example, they are asked to decide, "How might 'and' work to join the thoughts?" Students add the other words that are needed to construct a complete sentence. Oral and written renditions are combined, but students should do as much writing as possible. Possible target results are as follows:

- It was getting darker **and** the rain was coming down.
- Jim is tall **and** John is short.
- The lion growled **and** Bob ran in terror.
- Sally dreamed of growing up **and** becoming a famous doctor.

The activity is expanded with the addition of other connectives such as "because," "but," "and so," "and after that," "when," and "while" (see Appendix D) and new propositions. Students decide which of the conjunctions presented could replace the "and" in the sentences such as those shown above. They also decide which propositions would have to be resequenced or changed to create sentences that make sense. For example, it makes sense to say and write, "Bob ran in terror because the lion growled," but it does not make as much sense to say "The lion growled because Bob ran in terror." (In the appropriate context and in view of constructive comprehension themes, however, it might be possible to say that Bob's running did, in fact, cause the lion to growl, but it is not as probable an event without a context to support the sentence. For example, Bob was running from the tiger cage. The lion saw the movement. The lion growed. (See Bransford & Johnson's [1973] classic chapter that shows how "illogically sounding" sentences can make sense in the appropriate context.)

The Whys. Although we keep our eyes and ears focused on connected and academic discourse, we also recognize that syntactic knowledge is one of the micro pieces that forms the foundation for managing connected text. Students are going to be asked to comprehend, write, and edit sentences. Learning how to use connectives—the linguistic glue of language—on both sentence and text levels has been discussed many times in many different ways. To continue to beat the reiteration drum, we might add that using propositions from social studies and science contributes to the relevance of sentence-building tasks. For example, "the unfair tax/Boston Tea Party," "32 degrees/freezing," and "igneous rock/sedimentary rock" are phrases that can be used in sentence-building activities, among other concepts that come from classroom lessons and textbooks.

Remember: Syntactic and semantic elements of sentences form interesting interactions that students can be made aware of. It is important to help students understand the connection between form and meaning. For example, although all the sentences presented in activity nine represent the same syntactic structure—that is, they are coordinate sentences joined by "and"—they express different underlying semantic relations that are not always obvious on the surface. The darkness/rain sentence expresses a similarity of elements with the theme of a gloomy evening. The Jim/John sentence expresses comparison, and the lion/Bob sentence expresses causality. The Sally/doctor sentence has a temporal appropriateness (Athley, 1977). Discussions about the different ways we can use language form to express meanings is another aspect of meta awareness that can provide students with LLD with more stable and flexible language knowledge, skills, and strategies they can apply to both spoken and, especially, written language tasks.

Activity 10

Students use the science report frame shown in Figure 9-7. They review a science experiment that has taken place in class. Students write ideas they recall about the hands-on experiment in the appropriate frame bubbles. The frame serves as an organizational guide for what will become a complete report. The text on the right side of Figure 9-7 shows the complexity of science language and the level of organization, detail, lexical, and text knowledge required. The words *Purpose, Procedures, Results,* and *Conclusion* are written in the middle of the frame. These words can be color-coded to make the "main ideas" more predominant for the student. The questions on the left of the frame—*What did we do? What happened?* and *Why did it happen?*—serve as additional supports.

The Whys. Learning how to manage expository text is one of the challenges facing students with LLD. Science literacy, as we have seen, contributes to the task's complexity. Westby and Clauser (2005) remind us that science reports are constructed with a number of subgenres. For example, answering the "What did you do?" question requires a step-by-step recount of the important procedures involved in the experiment. "What happened?" requires a detailed description of things that occurred as a result of "what you did." And, finally, "Why did it happen?" involves a cause-effect explanation. Once again, say Westby and Clauser (2005), we see the density of specific scientific terminology in the mix, which creates a series of competing resources that may interfere with students' abilities to manage the task successfully (Lahey & Bloom, 1994).

Remember: The hands-on nature of experiments can certainly facilitate comprehension of the events. Helping students to manage the language that is superimposed on science, for example, is what intervention is about at school-age levels.

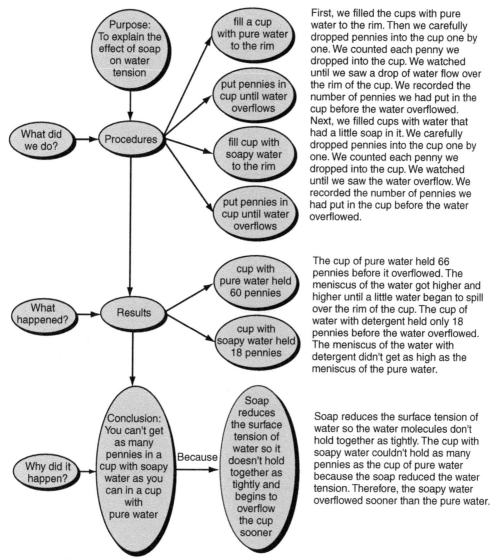

First, we filled the cups with pure water to the rim. Then we carefully dropped pennies into the cup one by one. We counted each penny we dropped into the cup. We watched until we saw a drop of water flow over the rim of the cup. We recorded the number of pennies we had put in the cup before the water overflowed. Next, we filled cups with water that had a little soap in it. We carefully dropped pennies into the cup one by one. We counted each penny we dropped into the cup. We watched until we saw the water overflow. We recorded the number of pennies we had put in the cup before the water overflowed.

The cup of pure water held 66 pennies before it overflowed. The meniscus of the water got higher and higher until a little water began to spill over the rim of the cup. The cup of water with detergent held only 18 pennies before the water overflowed. The meniscus of the water with detergent didn't get as high as the meniscus of the pure water.

Soap reduces the surface tension of water so the water molecules don't hold together as tightly. The cup with soapy water couldn't hold as many pennies as the cup of pure water because the soap reduced the water tension. Therefore, the soapy water overflowed sooner than the pure water.

Figure 9-7 ■ Activity 10: completed science report frame. *(Redrawn from Westby, C. E., & Clauser, P. S. [2005]. The right stuff for writing: Assessing and facilitating written language. In H. W. Catts & A. G. Kamhi [Eds.],* Language and reading disabilities *[2nd ed., p. 302]. Boston: Allyn & Bacon.)*

The science frame is one of many supportive tools that can help students begin to organize the written discourse of science. The activity can be used with additional scaffolds provided by clinicians. For example, clinicians can provide students with key words and phrases that they can copy and place in the appropriate sections. Clinicians may write parts of sentences and students complete them. A brainstorming session can serve as a warm-up before using the frame. Blachowicz's (1986, 1994) vocabulary knowledge checklist (see Figure 9-2) might also be used in conjunction with the science report frame.

Activity 11

Students participate in an exploration of ways to discuss and think about new words (Figure 9-8). Dictionary and other skills, including using background knowledge, are included in the word-learning activity. Similar to activity 10, students write their responses in the different bubbles. The A-F template,

Definition Diagram

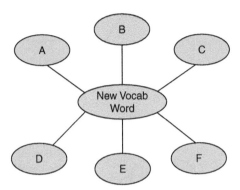

A) Dictionary definition
B) Important facts
C) Put the word in a sentence
D) Personal definition of the word—may be a drawing
E) Important facts you discovered
F) Negative definition

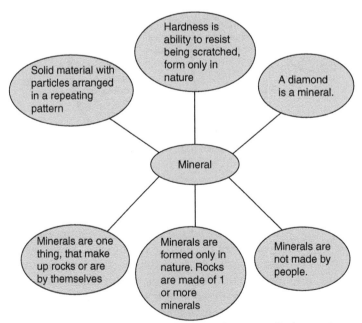

Figure 9-8 ■ Activity 11: definition diagram. *(Redrawn from Straits, W. [2005]. Mystery box writing.* Science and Children, *43, 35.)*

similar to the science report writing frame from the previous activity, reminds the student of ways to document the meanings of new words and some of the ways that words can be used. Spoken and written language are integrated into various aspects of the task. Word choices can vary.

The Whys. The activity is probably familiar to many clinicians and teachers who use semantic mapping activities with their students. Figure 9-8 presents an example from the science curriculum vocabulary. The definition diagram provides another scaffold for students with the addition of the A-F components. We have seen how dense and complex curricular language can be. Helping students make stronger connections to new words by using personal knowledge, dictionary renditions, and an understanding of "what words do *not* mean" (e.g., the "F" circle) provide them with additional skills and strategies for managing the curriculum. This activity and the diagram that accompanies discussions, word searches, and documenting meanings is another example of a way to help students begin to help themselves.

Remember: The last point is key—students may use the diagrams, science report forms, and other tools as reminders of "what to do." We often paste the visual maps and outlines in their notebooks. Eventually, however, our goal is to help students organize their work from the inside out as well as from the outside in (Lahey & Bloom, 1994).

Activity 12

Students are exposed to a number of word-recognition activities through sentence-completion or paragraph-completion tasks. In each of the tasks, students read the sentences and the word/phrase choices and then write their responses in the spaces provided. The scaffolding varies as needed. Discussions follow about the reason for students' choices. Examples are as follows:

1. Susan was so happy that she _____ through the park.*
   walked   trudged   skipped

2. Susan was so happy that she sk_____ through the park.*
   walked   trudged   skipped

3. George Washington who was the leader of the Continental army thought that his generals should _____ him.
   disobey   listen to   obey

4. Benedict Arnold had a reputation for being very fl_____ and consequently he made enemies with many of the other generals in Washington's army.
   show off   well-liked   flamboyant

The Whys. The scaffolding provided is aimed at combining word meaning, word recognition (decoding), and sentence structure knowledge in the activity. Pearson's classic (1982) and current works (e.g., Duke & Pearson, 2002) remind us that while students should be encouraged to make predictions about words in order to comprehend what authors are trying to say, they also have to be more precise about speech-to-print matches. Eventually, these matches become

9

more automatic as they are with proficient readers who stop to think only when there is a problem (e.g., an unfamiliar word). The examples in sentences 1 through 4 encourage students to *use context and print* to arrive at their answers in sentence completion tasks. We can see that some choices are more open-ended but logical (such as in sentences 1 and 3, with sentence 3 having two possible choices) whereas others are constrained by the letter/sound prompts shown in sentences 2 and 4. Any number of questions arise from the word choices. For example, why would "skipped" be a more precise or accurate choice than "walked?" Do students know the meaning of "flamboyant," and why might "being flamboyant" create enemies for Benedict Arnold? Finally, sentence structures such as the relative clause example (sentence 3) and the cause-effect example (sentence 4) provide models of literate forms for the students. Syntactic structures also make certain choices ungrammatical, as in "show off."

Remember: This activity is decontextualized and metalinguistic. But, clearly, many students with LLD have difficulties with decoding, semantic association and elaboration, and word retrieval, as noted earlier. The activity demonstrates how some of the elements of word knowledge, sentence structure, and decoding can be brought a bit closer together. We always want to keep some key points in mind, however, when embarking on activities such as these that "isolate" sentences and words on worksheets or blackboards: What is the purpose of reading? How can word-recognition/decoding activities facilitate comprehension and learning? How can fast and efficient decoding help students become proficient readers? Does facility with complex syntax have a role in school success? What does any of this have to do with the classroom?

Activity 13

Students are presented with the following paragraph, which comes from a Grade 5 social studies textbook (Boehm et al., 2000, p. 159):

Title

(We'll think of one after reading the passage)

The Spanish government _____ many of the conquistadors by giving _____ large areas of conquered land. Most of the _____ was in Mexico, which the Spaniards called New Spain. _____ became one of Spain's colonies in the Americas. A colony is a settlement ruled by another country. People who live in a colony are called settlers, or _____.

Students complete the paragraph by filling in the missing words. Similar to activity 12, the scaffolding provided may vary and the closure choices modified based on students' needs. For example, word choices may be listed for students, who then find appropriate slots in the paragraph. Choices are (in order of their appearance in the text) *rewarded, them, land, it, colonists.* As per activity 12, additional prompts may appear in the text in the form of first letters or oral prompts from the clinician. Likewise, word choice may appear under the blanks. The activity can focus on cohesion or other aspects of text that students need to understand. For example, cohesion questions would include the following: Do students understand that *conquistadors* and *them* "go together"? That *land*

and *land* are repeated for a reason, or that we could use another word, such as *area?* Do they know that *it* refers to *Mexico?* We could also consider helping students acquire morphological connections such as the one represented by *colony* and *colonists.*

The Whys. Tackling connected discourse, especially the discourse of school text, has been a recurring theme. Students with LLD have difficulty comprehending text that is high (or loaded) in content and complex in structure. The use of excerpts from textbooks in language intervention situations offers students the opportunity to "play with and manipulate" language with relevant materials. The inclusion of a title for the piece adds another dimension to the activity. As discussed elsewhere, titles help readers predict what's coming up in a text, but they can also be confusing. (Recall the example of a group session in Chapter 3, pp. 47–48). Encouraging students to create titles for texts is another way to introduce them to a strategy that they can use in other situations.

Remember: We have to consider the notion of competing resources when using classroom materials. Although students will be facing tough topics and dense textbook language, it is our responsibility to manipulate the scaffolding accordingly to help them work through the texts with an eye toward removing supports as intervention progresses.

> SLPs should manipulate scaffolding to help students work through texts with an eye toward removing those supports as intervention progresses.

Activity 14

Students are presented with a sentence, which they read or which is read to them:

> The skater was a top spinning on the ice.*

A brainstorming activity can precede the next step, which is deciding from a group of sentences which one matches the meaning of the target sentence. For example, as a first step, students participate in a discussion about ice skaters or the sport of ice skating. This taps into background knowledge (or lack thereof). Photos of Olympians and other skaters going through their moves on the ice complement the discussion. The next step involves picking out the "best" meaning from a choice of meanings, such as the following

A. The skater was twirling very fast.
B. She had a top next to her on the ice.
C. The skater was spinning so fast she looked like a toy.

Students are guided through discussions about the different possibilities. Some students may have the ability to participate in discussions about the differences between literal and nonliteral translations. The activity can be expanded on by using target sentences such as the one presented above in stories or expository pieces about the latest skating competition. Word knowledge can be reinforced by providing students with word pairs and discussing how they are alike and how metaphors and similes (using the word *like* to make the comparison) might be constructed. For example, consider the following pairs: hair/fire (her hair was like fire); eyes/marbles (his eyes looked like two blue marbles).

*From Nippold (1985, p. 9).

More abstract pairs would include words that may not be stated directly in the sentence but that connect to its overall meaning: anger/volcano (the teacher was a volcano, or the teacher's anger was like an erupting volcano); ice/unfriendly (the politician was like ice).

The Whys. "What else could a word mean?" Bashir's (1987) statement at the beginning of our "Word about Words" section reminds us that (1) words can have multiple and sometimes ambiguous meanings and (2) words often live in the world of figurative language where meanings move from literal to something more than their surface meanings suggest. When we say things such as "You're walking on thin ice," "Hold your tongue," and "He kicked the bucket," the meanings behind the statements move beyond the meanings of the individual words. Although statements such as "walking on thin ice" and "holding one's tongue" are closer to their actual meaning (e.g., walking on thin ice puts you in a dangerous situation), the origin and evolution of other statements, such as "kicked the bucket" to mean "he died," are less obvious. (See Milosky, 1994; Nippold, 1998; and van Kleeck, 1994; see also Owens, 2001, for a discussion on development in the area of figurative language.)

Using similes, metaphors, idioms, and puns and enjoying jokes and humor involves metalinguistic ability because it involves a student's understanding that language can be manipulated and that meaning goes beyond the individual parts of a sentence or textbook.

Working on various aspects of figurative language, a challenging aspect of language for students with LLD includes understanding and using similes, metaphors, idioms, and puns and enjoying jokes and humor (van Kleeck, 1994). This aspect of language learning is metalinguistic because it involves the understanding that language can be manipulated; it also involves the recognition that meaning goes beyond a text's or a sentence's individual parts. Older children learn that one word can have several different meanings (ambiguity), that two sentence forms can have the same meaning (synonymy), and that various combinations of words and sounds can serve to have different meanings altogether (figurative interpretations) (van Kleeck, 1994; Wallach & Miller, 1988).

These aspects of later language learning influence social as well as academic communication. Indeed, our everyday language, both spoken and written, is filled with idiomatic and metaphorical expressions, as well as other forms that require a more abstract level of comprehension. But, again, cautions Ehren (2006a), we should not veer too far away from curricular content. She suggests that we should avoid teaching students figurative forms they are unlikely to encounter. Rather, we should consider the metaphors, similes, and so on that they will face in their textbooks. For example, the statement from the "Emancipation Proclamation" (see Chapter 6, p. 158) that alluded to Lincoln (by one of his enemies) as "a wet rag" or another that refers to "George Washington as a rock" or "Benedict Arnold as a snake" are more relevant targets.

Remember: There are layers of learning involved in the mastery of figurative language. Figurative language evolves over many years from elementary to high school levels, with glimmers of this ability occurring as early as the preschool years (van Kleeck, 1994). A metaphor that expresses the relationship of an "ice skater as a top," according to Nippold (1985), has a perceptual base—that is, they both spin quickly. We can "see" the connection. By contrast, saying that "the politician was an iceberg" expresses a more abstract relationship—that is, he is cold, hard, and unmovable. Exposure to figurative forms in contextual situations (e.g., using stories that end with a figurative statement or that have characters using metaphors or idioms), followed by more perceptually based analyses (discussions of the relationship between a skater who spins and a top that spins), to more abstract connections (between cold and unfriendly and hard and inflexible) are among the suggestions to consider when including figurative work in language intervention programs (e.g., Milosky, 1994; Nippold, 1985, 1998).

Activity 15

Students are presented with passages that they read (or have read to them). The passages are organized so that a word with an ambiguous meaning occurs throughout the passage, as follows:

> We discovered a pit.
> We came across a pit while we were exploring a wilderness area.
> It looked as though it had been there for a long time.
> After finishing the fruit, some litterbug must have thrown it on the ground.*

Students are encouraged to stop at the end of each sentence and make an inference about what they think might be coming up in the text. After reading the first sentence, they talk about what the word "pit" could mean. As suggested by Bashir, they are encouraged to think about the question, "What else could it mean?" The decisions about the word's meaning will (or should) drive what students propose will follow. Each sentence provides clues that finally disambiguate the meaning of "pit." Students reread the passage and talk about "guesses" that worked and those that did not. Students (or the clinician) highlight or underline the words that really "give the meaning of 'pit' away" (e.g., fruit, litterbug, thrown, ground). Changes can be made in the text to create alternatives.

The Whys. The activity, although quite simple, integrates word knowledge, text, and inferential processing. Students work on double meanings within the context of connected text. This offers them the opportunity to learn how to use context, inferencing, and print to arrive at an author's meaning. Students also practice with linking words together from the text that contribute to comprehension of the "whole idea." As a bonus, students are exposed to more complex structures such as the "while" and "after" structures that appear in the passage.

Remember: The text and word choices can be altered as needed. It is important, however, not to overload the student with too much information, as we have discussed. If the text is overly complex and the word choices are well beyond a student's repertoire, the concept one wants to get across to the student—that you use what you know and validate your "guesses" with text—may be obscured.

Activity 16

Students are presented with pictures that have diagrams beneath them that represent the word's segments in this classic phonemic segmentation activity. Figure 9-9 shows the steps that can be used in the word-to-sound awareness task.

In the first step, students say the complete word, slowing their speech slightly, but not separating the word into its separate phonemes. At the same time, they place tokens in the boxes (with support as needed) to represent the phonemic segments within the word. For example, the word "man" is

---

*From Johnson and von Hoff Johnson (1986, p. 625).

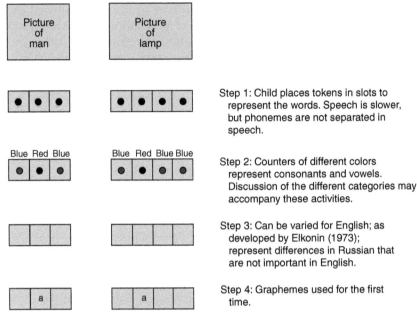

Figure 9-9 ■ Activity 16: phonemic segmentation format. (Modified from Wallach, G. P., & Miller, L. [1988]. *Language intervention and academic success.* Boston: Butterworth-Heinemann. Data from Elkonin, D. B. [1973]. U.S.S.R. In J. Downing [Ed.], *Comparative reading.* New York: Macmillan.)

represented by three tokens; the word "lamp" is represented by four. The word "ship" would represented by three tokens for /ʃ/, /I/, and /p/ even though it has four letters. In the second step, different-colored tokens may be used to represent consonants and vowels. In the last step, the graphemes are presented and placed in their appropriate slots. (The original method created by Elkonin [1973] showed four steps because there was an additional step in Russian that is not significant in English.) Students practice with the speech-to-print activities with different words. They manipulate the tokens to demonstrate knowledge of the number of sound segments in words. Adaptations are possible, and any number of higher-level segmentation abilities such as including morphophonemic work can be created for students who are ready for that level of analysis. For example, words such as "microorganism" can appear with a two-slot diagram and students can manipulate the parts and discuss their meanings.

The Whys. Phonemic segmentation activities have inundated language intervention programs for more than 25 years. In the approach described above, we can see the value of speech/spoken language leading the way to print so that students absorb the idea that meaning resides in spoken language and is ultimately superimposed on print. The encouragement of a "normal" production of words is also useful because when spoken words are "pulled apart" in unnatural ways, they can become unrecognizable. The artificial segmentation of words, common in formal phonics programs, can be especially confusing for children with LLD, who may have more limited word and metalinguistic skills. When a child says "bah-a-tuh" to represent the word "bat," he has actually produced five phonemes, not three. Thus the original idea of saying the whole word but recognizing its component parts is a useful one. Grounding students in the alphabetic principle and helping them manipulate tokens to represent that principle (i.e., letters "hook up" to sounds) is a core concept of activities such as the ones that grew out of Elkonin's (1973) and others' research (e.g., Blachman, 1994; see Troia, 2004, for a detailed review).

Remember: Phonemic segmentation activities such as the one presented are part of a much larger framework of teaching children to read. Elkonin-like activities seen every day in every classroom and clinic room may be useful, but they should be embedded in other literacy and comprehension-based activities that help students become proficient readers. In addition, many "pre" activities related to the acquisition of early phonological skills should be considered before more formal phonemic segmentation tasks are introduced. Finally, the research regarding the value of phonemic segmentation activities, especially those that stray too far from printed materials, is still in an evolutional phase (Troia, 2004).

Activity 17

Students participate in a three-phrase activity in a BEFORE reading, DURING reading, and AFTER reading format (adapted from McCrudden et al., 2005). As part of the BEFORE reading phase, students are guided through a discussion of some of strategies they can use when reading the story that will follow. These are outlined in a shorter version on a "Reading Strategies Reminder Board." Among the strategies are the following:

- BEFORE reading: Think about telling the story to a friend who has not heard it. What would you need to do to get your friend to understand the story (and tell it to someone else)? Look at the title to help you figure out what might be in the story (if there is a title). Look at pictures, charts, maps, and other items that accompany the story (if there are any).
- DURING reading: Create pictures in your mind as you read. Slow down and read carefully if you need to. If you don't understand something, try to figure it out before moving on. Check back to earlier sentences if you lose the meaning along the way.

After the discussion and a warm-up time, students read the following passage silently or take turns reading it aloud. The passage is read to those students who are poorer readers, who follow along with the text in front of them:

> Lawrence slowly got up from the mat, planning his escape. Things were not going well. What bothered him most was being held, especially since the charge against him had been weak. He considered his present situation. The lock that held him was strong, but he thought he could break it. Lawrence was aware that it was because of his early roughness that he had been penalized so severely. The situation was becoming frustrating; the pressure had been grinding on him too long. He was being ridden unmercifully. Lawrence was getting angry now. He felt ready to make his next move. He knew his success or failure would depend on

what he did in the next few seconds. (From Anderson et al. [1977, p. 376], as reported by McCrudden et al. [2005, p. 122] in their research with fourth graders)

- AFTER reading: Guided by their clinician, students participate in the AFTER reading portion of the activity: (1) Students summarize the story in their own words; (2) they check back to see if anything was confusing; (3) they talk about what they think the story was about; and (4) they suggest titles. An evaluation of the strategies that helped and did not help is discussed. In a final phase, the clinician offers two possible interpretations for the story: would an appropriate title be "The Prison Break" or "The Wrestling Match"?

The Whys. Our goal is to help our students become more active learners. Activities that engage them in text while building self-efficacy and getting students to take "ownership" of reading comprehension and other language learning strategies are among the key components of language intervention. The before, during, and after reading strategies are focused toward helping students become more involved in the reading (and listening) comprehension process. The idea that the "Rocky Passage," as it is called, is open to interpretation provides an interesting twist to the ways that a reader's background knowledge comes into play. Students with LLD should be encouraged to use their background knowledge, as well as decipher what an author's words are trying to tell them. (Recall the *In your Head* and *In the Text* discussion from Chapter 8, pp. 229–234, this text.) Discussions with students about how titles, pictures, and other supportive scaffolds might facilitate comprehension should be part of the language intervention goals and objectives. For example, would different titles—"The Wrestling Match" versus "The Prison Break"—facilitate comprehension in the same ways? A number of questions can form discussions about the text with students. For example, have students even been to or seen a wrestling match? Likewise, did students "visualize" a prison break during the reading of the passage? Key words and phrases can be highlighted to help students comprehend the passage. Other modifications can be added that may help students *use the strategies taught* and learn that comprehension, whether spoken or written, is an active process—like an intricate puzzle that includes finding and using clues and pulling the pieces of language together.

Remember: Think innovatively and keep questioning past and current practices.

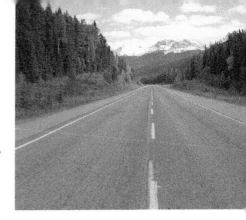

In conclusion, literacy learning as a collection of processing strategies and skills that continuously interweave with experiences can be thought of as an orchestra playing a symphony. Though they can function independently, each instrument and each part of the score contributes to the complex and dynamic sound of the whole concert. Harmony occurs when multiple instruments simultaneously produce individual yet related melodies. If one instrument is out of tune, the sound of the whole orchestra will be adversely affected.

(Silliman et al., 2004, p. 348)

10 The End Becomes a New Beginning

Coming Full Circle

SUMMARY STATEMENT ▰▰▰

At this writing, the New York Yankees, a baseball team with a long history of success, had just been eliminated from their divisional playoffs and a chance to go to the World Series by a team that was considered a huge underdog, the supposedly "lowly" Detroit Tigers. (No offense is meant to Tigers fans.) The fact that the Yankees had and still have the largest payroll in baseball, courting and hiring "big name stars" from every team who would release their players to the "evil empire," made the loss for the sixth straight year unacceptable to Yankee owners and fans alike. The New York

This chapter was inspired by a group of graduate students and clinicians-in-training from the Department of Communicative Disorders at the California State University at Long Beach, in Long Beach, California: Stephen Charlton, Julie Christie, Katie Kent, Robin Sprague, Lezlee Tamo, and Mehra Veremakis. I would also like to acknowledge Katie Kent and Mehra Veremakis for their outstanding work with "Michael" (not his real name) and for teaching me so much about what language intervention can and should be. This extraordinary group of students will, no doubt, carry the torch of superb and authentic speech and language services to the schools and students they serve with competence and enthusiasm. With them, I truly reached Nirvana as a teacher.

media rumor mill and the baseball world in general spread the word about whose heads would roll and what would happen within minutes of the last out in Detroit. What frustrated fans and baseball gurus were saying was that "something had to change!" Many among the collective "we" of Yankee loyalists continued voicing their grief by looking ahead and adding: "You can't keep doing the same thing year after year—like hiring ego-driven stars with inflated salaries, keeping the same manager, relying on hitting without solid pitching and in essence following the same game plan, etc.—and expect a different result" (Colin Cowherd, ESPN Radio, October 9, 2006). So although the Yankee organization has its work cut out for itself, so, too, do we, the New York Yankees of language learning disabilities. Can we keep doing the same things year after year with our students and expect different results? This chapter asks the collective "we" of school-based practitioners to consider this question as our exploration of alternative game plans continues with a look toward the future. Mini cases in the form of assessment and intervention scenarios serve as catalysts for summarizing key concepts from the text and encouraging discussions among practitioners. Keeping the symphonic view of language in mind, we reflect back on Apel's (1999) ideas from the first chapter of this text, that is, one's definition of language should drive what we do and what we do should include understanding the systemic, functional, and context-embedded nature of language.

KEY QUESTIONS

Following are the only two questions that underpin the one already asked in our introductory section:

1. Can we do better?
2. Are we willing to think outside the proverbial box?

INTRODUCTORY THOUGHTS

The answers to the questions raised in this chapter may seem obvious. Of course, we can always do better, and most of us on the front lines would agree that we have "done better" in our attempts to integrate current thinking into daily practice. Readers of this text and their colleagues who work in school settings and other settings such as private practices and clinics are always searching for more effective ways to treat the students in their care. Sometimes we look in places that lead us astray, and other times we find exciting, relevant, and evidence-based alternatives. We opened this text with the visual image of convention sites filled with the newest programs, kits, and texts. And although we all have moments of being enamored by glitzy packaging and overstated promises (such as the Randy Johnson acquisition for the Yankees), we know that the quick fixes and panaceas of today become the disappointments of tomorrow. Just one look at a history or science book—excerpts of which have weaved their way throughout this text—helps us appreciate the futility of adopting approaches to language intervention that have little to do with "Monday morning in the classroom."

For those of us who are school-based practitioners, we also know that we are often strapped by a system that may not make it easy for us to provide the best services for students. For example, in one school system that shall remain nameless, speech-language pathologists (SLPs) were told to "pick from a list of predetermined goals" for their students. In another, the administrator created a directive indicating to SLPs that "the students on their caseloads had to demonstrate *obvious* expressive language problems" or they could not be serviced by them. In yet another, the SLP was handed a book of idioms and metaphors and told to "work on these" with the adolescents on his caseload. And in still another school setting, the SLP was told to bring in an audiologist to "assess Max's central auditory processing abilities because he can't keep up with the Grade 6 social studies curriculum and he has trouble understanding instructions." The same school system that Max attends recommended adopting the LiPS Program (Lindamood Phoneme Sequencing Program, 2003) for *all* students with language learning/reading disabilities.

It gets even worse: In one middle school, a group of students with language learning disabilities (LLD) was observed in "speech" class blowing whistles and doing a number of odd-looking tongue exercises for reasons that remained unclear. And even worse than the last example is yet another one: The supervisor of a very large school system in Southern California who hired a recent, and exceptionally gifted, graduate in speech-language pathology said to her in no uncertain terms, "And we'll have none of that literacy stuff here!" Unfortunately, the examples could continue. They represent narrow and sometimes inaccurate ways of looking at language learning, language processing, and language intervention. The examples reflect a static "one size fits all" mentality and a disconnect between more relevant cause-effect factors and language proficiency, not to mention a misread about the evolving roles of SLPs.

Clearly, there are alternative scenarios that reflect innovative and cutting-edge thinking in many schools across this country. We see SLPs participating in in-class intervention, talking about "strategic" approaches to intervention, writing goals and objectives that are curriculum relevant, and integrating spoken and written language activities into their therapy plans, among other positive things they do every day. Indeed, available research and innovative practice have brought us quite far, so there is reason to remain optimistic. Nonetheless, we live in a world of constantly changing federal and state mandates, expanding cultural and linguistic differences among students, and a shifting of attention and resources toward the most severe among us (such as children with autism). These realities, among others mentioned throughout this text, continue to make meeting the needs of students with LLD a little tougher. The old adage of having "too many children to serve, too little time, and too much paperwork" couldn't be more relevant in today's climate (Creaghead, 2002). Likewise the doubled-edged sword of increasing demands on schools to produce results (known hereafter as the "Yankee factor") keeps us in "challenge mode" to be more effective. Yes, we will encounter roadblocks in systems that seemingly like keeping them in place. Nonetheless, we can find ways to overcome all of these challenges by steeping ourselves in current research, thinking in broader strokes (see Chapter 1), advocating for our students, and taking on leadership roles in our respective settings (Ehren, 2006a). Although systems cannot be changed overnight, taking small steps—for example, *implementing one specific idea* from a text and doing the same after attending the next curriculum-based intervention—are ways to start changing direction if directional changes are needed (Ehren, 2006a).

10

Engaging in some of the meta strategies we have talked about—that is, reflecting on what we are doing and why—underlies the path to reassessment and discovery. The scenarios presented in the following section provide us with additional opportunities to talk about some of the twists and turns in assessment and intervention directions that may be warranted. The scenarios are also a way to continue the process of summarization for the text. They are snapshots of behavior aimed at stimulating discussion with an understanding that more in-depth information would be needed to flesh out the cases and situations.

Returning to the principles from Chapter 1 that encouraged us to paint the canvas of language intervention in broader, more functional brush strokes, readers are asked to reflect on the following concepts as they read and discuss the scenarios with colleagues:

■ The connection between language performance (and intervention decisions) and the real world
■ The superficial versus deeper levels of a task's complexity
■ The interactions among context, language, text, and strategies
■ The "where" factor in language intervention—that is, asking if language intervention goals and objectives are taking students where they need to go

Pulling the Orchestra Apart: Targeting Ten Missed Notes

Scenario 1

Andrew is given a test or a series of tasks such as the one described. The test goes something like this: "Andy, I'm going to say two words. I want you to tell me if these two words sound the same or different." (*Note:* Andrew understands "same" and "different" and he has excellent articulation.) He also has normal hearing. Examples of the word pairs used are as follows:

■ thief-leaf
■ ship-sip
■ mitt-mat
■ mash-mash
■ lake-lake
■ king-ring

Andrew performs poorly on the test and other tasks similar to it.

Conclusion. This student has an auditory discrimination problem. He has problems perceiving the differences among sounds. It is recommended that intervention include work on auditory discrimination and possibly other listening activities.

Alternative Considerations. If Andrew has "excellent articulation" and he is speaking English, he has "discriminated" the sounds of his language on some level. The blanket statement that he has an "auditory discrimination problem" is premature and inaccurate. The task is more difficult than it appears to be on the surface. As noted in Chapter 1, *things are not always what they seem.* Far from being a straightforward discrimination task, this task requires metalinguistic ability (van Kleeck, 1994; Wallach, 2005b). Andrew is being asked to make a conscious judgment about language. Further, he is being asked to make a *phonemic judgment.* Phonemic judgments tend to be more difficult (and are later acquisitions) than semantic judgments (Blachman, 1994; Troia, 2004; van Kleeck, 1994).

Additional Discussion Points. Are the words within Andrew's spoken or written language repertoire? Is he a reader? Was Andrew asked *why* he made certain judgments? (For example, did he make a semantic judgment when he said that "lake-lake" are different because there are many different lakes in the United States, such as Lake Tahoe, Lake George, and Lake Michigan?) How does a task such as this relate to Andy's language learning or literacy problems? Does his performance (or difficulty) on the "auditory discrimination" task relate to his decoding issues? (Maybe [see Troia, 2004].) Is it irrelevant? (Possibly.) Clearly, we would always want to know more about the student— for example, his age and status linguistically and academically, and what provoked the choice to test this area in this way.

Scenario 2

Matthew is asked to sequence a number of disks with pictures of geometric designs painted on them. The disks are placed in a left-to-right sequence in front of him—circle, square, triangle, slanted line, trapezoid, and so on. He looks at six or seven disks for a few seconds. The disks are removed quickly and rearranged. Matthew is asked put them back in the original order. He sequences the disks incorrectly and shows confusion.

Conclusion. Matthew has a visual sequence/memory problem. That's why he missequences letters when he reads: "clam" for "calm," "lion" for "loin," and "was" for "saw." We must strengthen his visual memory skills as a foundational skill for better decoding.

Alternative Considerations. To use another metaphor, the conclusion about Matthew is an "apples-oranges" comparison. The sequencing of a series of geometric forms is the sequencing of geometric forms; the reading (or decoding) of real words is the reading (or decoding) of real words. Fortunately, we have moved far beyond the belief that visually based deficits are the cause of—or are related to—reading disorders (e.g., see Catts & Kamhi, 2005d). Further, Vellutino's classic works, among others (e.g., Fischer et al., 1978; Vellutino et al., 1973, 1975), have shown that reversal errors, like the oft-quoted "was" for "saw" example, constitute a very small percentage of children's overall errors and are natural occurrences when one is learning to read. In addition, Vellutino (1979) and Vellutino and colleagues (Vellutino et al., 1973, 1975) also remind us that when children make "stabs" at words they are reading (similar to what they do when listening; see Chapter 5), they usually substitute familiar words for unfamiliar words (e.g., "clam" for "calm"; "lion" for "loin"). These substitutions represent *linguistic intrusion errors*, as noted by Vellutino, and not "visual" errors.

> Reversal errors, such as using "was" for "saw," make up a very small percentage of children's overall errors and are natural when a person is learning to read.

Additional Discussion Points. What other clinical techniques have little or no relationship to language learning and academic success? (Think central auditory processing tasks; think oral-motor activities.) What strategies (or not) does Matthew use when trying to remember the geometric forms? For example, does he "name" the items to facilitate memory? Does he have the names of the geometric forms in his repertoire? Does Matthew have knowledge of the words he is being asked to read? On what level (conceptual, semantic, phonological; DeKemel, 2003d)? Does context help him decode unfamiliar words? What else

10

might we want to know about the strategies he uses to decipher the meaning of words in spoken and written text? What meta strategies does he have? What are the patterns of his so-called reversal errors? How might SLPs and reading specialists collaborate to help students such as Matthew? (Think of points made in the alternative considerations section.)

Scenario 3

Sydney is given a comprehension test. She is asked to follow these directions:
- Before picking up the red circle, touch the white square.
- After picking up the green circle, touch the red square.
- Feed the baby before putting her to bed.

Sydney has trouble with the first two sentences and others like them. However, she gets the last sentence correct (manipulating objects to demonstrate comprehension). Sometimes she leaves out a clause when following a command. Sometimes she missequences the items even though she "acts out" all of the actions.

Conclusion. Sydney has an auditory memory problem. Her ability to recall two-step commands is "inconsistent." (*Note:* Sydney understands the individual words. The verb changes are also not the issue.)

Alternative Considerations. The idea of counting clauses in a one-, two-, three-, and ten-"step" command format is an artificial, static, and literal way of looking at the processing and comprehending of complex syntactic forms and processing in general. There are a number of factors to consider, including the contextual and decontextual nature of the task and the sentences themselves. We can see that the last sentence (the feeding-bed events) has a level of predictability or real-world relevance that is absent from the first two sentences. (Recall our discussion of sentence types and strategies in Chapter 3.) The first two sentences are more decontextualized; one has to rely on syntactic cues and structure alone because there is no real-world relevance to facilitate comprehension. Looking further, we see that the first two sentences have different order-of-mention characteristics. The first sentence violates order-of-mention—that is, the way one has to complete the instruction is expressed in the opposite way the manipulation is completed; one has to touch the white square first and *then* pick up the red circle. The second sentence follows order-of-mention. Another factor in syntactic processing includes clause order. It may be more difficult, depending on the context and content, to process sentences when the subordinate clause appears in the first position.

Consequently, we should be cautious about oversimplifications and blanket statements about "memory" and "inconsistency." We need to consider the purpose of testing sentences in isolation (though we recognize the importance of syntactic ability), the nature of sentences being used, the strategies that Sydney employs to "get" the meaning, and the factors that *facilitate* comprehension. For example, does Sydney perform better on sentences such as the second one (*After picking up the green circle, touch the red square*) because she follows the order that is expressed? Additionally, the idea that learning the meanings of words (such as *before* and *after*) is a long process should be kept in mind. Sydney may understand these words on some level but may have difficulty when they are used in decontextualized and instruction-like situations.

We would certainly continue to investigate this student's syntactic knowledge of complex forms as it relates to the curricular and the classroom concerns.

Additional Discussion Points. Consider Lahey and Bloom's (1994) notion of competing resources when evaluating tasks such as the one facing Sydney. Ask yourself what some of the competing resources might be: content (familiar-predictable or not?), syntactic structure (clause order), sentence-strategy matches (order-of-mention matches order-of-meaning), and presence of potentially confusing connector words (before-after). We should also think, yet again, about the validity of tasks such as the one presented in this scenario. How does this task connect to Sydney's ability to follow classroom instructions?

Although we may glean some information from tests and subtests that tap syntactic processing, we must go to the actual source of difficulty (e.g., the social studies classroom) to fully understand instructional discourse. We must also think strategically. For example, might it help Sydney to become better at predicting the classroom routines so that the language used becomes embedded in a familiar context? At the very least, clinicians should question validity of "counting" clauses to make any statement about processing and comprehension. Consider how the complexity of sentence structure changes, especially in literate-style sentences such as embedded relatives, complements, and so on (see Eisenberg, 2006, and Chapters 8 and 9 of this text). Counting the number of words or clauses will not take us very far in understanding the interacting processes operating to get the message. It certainly helps to ask, again, the following questions: Where did this notion of "counting steps" come from? Does it "match" what we know about information processing and comprehension?

> Tests and subtests that tap syntactic processing can provide some information, but SLPs must dig deeper to the actual source of the student's difficulty to understand instructional discourse.

Scenario 4

Justin is given another comprehension test. He is asked to listen to sentences and then answer questions about them. The sentences are taken from Bransford and Johnson's (1973) classic chapter on constructive comprehension. Examples include the following:

1. The notes were sour because the seams were split.
   - *Question:* What were sour?
   - *Answer:* "the notes"
   - *Question:* Why were the notes sour?
   - *Answer:* "because the seams were split"
2. The haystack was important because the cloth ripped.
   - *Question:* What happened to the cloth?
   - *Answer:* "it ripped"
3. John was surprised when he saw Mary's hand with all the diamonds.
   - *Question:* Who was surprised?
   - *Answer:* "John"
   - *Question:* What might John say to Mary after seeing all the diamonds?
   - *Answer:* "Mary, I didn't know you were engaged!"

Justin performs quite well, as his responses suggest.

Conclusion. Justin's comprehension is excellent.

Alternative Considerations. We are pleased that Justin has comprehended the sentences—up to a point—and that he has completed the task successfully.

10

Before SLPs draw conclusions about students' comprehension abilities, they should explore inferential comprehension abilities across spoken and written domains.

But we must move beyond the literal level of comprehension reflected in the majority of questions and responses before making a judgment about excellent comprehension. Starting with the last example, however, we see that Justin is able to provide dialogue for John and make a reasonable inference about what he might say. He uses knowledge "in his head" and moves beyond the text alone to provide a response. Justin's response about Mary's engagement is a good one given the statement about her "hand" and "all the diamonds." However, if the John/Mary sentence appeared within the context of a card game, the dialogue would obviously be different. Likewise, if we consider the first two sentences as well as Justin's responses, we see that the questions and responses merely skim the surface and fail to get to the deeper meanings. Before drawing any conclusions about Justin's or any of our students' comprehension abilities, exploration of their inferential comprehension abilities across both spoken and written domains should be an integral part of our clinical and educational practices. Inferential processing is critical for literacy learning and for ultimate school success (Bransford et al., 1999; DeKemel, 2003c; Raphael & Au, 2005; Snyder et al., 2002; van Kleeck et al., 2006).

Additional Discussion Points. One might ask what Bransford and Johnson's (1973) sentence choices say to us about constructive and inferential comprehension. For example, do the sentences *The notes were sour because the seams were split* and *The haystack was important because the cloth ripped* make sense to readers who have never seen or heard them? What interpretation of the John/Mary/diamonds sentence came to mind? Did avid bridge players immediately think of diamonds, hearts, spades, clubs? Did Justin think "engagement ring" because he is more familiar with that scenario than he is with playing cards? It is clear that proficient readers can process the sentences presented in this scenario on a superficial, more literal level, just as Justin did, but full comprehension may elude them.

According to Bransford and Johnson (1973), providing a context enables the reader (or listener) to comprehend sentences at a deeper level. A listener or reader can also "create" a context "from his/her head" to facilitate comprehension (Raphael & Au, 2005). Thus creating or being given more contextual support influences one's interpretations. For example, consider sentences 1 and 2 in the following contexts:

1. Jim is a famous bagpipe player. He was looking forward to playing for the group. But on his way to the stage, the old instrument's material mysteriously started to came apart. He tried to play anyway but...(or some rendition thereof).

2. Matthew's wife was very nervous last Saturday. She wished Matthew would quit the skydiving club. She was right to be worried because Matt's parachute had a problem midair. Luckily, he landed on a farm and, even better for Matt...

We might consider the dynamic, integrated factors that influence and facilitate comprehension as our next scenario will also demonstrate. And, of course, as we have some fun with our colleagues by testing their ability to construct meaning from the Bransford and Johnson (1973) examples, we should also discuss the question of whether our current testing and intervention tools measure up.

Scenario 5

Carol is asked to read the following expository passage silently. She is told that she will be asked to reproduce the piece for the clinician (by restating the passage "in her own words") after reading the passage. She is also told that she should think of a title for the piece. The excerpt from a longer original rendition is from Bransford and Johnson (1973, p. 400):

> The procedure is actually quite simple. First, you arrange the items in two separate groups. Of course, one pile may be sufficient depending on how much there is to do. If you have to go somewhere else due to lack of facilities, that is the next step; otherwise you are pretty well set. It is important not to overdo things. That is, better to do a few things at once than too many. In the short run, this may not seem important, but complications can easily arise. A mistake can be expensive as well. At first, the whole procedure may be complicated. Soon, however, it will become just another facet of life. It is difficult to foresee any end to the necessity for this task in the immediate future, but one can never tell. After the procedure is completed one arranges the materials into different groups again. Then they can be put into their appropriate places.

Carol has difficulty with the task. She expresses some of the text's ideas to the clinician (e.g., "There's a problem. You can do too many things at once. You put things together."), but the ideas are out of sequence, disorganized, and filled with unclear references and ambiguous vocabulary (e.g., "things," "this," etc.). Carol fails to express a main idea although she talks about the fact that there can be "a problem with something." The title she picks for the passage is "Don't Make Mistakes." Carol produces three to four sentences with much prompting from the clinician.

Conclusion. Carol has poor reading comprehension skills complicated by a sequencing problem. Her ability to retain and recall "larger and longer chunks of information" needs work. There are too many sentences in the passage. Shorten the amount of information she is given.

Alternative Considerations. Carol may indeed have reading comprehension difficulties, but we would not jump to that conclusion before looking more closely at the materials being used. The statement that Carol also has a "sequencing" problem requires closer scrutiny. (Is this difficulty ordering events or details a "tip-of-the-iceberg" phenomenon as per Chapter 1?) The intervention suggestion of "shortening the amount of information given" is also open to question since length is not a sufficient explanation for Carol's difficulties with this task. Rather, other factors such as familiarity with the structure and content of text have a greater influence on what students retain and retell with accuracy, as many researchers and clinicians have noted (see, for example, Chapter 7).

It may be that some of Carol's difficulties lie within the text itself. Would starting with a macrostructure, such as presenting a title for this passage and some preparation, be helpful? Readers of this text who are unfamiliar with this passage might find their comprehension and retention facilitated when presented with the title and an understanding that the passage will be about "Washing Clothes." Although this is not the most engaging topic, listeners

10

and readers who bring background knowledge and the experience of washing clothes can use that schema, triggered by the title, to help them organize the details to come. As we have seen, titles can be helpful, but they can also be useless without an activation of background knowledge and an understanding of the vocabulary used in the titles. And although this classic passage may be an exaggerated version of a text that would be chosen for the task described in this scenario, it helps us to appreciate what connected, expository text sometimes "feels like" to students with LLD.

Additional Discussion Points. It is important to consider the complex nature of connected discourse and the interactions among context, content, and text structure, topics we have covered in this volume. As noted, this scenario asks us to consider the idea that the passage's lack of macrostructure (as a context) may be an influencing factor in comprehension, memory, and organization. This notion leads us to question the recommendation that we just "shorten" the amount of information presented. This is a simplistic and inappropriate solution to a complex problem. We have to help Carol manage connected text, not take connected text away from her. (This last statement reminds us of the Matthew effect, which was discussed by Stanovich, 1986. It is also known as the "rich get richer" phenomenon discussed earlier in this text, whereby better readers spend more time reading and are also exposed to more elaborated text. See Catts & Kamhi, 2005d, for additional information.

It is also important to recall the metaphor presented in Chapter 1 that encouraged us to view complex behaviors with a "two-way street" schema in mind. For example, the idea that Carol has an "inherent" sequencing problem is another simplistic conclusion. It is more likely that her sequencing difficulties are a result of, rather than a cause of, broader issues that relate to text structure knowledge and skills. "Sequencing" in itself is not a unitary, causal factor in discourse processing problems but it may, indeed, be a "tip-of-the-iceberg" phenomenon. Finally, we would also want to consider a student's lexical and syntactic knowledge as micro components that may or may not be issues. For example, what is Carol's understanding of words such as "procedure" and "complications"? Can she handle complex syntax, including *if* sentences? In sum: A key point that should be discussed among collaborators is that there are many interacting factors in discourse processing and production that create problems for students with LLD. Some of those factors reside within the student and others reside outside the student (Nelson, 2005).

> Sequencing by itself is not a unitary, causal factor in discourse processing problems; however, it may indicate deeper problems.

Scenario 6

A clinician is working with a young elementary school student with LLD. Danielle is in Grade 1. In this session, the clinician's goal is to help Danielle develop better narrative skills. The clinician and the student are looking at a series/sequence of four pictures. The first part of the session involves sequencing the pictures to form a complete story. After sequencing the pictures, Danielle is encouraged to "tell a story for the pictures." The student has difficulty with both activities.

Conclusion. Danielle has to learn how to sequence the pictures first and then develop the language to describe the pictures. It is noted that "her language is fragmented and unelaborated." In addition, "Danielle uses unclear referents like 'this' and 'that' while pointing to pictures when she tells the story to the clinician."

Alternative Considerations. Danielle may need help comprehending and producing narratives. And, as we have said, narrative ability is an important acquisition for lifelong and school success. Narratives form a link between oral and literate language; narratives entertain us and teach us things, and they expand our linguistic horizons by moving us from dialogue to monologue ability. Thus the clinician's decision to work on narratives with Danielle appears to be a reasonable one. What we want to evaluate, however, is the way the activity unfolds.

Pragmatically, when two people are looking at a picture (or series of pictures) together, there is no inherent reason for language to be elaborated. In other words, presupposition—assuming what your listener knows—comes into play. In the case of Danielle and her clinician, it may be the case that the principle of presupposition is operating, or at the very least, is interfering with the need to express relations explicitly. So although Danielle may not be consciously aware of the presupposition principle, she points and says "this" and "that" because the clinician is looking at the same pictures as she is. Hadley (1998) and others (see Chapter 7) have reminded us to consider using a "naïve listener" (one who has not heard the story) to encourage the need for more elaborated and specific language and to make the task more "natural" pragmatically. A second issue with the activity is the use of separate picture cards to represent one, unified story. Children have to integrate the pictures into a theme, make inferences across pictures, and understand that a continuous plot is represented by the pictures. Making these connections may be difficult for younger students with LLD.

Again, a "sequence problem" is not necessarily a "cause" of a child's narrative difficulties. In addition, "sequencing" is not a foundational skill for connected discourse proficiency. We tend to get better at "sequencing" the events in stories and the details in other types of connected text when we get better at comprehending and producing stories and other types of connected text. And, of course, we might consider what we mean by "sequencing"—the sequencing of what and why—and recognize that in some instances order is important (e.g., completing a science experiment) whereas at other times it is not (e.g., providing a description). Scenario 6 says that the activity, materials, and intervention direction require further scrutiny.

> A "sequencing problem" is not necessarily the cause of a child's narrative difficulties. Likewise, "better sequencing" may not be a foundational skill for connected discourse proficiency but, rather, *a result of* discourse proficiency.

Additional Discussion Points. What changes in this scenario would help make narrative intervention more meaningful for Danielle and students like her? Consider some of the suggestions by Gillam and colleagues (2006), among others that were discussed in Chapter 6. Think about how the content of the sequence pictures might change the result. For example, among the questions one might raise are the following:

- Do the pictures represent a temporal or causal sequence of events?
- Are the characters and their actions clearly identifiable?
- Is the theme familiar or unfamiliar to the child?

10

Other questions relate to the monologue "practice" that children such as Danielle have had in their preschool years (Westby, 1994), as follows:

■ Have they brought sufficient connected discourse and other preliteracy experiences to the activities described in the scenario?

■ Would icons or printed information about the key elements represented by the sequence cards (if we continued to use them) offer additional and appropriate scaffolding (Justice & Ezell, 2004)?

There are many directions one can take to improve the techniques outlined in the scenario. Discussions between SLPs and teachers who share responsibilities in literacy can set the wheels in motion and offer children some reasonable alternatives to "doing what we've always done."

Scenario 7

A language intervention session is taking place with four students who have LLD and suspected auditory processing problems. They are between 9 and 10 years old. The students have disks of varying colors in front of them. The clinician tells the students to listen to what she is saying and put the disks in the correct order. The instructions go something like this: "Ready, listen carefully: red, blue, orange, yellow, purple, black." The activity proceeds like this for awhile, with corrections and repetitions made for students as needed. The next activity goes something like this: "Listen carefully. You're going to follow my two- and three-step commands. Remember we talked about the 'step' commands"? Students take turns following the clinician's instructions and they accumulate points for correct responses. "Ready, Kyle, you go first: 'Go to the door, turn around three times, and then pick up the red book in the corner.'" The activity continues with another student. "Good! Next, Cal: 'Clap five times, go to the bookshelf, and pick out a book that does not have a brown cover.'"

Conclusion. These activities help students acquire better auditory memory and processing skills.

Alternative Considerations. It is questionable to think that these types of activities have any direct connection to the core of these students' language learning and academic issues. Although they may, indeed, have spoken and written comprehension problems that are affecting their academic success, the "literalness" of this intervention session requires some well-deserved skepticism. The last instruction, with its negation and relative clause structure that ends with "pick out a book that does not have a brown cover," may be a more relevant choice to include in *comprehension* activities than any of the other examples in this scenario. This complex structure would work even better if the clinician chose curriculum-based or classroom content.

Certainly, helping students learn how to process complex syntactic forms can prove to be a useful part of language intervention. But as we saw with Sydney in Scenario 3, we do not merely count clauses to arrive at a decision about processing load or difficulty. The "book/brown cover" sentence—part of a supposedly "three-step command"—consists of two clauses, so it is difficult to say what the clinician was "getting at" with its inclusion.

As we have discussed elsewhere in this text (see Chapter 5, for example), processing complexity, and more important, one's ability to *understand what was said or read*, is influenced by many factors, including structure, content, and contextual variables. Counting "steps" is an inaccurate and simplistic route to take. Further, when the "steps" become so isolated from each other that they make little sense, the activity becomes meaningless. Even if "steps" are added, they fail to form a unit of connected discourse. As we know, connected discourse takes on a structure all its own. (And how may "steps" does it take before the commands qualify for connected discourse status?) In the same vein, counting the number of sentences in a paragraph to judge complexity is also a questionable tact to take, as scenario 5 suggests.

Additional Discussion Points. Think about the functionality of activities such as those that require the sequencing of different-colored disks. Where can this activity take students with LLD? This auditory memory task is similar to the visual sequencing task described in scenario 2. We have to get beyond thinking that processing language is a linear event like the sequenced beads on a rosary or an abacus. More important, we have to be more focused on the distinction between testing students and facilitating language. What strategies have the students in scenario 7 acquired? What did the clinician say or do (except "listen") to help the students understand classroom instructions, test language, and social studies, science, and other subjects' language requirements? (See Scenario 10 for an alternative.) Again, we should keep our eyes and ears focused on creating functional linguistic and metalinguistic intervention goals and thinking of authentic ways to operationalize those goals. We should also exercise caution when using words such as "memory" and "processing" because they mean different things to different professionals.

> SLPs must go beyond thinking that processing language is a linear event.

Scenario 8

Robert, a fifth grader with LLD, is working with his speech-language clinician. The clinician is focused on helping Robert acquire more effective strategies for "finding the main idea." She has exposed Robert to various types of expository text structures and has guided him through some of the particular structures that he may encounter in his textbooks. Frequently, however, he misses the main point of a story or an explanatory piece. His organizational abilities and his lexical repertoire (his knowledge and use of elaborated vocabulary) are also below grade level. He is described as being approximately 2 years behind in reading.

The clinician decides to have Robert participate in various semantic mapping activities. She uses themes such as sports, foods, and television as a start. The semantic map consists of a large circle with spokelike bubbles coming out of it. Words are added to the bubbles that connect to the topic. For example, the word "baseball" appears in the large circle in the center. Words and phrases such as *catcher, home run, nine members,* and so on are added by Robert, along with a structured discussion with his clinician.

Conclusion. The semantic mapping activity will help Robert "see" a main idea (e.g., baseball) and the details that relate to that idea. The activity will also strengthen his vocabulary knowledge by having him participate actively in the mapping of semantic connections.

10

Alternative Considerations. The clinician is on the right track by choosing an aspect of comprehension—finding the main idea—that is problematic for many students with LLD. Having Robert participate actively in the task by writing in the words and using the map as a prompt also makes sense. But we might look in two directions to consider some other possibilities: (1) using a better semantic map for Robert and (2) using curricular content.

Regarding the first consideration, we might recall Singer and Bashir's (2004) suggestion that we find maps that are better matched to our intervention goals (see, for example, Figures 8-1 and 8-2, pp. 227 and 228). Semantic mapping is a fine idea, but using a framework that makes the connection between main ideas and details more explicit is warranted. Similar to Singer and Bashir's (2004) suggestion, Ehren (2006a) says that the popular semantic maps with circles and supporting bubbles may be useful in some situations, but they can also be confusing for students with LLD. She says that (1) we should use an outline that looks like what might be on the written page and (2) we should include sentence frames (**in bold**) that specify the following:

(1) **The passage is about:** *George Washington.* (2) **It tells me that (this is the main idea):** *George Washington was a great leader of the newly independent United States* (3) **because** *he won significant battles; he showed his courage in Valley Forge; he inspired the colonists;* and so on **(these are the details/supporting facts).**

Students complete the sentence frames (the *italicized parts*) by writing in or talking about the different aspects of the topic (Ehren, 2006a).

Additional Discussion Points. The value of starting with topics that students know and like should be part of our discussion points. Familiarity with a topic (such as baseball for some students) decreases the possibility of competing resources (Lahey & Bloom, 1994). It is important, however, to teach students how to apply the strategies learned with familiar content to curricular content. In addition, we should consider Ehren's (2006b) main point—that is, be explicit when helping students appreciate that some ideas are bigger than others. Moving from bigger to smaller ideas—for example, using bigger and smaller boxes in vertical arrangements on a page—may be an excellent alternative to explore.

Scenario 9

The clinician is working with a small group of 11- and 12-year-old students with LLD. The students attend a Special Day Class (SDC) in a large school system in Southern California. They, like many other students with LLD, have "come a long way" toward overcoming some of their early language disorders. (A younger first-grade child is profiled in the next scenario.) The students have reasonable conversational and spoken narrative abilities. Topics that are familiar to them are expressed more enthusiastically and coherently. (They have some proficiency reporting on the plots of Adam Sandler and Owen Wilson movies.) The students have lingering decoding difficulties (especially decoding multisyllabic words) and more significant reading comprehension difficulties. One problem they share is "limited vocabulary knowledge." They don't make connections among words and have difficulty learning new words. They demonstrate a limited ability to provide synonyms and antonyms for words when expressing themselves in spoken and written text. Figurative language is especially difficult for them.

The clinician uses several techniques to help the students acquire more elaborated semantic repertoires. One focus of intervention has included work on double meanings and nonliteral meanings of words. For example, she uses metaphors that have perceptually salient characteristics such as "The skater was a top on the ice." She also uses context, for example, presenting paragraphs describing a stormy night that end with a character saying, "It's raining cats and dogs."

Conclusion. Working on figurative language will help the students develop an appreciation for some of the ways that word meanings can change. These activities will benefit their overall comprehension and metalinguistic development.

Alternative Considerations. The use of perceptual characteristics to help students comprehend the relationships being expressed is a reasonable way to proceed. As noted in Chapter 9, the image of a top and an ice skater spinning makes the metaphor more transparent (Milosky, 1994; Nippold, 1985; van Kleeck, 1994). The perceptual salience helps students relate to the ideas because they have a concrete tenor to them. In addition, the inclusion of contextual support for figurative language forms is quite appropriate because figurative language usually occurs within a context that disambiguates its meaning. However, we would like to know more about how the students are being "taught" to find and express meanings, and most important, we would also want to consider the choice of metaphors (or other figurative forms). Again, using familiar situations (e.g., the students know something about ice skating) may provide a starting point, but we might use our time more effectively by looking toward the curriculum and discovering the figurative forms that students are more likely to encounter. Metaphors such as "Washington was a rock," "George III was a blown volcano," and "The Civil War tore the fabric of the new country apart" might be better choices. The random choice of idioms, metaphors, similes, and other forms from a workbook requires a second look.

Additional Discussion Points. Think about the kinds of idioms and other forms of figurative language that occur each day. Our language is more idiomatic and figurative than we may think it is at first glance. Looking through students' textbooks for clues to the types of nonliteral forms that occur may be a more direct route to take, as mentioned in the previous section. Practitioners might also consider some of the contexts that help facilitate nonliteral comprehension. For example, Milosky (1994) presents an excellent summary of the different degrees of linguistic context that facilitate idiom and metaphor comprehension interpretation. Among the contexts she outlines include those that build on one another until the idiom's meaning is embedded in the surrounding language, as follows:

- *Metalinguistic task* (What does "spill the beans" mean?)
- *Animate agent* (<u>The man</u> spilled the beans.)
- *State of mind of agent* (The <u>nervous</u> man spilled the beans.)

Using familiar situations may provide a starting point in helping students to comprehend nonliteral texts, but SLPs would be wise to look toward the curriculum to discover the figurative forms students will encounter to ensure authentic intervention.

10

- *Event* (The nervous man spilled the beans <u>about the birthday party.</u>)
- *Mention of contrasting state* (The woman's friends wanted to throw a surprise birthday party for her. They worked hard to <u>keep it a secret.</u> A nervous man spilled the beans about the <u>surprise</u> birthday party.)

Milosky's suggestions continue with linguistic markers added to text such as *but* and *accidentally* that make the relations among the words even tighter. For example, a sentence would read, "They worked hard to keep it a secret *but* the nervous man spilled the beans about the surprise party *accidentally*." Milosky (1994) follows by presenting more detailed examples that show how the meaning of "spilled the beans" can be made even more explicit by adding sentences and dialogue to paragraphs. In summary, there is much to learn about figurative language, including its long course of development into the adolescent years, its prevalence in language, and the many techniques available for its facilitation.

Scenario 10

The Way It Sometimes "Plays Out" for Our Children. A first grader with a history of preschool LLD has come a very long way linguistically but is not out of the woods. (Maybe we're back in the proverbial forest?) Michael is a completely engaging, funny, and creative individual. He enjoys communicating, can tell fairly integrated stories, loves words and wordplay, and is basically a wonderful conversationalist. He has overcome most of his earlier syntactic, semantic, and pragmatic difficulties. He participated in intensive speech-language therapy from 2 until 5 years old. His home life is rich, warm, and supportive.

He is currently 6½ years old and having trouble in Grade 1. He is described by his school as "possibly having ADD, or an auditory processing disorder, or a learning disability." Michael has trouble following the teacher's directions and is behind the other children in reading and writing. He sometimes needs more time to respond to her directions and "turns his head away," informing the speaker that he needs some time to think. Speech-language intervention has been reinstated in a setting outside of school. The clinicians at the center are versed in curriculum-based assessment and intervention. A typical homework assignment for Michael is to write five complete sentences for given words. This assignment, among others like it, is difficult for him.

Conclusion. Additional testing, identification, and placement in special education is in the cards for Michael.

Alternative Considerations. The speech-language clinicians (a team of two) are helping Michael develop language skills and strategies that will facilitate his ability to thrive and survive in the classroom. They are also working closely with Michael's teacher, who is described as a more seasoned, structured, traditional Grade 1 teacher. She moves fairly quickly through the curriculum. Although Michael has been successful in language intervention, picking up concepts quickly and being highly motivated, first grade is still a challenge for him. Fortunately, he still loves learning and has some good foundational metalinguistic abilities that work to his advantage. He also has a rich family life, as mentioned, so that he brings some excellent background knowledge to the tasks he faces.

Intervention is focused on expanding his "meta" strategies with a semantic thrust that includes identifying words he doesn't understand and asking for clarification about word meanings, assignments, and instructions. For example, the clinicians have Michael participate in a number of instructional language games that challenge him. The instructions contain "tricky words or phrases" such as *in between, in the center, to the left of,* and so on. He listens, asks a question (if needed), and follows the command (Kent & Veremakis, 2006). Reminders (listen, question, do it) are written on a card. They contain icons and printed words. The clinicians role-play following commands and asking for clarification or repetition as needed. Michael is encouraged to ask one of his clinicians questions such as "What does the *center* mean?" or "Can you say that again?" or "Is center like the middle?" (His Grade 1 teacher has reviewed the strategies with the clinicians, and she is encouraging Michael to use them in the classroom. This collaboration is a critical key to intervention success.) His SLPs are also working on segmentation skills, including sentence, word, and sound segmentation, and other literacy skills, including decoding and reading comprehension, within the contexts of spoken and written narrative and expository discourse. His improving segmentation skills have had a positive effect on his ability to "pick out" words of which he is unsure.

Although covering a number of areas, the clinicians view the "meta" focus as weaving its way through all the other goals and objectives. They see spoken and written language and receptive and expressive language as integrated pieces of Michael's intervention program. The parents, teacher, and speech-language pathologist have formed a tight-knit team to provide Michael with the additional support he needs to stay in the mainstream where he belongs. Although the Grade 1 teacher is not as sure about Michael's long-term placement in regular education, she is supportive of current efforts. The clinicians and parents are more mainstream focused for him. The team has discussed responsiveness to intervention (RTI) models (see Chapter 2) and everyone agrees that there may be several rungs of service available to Michael at this time.

Additional Discussion Points. Practitioners who work both in and outside of the classroom might ask themselves if the Grade 1 curriculum is what Grade 2 used to be. They might also discuss the idea that perhaps too many children may be headed for special education too soon (see Troia's [2005] discussion of RTI models and Chapter 2 of this text). We might also consider the level of "meta" required for many homework assignments as early as first grade. For example, what knowledge is assumed to be intact to "write a complete sentence"? Michael needed help in this area because he wasn't sure how to make this syntactic judgment. He uses complete and often complex sentences in his spoken language but does not yet have the level of "meta" ability to make the determination of syntactic correctness. It is unclear where the majority of children in his class fared with this assignment, but it is probable that the readers and writers performed better on the sentence writing and other "meta" tasks. An observation and understanding of the Grade 1 curriculum is clearly a worthwhile endeavor for SLPs and those professionals who work outside of the regular education framework.

10

Another area ripe for discussion is the question of whether attention-deficit disorder (ADD), learning disable (LD), or any other "new" label is appropriate for Michael. As noted in Chapter 2, these labels may not represent distinct populations. Michael is a child with *language* disorders who is getting older. And language disorders are pervasive, as we have discussed. Michael's language disorders have changed over time, and they "look different" but are still present. It would be inaccurate to say he has a language disorder *and* a learning disability—suggesting that he has acquired something new. This is a critical discussion point for practitioners, especially when intervention or placement goes in a different direction from the one a child actually needs. Similarly, Michael may appear to be "inattentive" in class when he is actually struggling to comprehend the message.

His clinicians are helping him develop strategies that are more effective—and appreciated by the teacher—than turning his head (to think) when the teacher is talking and requiring that all eyes remain on her. And, finally, it is important to reiterate the idea that the SLPs are not helping Michael complete his homework assignments. Rather, they are using the language assignments from Grade 1 as a backdrop for language intervention. They are uncovering the language knowledge and skills that underlie Michael's assignments and other curricular demands. And, so, in closing, although we do not know what the future holds for Michael, we do know that the system can "do better" for Michael and other children like him who have language learning and academic difficulties.

The Symphony Comes Together: Ending on a Positive Note

At a recent conference of speech and language professionals, Ehren and colleagues (2007) used the title: "Nirvana or Bust: Quality Services in Schools—Settle for No Less." In their presentation, whose title was suggested by Ehren (2006, personal communication), the authors used the concept of Nirvana to hypothesize about what it could be like to serve children and adolescents in a "perfect world" where harmony and stability exist and enlightenment rules. Although both the authors and the attendees alike recognized that the world of schools is indeed imperfect, they also recognized that taking steps toward creating a Nirvana of quality services means recognizing that the process of change is a long and gradual one of discovery, acceptance, and growth. From Buddhist and Hindu perspectives, moving toward Nirvana in life (and in schools) also means "letting go" of unhealthy practices along the way. And although this last piece—the letting go—is no easy task, we do have the knowledge, skills, and strategies to do so. This reality is brought home to us, yet again, through the words of wisdom of a current sage: "You've got to leave the past behind, even if it provides you with a level of comfort, before you can move forward and see change" (Colin Cowhead, ESPN radio, October 26, 2006). Thus, in settling for no less than the best in schools, we might consider the reminders summarized in Box 10-1.

In closing, then, we will leave readers with the following thoughts. Although we have integrated some of the critical components of language intervention at school-age levels in this text, we have merely scratched the surface of possibilities. The references documenting the many excellent works of our colleagues from

BOX 10-1 | *How to Ensure Quality Service in Schools*

1. Stay focused on the real world of students and think logically.
2. Create language intervention goals and objectives that are authentic and curriculum relevant.
3. Paint language intervention canvases with broad brush strokes that keep the horizon in focus.
4. Think strategically and help children do the same.
5. Take on leadership roles in language and literacy.
6. Be brave! Be a "meme breaker."
7. Believe that change is possible even in an imperfect world.

speech and language, early literacy, reading acquisition and disorders, regular and special education, and curriculum design, among others, must continue to enrich us and the students we serve. The work of others in the area of spelling, for example, was not covered in detail in this volume but is available to practitioners who wish to explore the other side of the decoding coin by taking a strong linguistic approach that breaks the mold of traditional practices (see Masterson & Apel, 2000; Masterson et al., 2002; Wasowicz et al., 2003).

Indeed, before the metaphorical ink is dry on this publication, there will be many other contributions that add to our body of knowledge. But we, as consumers, must always be vigilant. So although there may be a long road to Nirvana ahead of us in the world of school-age language disorders, we must maintain our optimism on the path to achieving a higher standard for our students. Maybe the small successes on that road to language learning and academic success are the real Nirvana. When we see Michael, our first grader from Scenario 10, say "I get it now! I really get it!" with excitement in his eyes, we know we're getting there. When he uses a strategy learned in a language intervention session in his classroom successfully, we know we've made a significant contribution to his life as a student and beyond. Creating and appreciating the small victories may be as important as the end result, as Kahlil Gibran, Lebanese mystical poet, philosopher, and painter, points out:

> Yes. There is a Nirvana; it is in leading your sheep to a green pasture, and in putting your child to sleep, and in writing the last line of your poem.

Indeed, getting to the last line of a book is a very good thing. It reminds us that Nirvana is all around us if we choose to embrace it. It is possible to change a little piece of our world. It is possible to create a different outcome for our students. It is even possible to think that in the not-so-distant future, the New York Yankees will win that elusive twenty-seventh World Series and that, through our individual efforts, schools will become a happier place for children and adolescents with LLD.

10

Appendix A: Examples of Scripts at Each Level Using the Book-Sharing Intervention

Levels and Questions	Prompts and Responses

Level I (literal)
"What's that?" (pointing to a candle in the picture)
	1. *Candle.* Yes, that's a candle.
	2. *Light.* Yes, it is a kind of light. It's a kind of light called a (using rising intonation on "a" that indicates "you finish the sentence") _____.
	  a. *Candle.* Yes, it's a candle.
	  b. *Inappropriate response; no response; I don't know.* It's a kind of light called a candle. (Point to candle and then the flame.) See, this is a candle and here's the flame of the candle that gives it a little light (circle finger around the halo of light).
	3. *Inappropriate response; no response; I don't know.* It's called a _____ (pause, and if no response) a can (prolong saying "can") _____.
	  a. *Candle.* Yes, it's a candle.
	  b. *Inappropriate response; no response; I don't know.* That's called a candle. (Point to candle and then the flame.) See, this is a candle and here's the flame of the candle that gives it a little light (circle finger around the halo of light).

Level II (literal)
"What's Bear doing here?"
	1. *He's waving.* Yes, he's waving good-bye to Little Bird.
	2. *Inappropriate response; no response; I don't know.* He's waving good-bye to_____.
	  a. *Little Bird.* Yes, he's waving good-bye to Little Bird.
	  b. *Inappropriate response; no response; I don't know.* Little Bird. He's waving good-bye to Little Bird, isn't he?

Note. Adult script is in regular font; potential kinds of child responses or nonresponses are indicated in *italics*.
From van Kleeck, A., Vander Woude, J., & Hammett, L. (2006). Fostering literal inferential language skills in Head Start preschoolers with language impairment using scripted book-sharing discussions. *American Journal of Speech-Language Pathology, 15,* 95.

Continued

Levels and Questions	Prompts and Responses

Level III (inferential)
"How do you think Bear feels because his friend Little Bird is leaving?"
	1. *Sad.* Yes, I think he feels sad because he won't see his friend for a long time. Do you ever feel sad when you won't see someone for a long time?
	2. *Inappropriate response; no response; I don't know.* I think he maybe feels sad because he won't see (pointing to Little Bird)_____.
	   a. *Child's appropriate response (Little Bird; his friend; etc.).* Yes, Bear's sad because he (repeat child's reason if appropriate).
	   b. *Inappropriate response; no response; I don't know.* His friend for a long time. Bear is sad because he won't see his friend for a long time. Do you ever feel sad when you won't see someone for a long time?

Level IV (inferential)
"What do you think Bear's gonna do with his arrow with the spoon on it?"
	1. *Try to shoot it at the moon; other appropriate response.* I think so, too! I think he wants to see how the moon tastes, so he's going to try to shoot his arrrow all the way to the moon. Shall we keep reading and see?
	2. *Inappropriate response; no response; I don't know.* He wants to see how the moon tastes, remember? So, I think he's going to try to shoot his arrow all the way to the (pointing to the moon) _____.
	   a. *Moon.* Yes, I think so, too! I think he wants to see how the moon tastes, so he's going to try to shoot his arrow all the way to the moon. Shall we keep reading and see?
	   b. *Inappropriate response; no response; I don't know.* Moon. I think maybe he's going to try to shoot his arrow all the way to the moon. Shall we keep reading and see?

Appendix B: Suggested Sequence of Literature-Based Intervention Activities

A. **Prestory Knowledge Activation**
1. Graphic organizer
2. Prestory discussion
   a) Use linguistic facilitations (e.g., semantic expansion) to make the student's language more complete and complex.
   b) Discuss the pictures on every page, using questions to help guide the student through the main story line.

B. **Shared Reading of the Entire Story**
   Read the book aloud, stopping occasionally to comment or discuss concepts, sentence structures, or plot elements.

C. **Post-Story Comprehension Discussion**
   Use general comprehension and story grammar questions.
1. Who are the most important characters in this story?
2. What do we know about them?
3. Describe what they look like, their personalities, their values, etc.
4. How do we know that?
5. What did (name of main character) do?
6. Why did he/she do that?
7. What happened after he/she (name the main activity)?
8. What was the main problem in the story?
9. How was the problem solved?
10. What is the main point of this story?

D. **Focused Skill Activities**
1. Semantic activities
   a) Select vocabulary from the story and/or related vocabulary.
   b) Make a New Word Book that lists words from the story.
   c) Define and discuss the words in student-friendly language.
   d) Create a wall chart and encourage use of the target words in other activities.
2. Syntax Activities
   a) Select a sentence pattern that is repeated throughout the book.
   b) Read the sentences with the student.
   c) Place the noun and verb phrases onto sentence strips that students can manipulate.
   d) Have students draw pictographs to represent the sentences.
   e) Match the sentence strips to the sentences.
   f) Retell the story with an added focus on using the target sentence pattern.
3. Narrative Activities
   a) Retell through pictography.
   b) Create a retold book.
   c) Create a parallel story.

4. Pragmatics activities
   a) Select a pragmatic ability represented within the story (e.g., politeness, requesting, topic shifting, restating, justifying).
   b) Discuss how the characters used language to handle a situation in the story.
   c) Create parallel situations.
   d) Discuss how language could be used in these situations.
   e) Act out the situations.
   f) Apply one of the created situations and the pragmatic usage in the parallel stories.

E. **Book as Model for Parallel Story**
   1. Discuss the original graphic organizer and revise it if necessary.
   2. Review the vocabulary in the student's New Word Book.
      a) Find the target vocabulary in the original book.
      b) Read the sentences containing the target vocabulary.
      c) Create new parallel sentences containing the vocabulary.
   3. Review the retold story book.
   4. Create another parallel story or revise the earlier ones.
   5. Share the parallel stories and review the target skills learned.

From Gillam, R. B., & Ukrainetz, T. A. (2006). Language intervention through literature-based units. In T. A. Ukrainetz (Ed.), *Contextualized language intervention* (pp. 72–73). Eau Claire, WI: Thinking Publications.

Appendix C: Eliciting Conversation, Narrative, and Expository Samples of Connected Speech and Eliciting Story Retelling/Generation

Instructions: *We're going to talk for a while. I'll ask you some questions about your family and things you like to do, so I can get to know you better. You can ask me questions too. I'm going to use this stopwatch to help me remember when it's time to do something new.*

Block 1: You and Your Family		Child Information
	Topic 1. How old are you? a. When is your birthday? b. If recent or imminent: What did/will you do for your birthday?	_____ (age) _____ (birth date) Siblings Age _____ _____ _____
Tell a personal story about you and your siblings…	Topic 2. Do you have any brothers or sisters? a. What are their names? b. How old are they?	
	c. Have you ever done something like that to your brother or sister? Tell me about that. Tell me what you like to do with your brother or sister.	
	Topic 3. Do you have any pets? a. What kind? b. Tell me how you take care of _____.	_____ (kind of pet) _____ (pet's name)
Tell a personal story about a pet…	c. Has _____ ever done something like that? Tell me about that. Tell me about what you do with _____.	
	d. What happens to _____ when he/she does that?	

Block 2: Favorite Things to Do (Begin around 4 min mark)

Tell child about how you spend your free time. Tell about a game/sport you like and how you play it.	Topic 4. What's your favorite thing to do when you're at home? a. Do you play games like _____ (game, sport) with your _____ (brother, sister, friends)? b. If game, tell me how you play that game. c. If sport, tell me how you play/do that.	_____ (favorite game) _____ (favorite sport)
I know you are in/just finished _____ grade. *Tell a personal story about something you liked about school.*	Topic 5. What is/was your favorite part of _____ grade? a. Tell me why you liked _____ so much.	_____ (grade)

Block 3: Favorite Stories, TV Shows, Movies (Begin around 8 min mark)

I like to read good books and go to movies. This _____ (season) I saw _____ (movie).	Topic 6. Have you seen any good movies lately? a. I haven't seen that movie. What is it about?	_____ (recent movie)
Tell briefly about the characters, plot, and why you liked it.	Topic 7. Do you have a favorite book? a. Who is that book about? b. Tell me what happens to _____ in that book.	_____ (favorite book)
	Topic 8. Do you have a favorite TV show? a. Who is that show about? b. Tell me what happened to _____ on the last show.	_____ (favorite show)

From Hadley, P. A. (1998). Language sampling protocols for eliciting text-level discourse. *Language, Speech, and Hearing Services in Schools, 29,* 132–147.

Instructions for Eliciting Story Retelling/Regeneration

Materials needed: tape recorder; microphone; audiotape; comprehension query checklist for story grammar elements; pencil; *Frog, Where Are You?* video set to the title frame on video player; frog title page; basket containing large pencil, colored markers, storytelling paper, and stapler

Step 1: Story Retelling

We're going to watch a story on TV together. It's a story about a frog [point to frog on the title page of the booklet]. *This is a different kind of story. This story doesn't have any words. After you watch the story, you will get to tell the story in your own words! And then I'll have you tell the story to _____ (mom, dad, ...). So...*

First, we'll watch the story. Next, you'll practice telling the story in your own words with me. And then, you can tell _____ (your mom, dad) all about your story. What are we going to do?

This serves as a comprehension check to see if the child understand the directions. If the child cannot recite the three steps, use the following prompts.

First...   *Next...*   *Then...*

If these prompts are not effective, repeat the instructions and check again. If the child still does not understand the task, this protocol may not be appropriate for the child and an alternative protocol should be used.

Ok, watch the story carefully. When it ends, you will tell me the story in your own words.

Turn on the videotape. Watch the videotape with the child, but do not initiate any conversation at this time. If the child says something to you during the viewing, respond with minimal, but appropriate, back channel responses. (e.g., *uhhuh, yeah, oh, hmm*). You will stop the video after the boy goes to sleep and the frog is contained in the jar.

Did you like that story? Let's give your story a title.

Prepare to write title and author (child's name) on title page. If child does not provide title,

Title Prompt: *What should we call your story?*
Author Prompt: *by....*

Ok, now tell me the story in your own words.

Allow the child to retell the story. The following prompts should be used, if necessary.

Story Retelling Prompts:

Prompt 1: This is for children who have difficulty getting started. Once the child begins talking, clinician should use only backchanneling acknowledgments.

What happened in the story?

Prompt 2: This is for children who get started, but stop 2 or 3 utterances into the retelling.

Tell me more. I want to hear your whole story.

Prompt 3: If the second prompt does not elicit a continuous narrative, give one additional prompt.

Then what happened? Tell me more.

Step 2: Comprehension Queries (if information is missing from retelling)

While you listen to the retelling, check to see if the child includes these important elements. If not, you will use the comprehension probes on the far right to have the child rehearse this information before retelling to a parent. Help the child to understand that the listener has not seen the movie and it is his/her job to help the listener understand the whole story. Pretend to be the listener and try to tell the child's story back to him. When you identify missing information, use the following comprehension queries to make sure the child has practiced a coherent and cohesive narrative before the retelling with the unfamiliar listener.

1. Characters	frog		*Who was the story about?*
	boy, mom, dog		*Were there any other important characters?*
2. Setting	yard-kitchen-bedroom		*Where does the story take place?*
3. Events	frog dives in pool		*How does the story begin?*
	boy brings frog inside		*How does the frog get inside the house?*
	frog jumps into pie		*What funny thing does the frog do?*
	mom pokes frog		*How does the mother find the frog?*
	frog gets put in jar		*What happens to the frog?*

Step 3: Story Generation

Let's watch just a little bit more to see what happens next.

Show portion of video where the frog escapes. This is used to prompt the generation of a new episode.

Oh my, the frog got out of the jar. That's where the movie stopped. What do you think happens next? How do you think the story ends?

If the child is unable to make up a new episode/ending, provide the following starter idea for the story generation component of this task.

Prompt: *I wonder where the frog went. Can you make up your own ending to the story?*

Step 4: Story Retelling to Parent (Listener unfamiliar with story)

What a great story! Let's tell your story to _____ (mom, dad, friend). She/he didn't get to see the movie. I know _____ will love to hear your story! I'll go ask him/her to come in.

Place title page and basket of bookmaking materials in front of child and parent.

To parent: _____ *(child) just saw a movie about a little boy and his frog.*
_____ (child) just told me the story in his/her own words and called
his/her story _____ (title). I need to talk to _____
for a little while. Here are some markers for coloring and some pencils
for writing. You'll have 10 or 15 minutes to work together to finish
_____'s (child) book, so _____ (child) will have something
to take home after all his/her hard work today.

To child: *Now you tell _____ (your mom, dad) the story and he/she can help*
you finish your book.

Appendix D: List of Connecting Words and Their Definitions and Words with Similar Meanings

Connecting Words	Definition	Words with Similar Meaning
Coordinating Connectors: Link Independent Clauses		
and	plus together with occurring at the same time	in addition as well as
or	tells us we have a choice	no true synonyms; in some contexts *optionally, alternatively,* or *on the other hand* may be substituted
but	contrary to expectations	on the contrary however yet still nevertheless except that
hence	as a result from this time	therefore as a result from now on
therefore	for that reason	consequently hence
yet	means the same as but	but however nevertheless still except that
Subordinating Connectors: Link Dependent Clauses		
after	following the time that	
although/though	in spite of the fact	even though even if supposing that
as	to the same degree that in the same way that	while because

From Westby, C. E., & Clauser, P. S. (2005). The right stuff for writing: Assessing and facilitating written language. In H. W. Catts & A. G. Kamhi (Eds.), *Language and reading disabilities* (2nd edition, pp. 310–311). Boston: Allyn & Bacon.

Continued

Connecting Words	Definition	Words with Similar Meaning
Subordinating Connectors: Link Dependent Clauses—cont'd		
because	for the reason that since	for in view of the fact inasmuch as taking into account that
before	in advance of the time when	prior to
if	in the case that in the event that whether	granting that on condition that
meanwhile	during or in the intervening time at the same time	
since	from the time that (preferred meaning) continuously from the time when as a result of the fact that	inasmuch because for
so that/in order that	for the purpose of	so with the wish that with the purpose that with the result that
than	compared to the degree that	
unless	except on the condition that	
until	up to the time that to the point or extent that	
when/whenever	at the time that	as soon as if while (although not synonymous)
where/wherever	at what place in a place that to a place that	
while	during the time that at the same time that although	as long as

Bibliography

Abedi, J., & Lord, C. (2001). The language factor in mathematics tests. *Applied Measurement in Education, 14,* 219-234.

Alexander, P. A. (2000). Toward a model of academic development: Schooling and the acquisition of knowledge. *Educational Researcher, 29,* 29-33, 44.

Alvermann, D. E., & Phelps, S. (2002). *Content reading and literacy: Succeeding in today's diverse classroom* (3rd edition). Boston: Allyn & Bacon.

American Speech-Language-Hearing Association Committee on Language Learning Disabilities (1982). The role of the speech-language pathologist in learning disabilities. *ASHA, 24,* 937-944.

American Speech-Language-Hearing Association Committee on Language (1983, June). A definition of language. *ASHA, 24,* 44.

American Speech-Language-Hearing Association (ASHA) (2001). Position statement on the roles and responsibilities of speech-language pathologists with regard to reading and writing in children and adolescents (position statement, executive summary of guidelines, technical report). *ASHA Supplement, 21,* 17-27.

American Speech-Language-Hearing Association (ASHA) (2003). *A workload analysis approach for establishing speech-language caseload standards in the schools: Implementation guide.* Rockville, MD: Author.

American Speech-Language-Hearing Association (ASHA) (2005). *Literacy and communication: Expectations from kindergarten through fifth grade.* Rockville, MD: Jointly published by the Association's Division 1, Language Learning and Education & Division 16, School-based Issues.

Anderson, R. C., Reynolds, R. E., Schallert, D. L., & Goetz, E. T. (1977). Framework for comprehending discourse. *American Educational Research Journal, 14,* 376-382.

Apel, K. (1999). Checks and balances: Keeping science in our profession. *Language, Speech, and Hearing Services in Schools, 30,* 98-107.

Apel, K., Masterson, J. J., & Hart, P. (2004). Integration of language components in spelling: Instruction that maximizes students' learning. In E. R. Silliman & L. C. Wilkinson (Eds.), *Language and literacy learning in schools* (pp. 292-315). New York: Guilford Press.

Applebee, A. (1978). *The child's concept of story: Ages two to seventeen.* Chicago: University of Chicago Press.

Aram, D. M. (1991). Comments on specific language impairment as a clinical category. *Language, Speech, and Hearing Services in Schools, 22,* 66-87.

Aram, D. M., & Hall, N. (1989). Longitudinal follow-up of children with preschool communication disorders. *School Psychology Review, 18,* 487-501.

Asch, F. (1987). *Mooncake.* New York: Scholastic.

Asch, F. (1990). *Skyfire.* New York: Scholastic.

Athey, I. (1977). Syntax, semantics, and reading, In J. Guthrie (Ed.), *Cognition, curriculum, and comprehension* (pp. 71-98). Newark, DE: International Reading Association.

Baddeley, A., Gathercole, S., & Papagno, C. (1998). The phonological loop as a language learning device. *Psychological Review, 105,* 158-173.

Baker, S., Gersten, R., Lee, D. S. (2002). A synthesis of empirical research on teaching mathematics to low-achieving students. *Elementary School Journal, 103,* 51-73.

Barton, K. (1997). "I just kinda know": Elementary students' ideas about historical evidence. *Theory and Research in Social Education, 24,* 407-430.

Bashir, A. S. (1987, June). Language and the curriculum. Workshop presented at the Emerson College Language Learning Disabilities Institute, Boston.

Bashir, A. S. (1989). Language intervention and the curriculum. *Seminars in Speech and Language, 10,* 181-191.

Bashir, A. S., Conte, B. M, & Heerde, S. M. (1998). Language and school success: Collaborative challenges and choices. In D. D. Merritt & B. Culatta, *Language intervention in the classroom* (pp. 1-36). San Diego, CA: Singular Publishing Group.

Bashir, A. S., Kuban, K. C., Kleinman, S., & Scavuzzo, A. (1984). Children with language disorders: Considerations of cause, maintenance, and change. *ASHA Reports, 12,* 92-106.

Bashir, A. S., & Scavuzzo, A. (1992). Children with language disorders: Natural history of academic success. *Journal of Learning Disabilities, 25,* 53-65.

Bashir, A. S., & Singer, B. D. (2006). Assisting students in becoming self-regulated writers. In T. A. Ukrainetz (Ed.), *Contextualized language intervention* (pp. 565-598). Eau Claire, WI: Thinking Publications.

Beck, A., & Knoll, C. (2006, May). Curriculum-based and collaborative language intervention. Paper prepared for the Department of Communicative Disorders at California State University at Long Beach, Long Beach, CA.

Beck, I. L., McKeown, M. G., Sinatra, G. M., & Loxterman, J. A. (1991). Revised social studies text from a text-processing perspective: Evidence of improved comprehension. *Reading Research Quarterly, 26,* 251-276.

Beck, I. L., McKeown, M. G., & Worthy, J. (1995). Giving text a voice to improve students' understanding. *Reading Research Quarterly, 30,* 220-234.

Berlin, L. J., Blank, M., & Rose, S. A. (1980). The language of instruction: The hidden complexities. *Topics in Language Disorders, 1,* 47-58.

Best, R. M., Rowe, M., Ozuru, Y., & McNamara, D. S. (2005). Deep-level comprehension of science text: The role of the reader and the text. *Topics in Language Disorders, 25,* 65-83.

Bever, T. (1970). The cognitive basis of linguistic structures. In J. R. Hayes (Ed.), *Cognition and the development of language* (pp. 279-362). New York: Wiley.

Bird, J., Bishop, D., & Freeman, N. H. (1995). Phonological awareness and literacy development in children with expressive phonological impairments. *Journal of Speech and Hearing Research, 38,* 446-462.

Bishop, D. V. M., & Adams, C. (1990). A prospective study of the relationship between specific language impairment, phonological disorders and reading impairment. *Journal of Child Psychology and Psychiatry, 31,* 1027-1050.

Bishop, D. V. M., Carlyon, R. P., Deeks, J. M., & Bishop, S. J. (1999). Auditory temporal impairment: Neither necessary nor sufficient for causing language impairment in children. *Journal of Speech, Language, and Hearing Research, 42,* 1295-1310.

Bittel, K., & Hernandez, D. (2006). Kinesthetic writing of sorts. *Science Scope, 29,* 37-39.

Blachman, B. (1994). Early literacy acquisition: The role of phonological awareness. In G. P. Wallach & K. G. Butler (Eds.), *Language learning disabilities in children and adolescents: Some principles and applications* (pp. 253-269). Boston: Allyn & Bacon.

Blachowicz, C. L. Z. (1986). Making connections: Alternatives to the vocabulary notebook. *Journal of Reading, 29,* 643-649.

Blachowicz, C. L. Z. (1994). Problem-solving strategies for academic success. In G. P. Wallach & K. G. Butler (Eds.), *Language learning disabilities in school-age children and adolescents: Some principles and applications* (pp. 304-322). Boston: Allyn & Bacon.

Blachowicz, C. L. Z., & Fisher, P. (2004). Building vocabulary in remedial settings: focus on word relatedness. *Perspectives: Newsletter of the International Dyslexia Association, 30,* 24-31.

Blank, M. (1986 June). Natural language exchanges and coding techniques. Workshop presented at the Language Learning Disabilities Institute, Emerson College, Boston.

Blank, M. (2002). Classroom discourse: A key to literacy. In K. G. Butler & E. R. Silliman (Eds.), *Speaking, reading and writing in children with language learning disabilities: New paradigms in research and practice* (pp. 151-173). Mahwah, NJ: Erlbaum.

Blank, M., & Marquis, A. M. (1987). *Teaching discourse.* Tucson, AZ: Communication Skill Builders.

Blank, M., Marquis, A. M., & Klimovitch, M. (1994). *Directing school discourse.* San Antonio, TX: Communication Skill Builders.

Blank, M., Marquis, A. M., & Klimovitch, M. (1995). *Directing early discourse.* San Antonio, TX: Communication Skill Builders.

Blank, M., Rose, S., & Berlin, L. (1978). *The language of learning: The preschool years.* New York: Grune & Stratton.

Blank, M., Rose, S., & Berlin, L. (2003). *Preschool Language Assessment Instrument—2.* Austin, TX: Pro-Ed.

Bloom, L., & Lahey, M. (1978). *Language development and language disorders.* New York: Wiley.

Boehm, R. G., Hoone, C., McGowan, T. M., McKinney-Browning, M. C., Miramontes, O. B., & Porter, P. H. (2000). *Early United States: Harcourt Brace social studies.* New York: Harcourt Brace & Co.

Boudreau, D. (2005). Use of a parent questionnaire in emergent and early literacy assessment of preschool children. *Language, Speech, and Hearing Services in Schools, 36,* 33-47.

Boudreau, D., & Hedberg, N. L. (1999). A comparison of early literacy skills in children with specific language impairment and their typically developing peers. *American Journal of Speech-Language Pathology, 8,* 249-260.

Bransford, J. D., Brown, A. L., & Cocking, R. R. (1999). *How people learn: Brain, mind, experience, and school.* Washington, DC: National Academic Press.

Bransford, J. D., & Johnson, M. (1973). Considerations of some problems in comprehension. In W. Chase (Ed.), *Visual information processing* (pp. 383-438). New York: Academic Press.

Brock, C. H., & Raphael, T. E. (2003). Guiding three middle school students in learning written academic discourse. *Elementary School Journal, 103,* 481-502.

Burns, M. (2004). Writing in math. *Educational Leadership, 62,* 30-34.

Butler, K. G. (Ed.), & Venable, G. P. (Issue Ed.). (2003). Readability in classroom and clinic: New perspectives. *Topics in Language Disorders,* Issue 23.

Caccamise, D., & Snyder, L. (2005). Theory and pedagogical practices of text comprehension. *Topics in Language Disorders, 25,* 5-20.

Cain, K. (2003). Text comprehension and its relation to coherence and cohesion in children's fictional narratives. *British Journal of Developmental Psychology, 21,* 335-351.

Carle, E. (1979). *The very hungry caterpillar.* New York: Philomel Books.

Carlson, J., Gruenewald, L. J., & Nyberg, B. (1980). Everyday math is a story problem: The language of the curriculum. *Topics in Language Disorders, 1,* 59-70.

Carr, E., & Ogle, D. (1987). K-W-L plus: A strategy for comprehension and summarization. *Journal of Reading, 30,* 626-631.

Carver, R. P. (1992). Effects of prediction activities, prior knowledge, and text type upon amount comprehended: Using Rayding theory to critique schema theory research. *Reading Research Quarterly, 27,* 165-173.

Catts, H. W., Fey, M. E., Zhang, X., & Tomblin, J. B. (1999). Language basis of reading and reading disabilities: Evidence from a longitudinal investigation. *Scientific Studies of Reading, 3,* 331-361.

Catts, H. W., Fey, M. E., Zhang, X., & Tomblin, J. B. (2001). Estimating the risk of future reading difficulties in kindergarten children: A research-based model and its clinical implications. *Language, Speech, and Hearing Services in Schools, 32,* 38-50.

Catts, H. W., & Kamhi, A. G. (2005a). *Language and reading disabilities* (2nd edition). Boston: Allyn & Bacon.

Catts, H. W., & Kamhi, A. G. (2005b). Language and reading: Covergences and divergences. In H. W. Catts & A. G. Kamhi, *Language and reading disabilities* (2nd edition, pp. 1-25). Boston: Allyn & Bacon.

Catts, H. W., & Kamhi, A. G. (2005c). Classification of reading disabilities. In H. W. Catts & A. G. Kamhi, *Language and reading disabilities* (2nd edition, pp. 72-93). Boston: Allyn & Bacon.

Catts, H. W., & Kamhi, A. G. (2005d). Causes of reading disabilities. In H. W. Catts & A. G. Kamhi, *Language and reading disabilities* (2nd edition, pp. 94-127). Boston: Allyn & Bacon.

Catts, H. W., & Kamhi, A. G. (2005e). Defining reading disabilities. In H. W. Catts & A. G. Kamhi, *Language and reading disabilities* (2nd edition, pp. 50-71). Boston: Allyn & Bacon.

Charlton, S., & Christie, J. (2006, May). Language intervention for elementary history. Paper prepared for the Department of Communicative Disorders at California State University at Long Beach, Long Beach, CA.

Chomsky, N. (1965). *Aspects of a theory of syntax*. Cambridge, MA: MIT Press.

Christensen, C. A. (1992). Discrepancy definitions of reading disability: Has the quest led us astray? A response to Stanovich. *Reading Research Quarterly, 27,* 276-278.

Christie, J. (2006, November). Report prepared for CD 669C, Child Language Clinic. Department of Communicative Disorders. California State University at Long Beach, Long Beach, CA.

Cirrin, F. (2000). Assessing language in the classroom and curriculum. In J. B. Tomblin, H. L. Morris, & D. C. Spriestersbach (Eds.), *Diagnosis in speech-language pathology* (2nd edition, pp. 283-314). San Diego, CA: Singular Publishing Group.

Creaghead, N. (1992). Classroom interactional analysis/script analysis. In W. A. Secord & J. S. Damico (Eds.), *Best practices in school speech* (pp. 65-72). Austin, TX: Psychological Corporation.

Creaghead, N. A. (2002). Healthcare and school service: More coalitions and collaborations. *ASHA, 7*(14), 35.

Culatta, B., Horn, D. G., & Merritt, D. D. (1998). Expository text: Facilitating comprehension. In D. D. Merritt & B. Culatta (Eds.), *Language intervention in the classroom* (pp. 215-276). San Diego, CA: Singular Publishing Group.

Culatta, B., & Merritt, D. D. (1998). Enhancing comprehension of discourse. In D. D. Merritt & B. Culatta (Eds.), *Language intervention in the classroom* (pp. 175-214). San Diego, CA: Singular Publishing Group.

Dale, P. S., Crain-Thoreson, C., Notari-Syverson, A., & Cole, K. (1996). Parent-child book reading as an intervention technique for young children with language delays. *Topics in Early Childhood Special Education, 16,* 213-235.

Daneman, M., & Carpenter, P. (1983). Individual differences in integrating information between and within sentences. *Journal of Experimental Psychology: Learning, Memory, and Cognition, 9,* 561-584.

DeKemel, K. (2003a). *Intervention in language arts: A practical guide for speech-language pathologists*. Philadephia: Butterworth-Heinemann.

DeKemel, K. (2003b). Dealing with the dismissal dilemma and long-term follow up of language learning disabled students. In K. DeKemel, *Intervention in language arts: A practical guide for speech-language pathologists* (pp. 127-138). Philadelphia: Butterworth-Heinemann.

DeKemel, K. (2003c). Memory, inferences, and the comprehension of narrative discourse. In K. DeKemel, *Intervention in language arts: A practical guide forspeech-language pathologists* (pp. 1-16). Philadelphia: Butterworth-Heinemann.

DeKemel, K. (2003d). Building a power lexicon: Vocabulary acquisition in language-learning disabled students. In K. DeKemel, *Intervention in language arts: A practical guide for speech-language pathologists* (pp. 79-94). Philadelphia: Butterworth-Heinemann.

De Temple, J. M. (2001). Parents and children reading books together. In D. K. Dickinson & P. O. Tabors (Eds.), *Beginning literacy with language* (pp. 31-51). Baltimore: Paul H. Brookes.

DiCecco, V., & Gleason, M. (2002). Using graphic organizers to attain relational knowledge from expository text. *Journal of Learning Disabilities, 35,* 306-320.

Dickinson, D. K., De Temple, J., Hirschler, J., & Smith, M. (1992). Book reading with preschoolers: Coconstruction of text at home and at school. *Early Childhood Research Quarterly, 7,* 323-346.

Dickinson, D. K., & Tabors, P. O. (2001). *Beginning literacy with language.* Baltimore: Paul H. Brookes.

Dickinson, S. V., Simmons, D. C., & Kameenui, E. J. (1998). Text organization: Research bases. In D. C. Simmons & E. J. Kameenui (Eds.), *What reading research tells us about children with diverse learning needs: Bases and basics* (pp. 239-277). Mahwah, NJ: Erlbaum.

Donahue, M. L., & Foster, S. K. (2004). Integration of language and discourse components with reading comprehension: It's all about relationships. In E. R. Silliman & L. C. Wilkinson (Eds.), *Language and literacy learning in schools* (pp. 175-198). New York: Guilford Press.

Donahue, O., Daane, M., & Grigg, W. (2003). *The nation's report card: Reading highlights 2003* (NCES 2004-452). Washington, DC: National Assessment of Educational Progress.

Donnelly, J. (1989). *Moonwalk: The first trip to the moon.* New York: Random House.

Duke, N. K. (2000). 3.6 minutes per day: The scarcity of informational text in first grade. *Reading Research Quarterly, 35,* 202-224.

Duke, N. K., & Pearson, D. P. (2002). Effective practices for developing reading comprehension. In A. E. Farstrup & S. J. Samuels (Eds.), *What research has to say about reading instruction* (2nd edition, pp. 205-242). Newark, DE: International Reading Association.

Dymock, S. (2005). Teaching expository text structure awareness. *Reading Teacher, 59,* 177-182.

Ehren, B. J. (2000). Maintaining a therapeutic focus and shared responsibility for student success: Keys to in-classroom speech-language services. *Language, Speech, and Hearing Services in Schools, 31,* 219-229.

Ehren, B. J. (2003, October). Helping students with language impairments construct meaning from print. Workshop presented at the Kansas Speech-Language-Hearing Association Convention, Wichita, KS.

Ehren, B. J. (2004, March). Pinning down the language underpinnings of curriculum: Defining the SLP's contribution in collaboration. Workshop presented at the California Speech-Language-Hearing Association Convention, Long Beach, CA.

Ehren, B. J. (Issue Ed.). (2005a). Responsiveness to intervention and the speech-language pathologist. *Topics in Language Disorders, 25,* 89-185.

Ehren, B. J. (2005b). Looking for evidence-based practice in reading comprehension instruction. *Topics in Language Disorders, 25,* 310-321.

Ehren, B. J. (2006a, October). Curriculum-based intervention. Workshop presented for Region 10 of the Corona-Norco Unified School System, Norco, CA.

Ehren, B. J. (2006b). Partnerships to support reading comprehension for students with language impairment. *Topics in Language Disorders, 26,* 42-54.

Ehren, B. J., Lenz, B. K., & Deshler, D. D. (2004). Enhancing literacy proficiency in adolescents and young adults. In A. Stone, E. Silliman, B. Ehren, & K. Apel (Eds.), *Handbook of language and literacy* (pp. 600-625). New York: Guilford Press.

Ehren, B. J., & Nelson, N. W. (2005). The responsiveness to intervention approach and language impairment. *Topics in Language Disorders, 25,* 120-131.

Ehren, B. J., Wallach, G. P., Bashir, A. S., & Gillam, R. (2007, March). Nirvana or bust: Quality services in schools—Settle for no less. Seminar presented at the California Speech-Language-Hearing Association Convention, Long Beach, CA.

Eisenberg, S. L. (2006). Grammar: How can I say that better? In T. A. Ukrainetz (Ed.), *Contextualized language intervention* (pp. 145-194). Eau Claire, WI: Thinking Publications.

Elkonin, D. B. (1973). U.S.S.R. In J Downing (Ed.), *Comparative reading.* New York: MacMillan.

Ellis, E. (1997). Watering up the curriculum for students with disabilities: Goals of the knowledge dimension. *Remedial and Special Education, 18,* 326-347.

Englert, C. S., Raphael, T. E., Anderson, L. M., Anthony, H. M., Fear, K. L., & Gregg, S. L. (1988). A case for writing intervention: Strategies for writing informational text. *Learning Disability Focus, 3,* 98-113.

Ezell, H. K., & Justice, L. M. (2000). Increasing the print focus of adult-child shared book reading through observational learning. *American Journal of Speech-Language Pathology, 9,* 36-47.

Fang, Z. (2004). Scientific literacy: A systematic functional linguistics perspective. *Science Education, 89,* 335-347.

Fey, M. E., Catts, H. W., and Larrivee, L. S. (1995). Preparing preschoolers for the academic and social challenges of school. In M. E. Fey, J. Windsor, and S. F. Warren (Eds.), *Language intervention: Preschool through elementary years* (pp. 3-37). Baltimore: Paul H. Brookes.

Fincher-Kiefer, R. (1992). The role of prior knowledge in inferential processing. *Journal of Research in Reading, 15,* 12-27.

Fischer, F. W., Liberman, I. Y., & Shankweiler, D. (1978). Reading reversals and developmental dyslexia: A further study. *Cortex, 14,* 496-510.

Friel-Patti, S. (1994). Auditory linguistic processing and language learning. In G. P. Wallach & K. G. Butler (Eds.), *Language learning disabilities in school-age children and adolescents: Some principles and applications* (pp. 373-392). Boston: Allyn & Bacon.

Frith, U. (1985). Beneath the surface of developmental dyslexia. In K. Patterson, J. Marshall, & M. Coltheart (Eds.), *Surface dyslexia* (pp. 301-330). London: Lawrence Erlbaum.

Geddes, C. R., & Fukumoto, A. K. (2005, Spring). Sampling adolescents' language abilities across conversational, narrative, and expository discourse genres. Paper completed in the Department of Communicative Disorders at the California State University at Long Beach, Long Beach, CA.

Gerber, M. M. (2005). Teachers are still the test: Limitations of response to instruction strategies for identifying children with learning disabilities. *Journal of Learning Disabilities, 38,* 516-524.

German, D. J. (1987). Spontaneous language profiles in children with word finding problems. *Language, Speech, and Hearing Services in Schools, 18,* 217-230.

German, D. J. (1990). *Test of adolescent/adult word finding.* Austin, TX: Pro-Ed.

German, D. J. (1991). *Test of word finding in discourse.* Austin, TX: Pro-Ed.

German, D. J. (1992). Word finding intervention in children and adolescents. *Topics in Language Disorders, 13*(1), 33-50.

German, D. J. (1994). Word finding difficulties in children and adolescents. In G. P. Wallach & K. G. Butler (Eds.), *Language learning disabilities in school-age children and adolescents: Some principles and applications* (pp. 323-347). Boston: Allyn & Bacon.

German, D. J. (2000). *Test of word finding* (2nd edition). Austin, TX: Pro-Ed.

German, D. J. (2001). *It's on the tip of my tongue: Word-finding strategies to remember names and words you often forget*. Chicago: Word Finding Materials.

Gillam, R. B., & Gorman, B. K. (2004). Language and discourse contributions to word recognition and text interpretation: Implications of a dynamic systems perspective. In E. R. Silliman & L. C. Wilkinson (Eds.), *Language and literacy learning in schools* (pp. 63-97). New York: Guilford Press.

Gillam, R. B., Hoffman, L. M., Marler, J. A., & Wynn-Dancy, M. L. (2002). Sensitivity to increased task demands: Contributions from data-driven and conceptually-driven information processing deficits. *Topics in Language Disorders, 22*, 30-48.

Gillam, R. B., & Pearson, N. (2004). *Test of narrative language*. Austin, TX: Pro-Ed.

Gillam, R. B., Pena, E. D., & Miller, L. (1999). Dynamic assessment of narrative and expository discourse. *Topics in Language Disorders, 20*, 33-47.

Gillam, R. B., & Ukrainetz, T. A. (2006). Language intervention through literature-based units. In T. A. Ukrainetz, *Contextualized language intervention* (pp. 59-94). Eau Claire, WI: Thinking Publications.

Ginsberg, M. (1974). *Mushroom in the rain*. New York: Macmillan.

Golder, C., & Coirier, P. (1994). Augmentative text writing: Developmental trends. *Discourse Processes, 18*, 187-210.

Gorrell, P. (1998). Syntactic analysis and reanalysis in sentence processing. In J. D. Fodor & F. Ferreira (Eds.), *Reanalysis in sentence processing* (pp. 201-246). Norwell, MA: Kluwer Academic.

Graner, P. S., Faggella-Luby, M. N., & Fritschmann, N. S. (2005). Overview of responsiveness to intervention: What practitioners out to know. *Topics in Language Disorders, 25*, 93-105.

Gruenewald, L. J., & Pollak, S. (1990). *Language interaction in the curriculum and instruction* (2nd edition). Austin, TX: Pro-Ed.

Hadley, P. A. (1998). Language sampling protocols for eliciting text-level discourse. *Language, Speech, and Hearing Services in Schools, 29*, 132-147.

Hall, K., Markham, J. C., & Culatta, B. (2005). The development of the early expository comprehension assessment (EECA): A look at reliability. *Communication Disorders Quarterly, 26*, 195-206.

Halliday, M. A. K. (1993). Some grammatical problems in scientific English. In M. A. K. Halliday & J. R. Martin (Eds.), *Writing science: Literacy and discursive power* (pp. 69-85). London: Falmer.

Hansen, L. (2006). Strategies for ELL success. *Science and Children, 43*, 22-25.

Hayes, S. (1990). *Nine ducks nine*. Cambridge, MA: Candlewick Press.

Hegde, M. N., & Maul, A. (2006). *Language disorders in children: An evidence-based approach to assessment and treatment*. Boston: Pearson.

Hennings, D. G. (1993). On knowing and reading history. *Journal of Reading, 36*, 362-370.

Hight, G. L. (2005). Teachers' knowledge and perceptions of dyslexia. Thesis completed in the Department of Communicative Disorders. California State University at Long Beach, Long Beach, CA.

Hoffman, M. (1984). *Animals in the wild: Elephant*. New York: Random House. (Original work published in 1945.)

Hutson-Nechkash, P. (2004). *"Help me write."* Eau Claire, WI: Thinking Publications.

Individuals with Disabilities Education Act of 1997. Public Law no. 105-117 (June 4, 1997).

Individuals with Disabilities Education Improvement Act of 2004. Public Law no. 108-446 (December 3, 2004).

Johnson, D. D., & van Hoff Johnson, B. (1986). Highlighting vocabulary in inferential comprehension. *Journal of Reading, 29*, 622-625.

Johnston, R. (1999). Cognitive deficits in specific language impairments: Decision in spite of uncertainty. *Journal of Speech-Language Pathology and Audiology, 23,* 1165-1172.

Justice, L. M., Bowles, R. P., Kaderavek, J. N., Ukrainetz, T. A., Eisenberg, S. L., & Gillam, R. B. (2006). The index of narrative microstructure: A clinical tool for analyzing school-age children's narrative performance. *American Journal of Speech-Language Pathology, 15,* 177-191.

Justice, L. M., & Ezell, H. K. (2004). Print referencing: An emergent literacy enhancement strategy and its clinical applications. *Language, Speech, and Hearing Services in Schools, 35,* 185-193.

Kaderavek, J., & Justice, L. M. (2002). Shared storybook reading as an intervention context: Practices and potential pitfalls. *American Journal of Speech-Language Pathology, 11,* 395-406.

Kaderavek, J. N., Gillam, R. B., Ukrainetz, T. A., Justice, L. M., & Eisenberg, S. N. (2004). School-age children's self-assessment of oral narrative production. *Communication Disorders Quarterly, 26*(1), 37-48.

Kail, R., & Leonard, L. B. (1986). Word-finding abilities in language-impaired children. *ASHA Monographs, 25.*

Kamhi, A. G. (1997). Three perspectives on comprehension: Implications for assessing and teaching comprehension problems. *Topics in Language Disorders, 17,* 62-74.

Kamhi, A. G. (1999). To use or not to use: Factors that influence the selection of new treatment approaches. *Language, Speech, and Hearing Services in Schools, 30,* 92-98.

Kamhi, A. G. (2004). A meme's eye view of speech-language pathology. *Language, Speech, and Hearing Services in Schools, 35,* 105-111.

Kamhi, A. G. (2006). Prologue: Research and reason to make treatment decisions. *Language, Speech, and Hearing Services in Schools, 37,* 255-256.

Kamhi, A. G., & Catts, H. W. (2005). *Reading development.* In H. W. Catts & A. G. Kamhi, *Language and reading disabilities* (2nd edition, pp. 26-49). Boston: Allyn & Bacon.

Katz, B. (1998). *American history poems.* N.Y.: Scholastic.

Kent, K., & Veremakis, M. (2006 May). Report prepared for Child Language Clinic. Department of Communicative Disorders. California State University at Long Beach, Long Beach, CA.

Killgallon, D., & Killgallon, J. (2000). *Sentence composing for elementary school: A work text to build better sentences.* Portsmouth, NH: Heinemann.

Kim, A., Vaughn, S., Wanzek, J., & Wes, J. (2004). Graphic organizers and their effects on the reading comprehension of students with LD: A synthesis of research. *Journal of Learning Disabilities, 37,* 105-118.

Kinder, D., Bursuck, W. D., & Epstein, M. H. (1992). An evaluation of history textbooks. *Journal of Special Education, 25,* 472-491.

Kintsch, E. (2005). Comprehension theory as a guide for the design of thoughtful questions. *Topics in Language Disorders, 25,* 51-64.

Kirk, S., McCarthy, J., & Kirk, W. (1968). *The Illinois Test of Psycholinguistic Abilities.* Urbana, IL: University of Illinois Press.

Lahey, M. (1990). Who shall be called language disordered? Some reflections and one perspective. *Journal of Speech and Hearing Disorders, 55,* 612-620.

Lahey, M., & Bloom, L. (1994). Variability in language learning disabilities. In G. P. Wallach & K. G. Butler (Eds.), *Language learning disabilities in school-age children and adolescents: Some principles and applications* (pp. 354-372). Boston: Allyn & Bacon.

Lahey, M., & Edwards, J. (1996). Why do children with specific language impairments name pictures more slowly than their peers? *Journal of Speech and Hearing Research, 39,* 1081-1098.

Laing, S. P. (2006). Phonological awareness, reading fluency, and strategy-based reading comprehension instruction for children with language learning disabilities: What does the research show? *Perspectives on Language Learning and Education, 13,* Rockville, MD: American Speech-Language-Hearing Association. Division 1, Newsletter.

Learning Disabilities Online (2005, September). *Important definitions of learning disabilities.* Retrieved on September 17, 2005, from http://www.ldonline.org/ld_in-depth/general_info/definitions.html.

Lee, P. J., & Ashby, R. (2000). Progression in historical understanding among students ages 7-14. In P. Stearns, P. Seixas, & S. Wineberg (Eds.), *Knowing and learning history: National and international perspectives* (pp. 199-222). New York: Academic Press.

Leonard, L. (1986, August). *Word finding abilities of language disabled children.* Workshop presented at the Emerson College Language Learning Disabilities Institute, San Diego, CA.

Levelt, W. J., Roelofs, A., & Meyer, A. S. (1999). A theory of lexical access in speech production. *Behavioral and Brain Sciences, 22,* 1-75.

Lindamood, C., & Lindamood, R. (1979). *Lindamood Auditory Conceptualization Test.* Allen, TX: DLM Teaching Resources.

Lindamood Phoneme Sequencing Program (LiPS) (2003). San Luis Obispo, CA: Lindamood-Bell Learning Processes.

Lof, G. L. (2003). Oral motor exercises and treatment outcomes. *Language Learning and Education, ASHA Division I Newsletter, 1*(1), 7-11.

Lyon, G. R., Shaywitz, S. E., & Shaywitx, B. A. (2003). A definition of dyslexia. *Annals of Dyslexia, 53,* 1-14.

MacDonald, W., & Cornwall, A. (1995). The relationship between phonological awareness and reading and spelling achievement eleven years later. *Journal of Learning Disabilities, 28,* 523-527.

Maestro, B., & Maestro, G. (1987). *A more perfect union: The story of the Constitution.* New York: Mulberry.

Mason, L. (2004). Explicit self-regulated strategy development versus reciprocal questioning: Effects on exposition reading comprehension among struggling readers, *Journal of Educational Psychology, 96,* 283-296.

Mason, L., Meadan, H., Hedin, L., & Corso, L. (2006). Self-regulated strategy development instruction for expository text comprehension. *Teaching Exceptional Children, 38,* 47-52.

Masterson, J. J., & Apel, K. (2000). Spelling assessment: Charting a path to optimal intervention. *Topics in Language Disorders, 20,* 50-65.

Masterson, J. J., Apel, K., & Wasowicz, J. (2002). *SPELL: Spelling assisted software, Grade 2-Adult.* Evanston, IL: Learning by Design.

Masterson, J. J., & Kamhi, A. G. (1991). The effects of sampling conditions on sentence production in normal and reading disabled, and language-learning disabled children. *Journal of Speech and Hearing Research, 34,* 549-558.

Mastropieri, M. A., & Scruggs, T. E. (2005). Feasibility and consequences of responsiveness to intervention: Examining the issues and scientific evidence as a model of identification of individuals with learning disabilities. *Journal of Learning Disabilities, 38,* 525-531.

Mathematics (2002). California Edition. Grade 2. Boston: Houghton Mifflin.

Mathematics (2002). California Edition. Grade 6. Boston: Houghton Mifflin.

May, C. H. (1994). *Conversations with conjunctions.* Tucson, AZ: Communication Skill Builders.

Mayer, M. (1969). *Frog, where are you?* New York: Dial Books.

Mayer, M., & Mayer, M. (1971). *A boy, a dog, a frog and a friend*. New York: Dial Books.

Mayer, M., & Mayer, M. (1975). *One frog too many*. New York: Dial Books.

McCrudden, M. T., Perkins, P. G., & Putney, L. G. (2005). Self-efficacy and interest in the use of reading strategies. *Journal of Research in Childhood Education, 20*, 119-131.

McDougal, L. (2002). *Grade seven textbook series for literature and language arts*. Evanston, IL: Houghton-Mifflin.

McFadden, T. U. (1998). The immediate effects of pictographic representation on children's narratives. *Child Language Learning and Teaching, 14*, 51-67.

McKeown, M., Beck, I. I., Sinatra, G. M., & Loxterman, J. A. (1992). The contribution of prior knowledge and coherent text to comprehension. *Reading Research Quarterly, 27*, 79-93.

McLaughlin, S. (2006). *Introduction to language development* (2nd edition). Clifton Park, NY: Thomson Delmar Learning.

Medina, K. (2005). Building academic literacy through history. Paper presented at the meeting for the California History Social Science Project funded by the University of California at Irvine, Irvine, CA.

Meltzer, L. J., Roditi, B., Haynes, D., Biddle, K., Paster, M., & Taber, S. (1996). *Strategies for success: Classroom teaching techniques for students with learning problems*. Austin, TX: Pro-Ed.

Merritt, D. D., & Culatta, B. (Eds.) (1998). *Language intervention in the classroom*. San Diego, CA: Singular Publishing Group.

Merritt, D. D., Culatta, B., & Trostle, S. (1998). Narratives: Implementing a discourse framework. In D. D. Merritt & B. Culatta (Eds.), *Language intervention in the classroom* (pp. 227-330). San Diego, CA: Singular Publishing Group.

Miller, L. (1989). Classroom-based language intervention. *Language, Speech, and Hearing Services in Schools, 20*, 153-169.

Milosky, L. M. (1994). Nonliteral language abilities: Seeing the forest for the trees. In G. P. Wallach & K. G. Butler (Eds.), *Language learning disabilities in school-age children and adolescents: Some principles and applications* (pp. 275-303). Boston: Allyn & Bacon.

Moje, E. B., Ciechanowski, K. M., Kramer, K., Ellis, L., Carrillo, R., & Collazo, T. (2004). Working toward third space in content area literacy: An examination of everyday funds of knowledge and Discourse. *Reading Research Quarterly, 39*, 38-70.

Montgomery, J. W. (1995). Sentence comprehension in children with specific language impairment: The role of phonological working memory. *Journal of Speech and Hearing Research, 38*, 187-199.

Montgomery, J. W. (2000). Verbal working memory and sentence comprehension in children with specific learning impairment. *Applied Psycholinguistics, 21*, 117-148.

Montgomery, J. W. (2002). Information processing and language comprehension in children with specific language impairment. *Topics in Language Disorders, 22*, 62-84.

Myers, P. A. (2006). The Princess storyteller, Clara clarifier, Quincy questioner, and the Wizard: Reciprocal teaching adapted for kindergarten students. *Reading Teacher, 59*, 314-325.

Nail-Chiwetalu, B. J., & Ratner, N. B. (2006). Information literacy for speech-language pathologists: A key to evidence-based practice. *Language, Speech, and Hearing Services in Schools, 37*, 157-167.

Nation, K., Clarke, P., Marshall, C. M., & Durand, M. (2004). Hidden language impairment in children: Parallels between poor reading comprehension and specific language impairment. *Journal of Speech and Hearing Research, 47*, 199-211.

National Assessment Governing Board (2004). *Reading framework for the 2009 National Assessment of Educational Progress* (Contract no. ED-02-R-0007). Washington, DC: American Institute for Research.

National Joint Committee on Learning Disabilities (1991). Learning disabilities: Issues on definition. *ASHA, 33*(suppl 5), 18-20.

National Joint Committee on Learning Disabilities (2005). Important definitions of learning disabilities. Retrieved September 17, 2005, from http://ldonline.org/ld_indepth/general_info/definitions.html.

Nelson, N. W. (1994). Curriculum-based language assessment and intervention across the grades. In G. P. Wallach & K. G. Butler (Eds.), *Language learning disabilities in school-age children and adolescents: Some principles and applications* (pp. 104-131). Boston: Allyn & Bacon.

Nelson, N. W. (1998). *Childhood language disorders in context: Infancy through adolescence.* Boston: Allyn & Bacon.

Nelson, N. W. (2005). The context of difficulty in classroom and clinic: An update. *Topics in Language Disorders, 25*(4), 322-331.

Nelson, N. W., & Van Meter, A. M. (2006). Finding the words: Vocabulary development for young authors. In T. A. Ukrainetz, *Contextualized language intervention* (pp. 95-144). Eau Claire, WI: Thinking Publications.

Neufeld, P. (2006). Comprehension instruction in content area classes. *Reading Teacher, 59,* 302-312.

Nippold, M. A. (1985). Comprehension of figurative language in youth. *Topics in Language Disorders, 5,* 1-20.

Nippold, M. A. (1998). *Later language development: Ages nine through nineteen.* Austin, TX: Pro-Ed.

Nippold, M. A., Moran, C., & Schwarz, I. E. (2001). Idiom understanding in pre-adolescents; Synergy in action. *American Journal of Speech-Language Pathology, 10,* 169-179.

Nippold, M. A., Ward-Lonergan, J. M., & Fanning, J. L. (2005). Persuasive writing in children, adolescents, and adults: A study of syntactic, semantic, and pragmatic development. *Language, Speech, and Hearing Services in Schools, 36,* 125-138.

Nittrouer, S. (1999). Do temporal processing deficits cause phonological processing problems? *Journal of Speech, Language, and Hearing Research, 42,* 925-942.

Nittrouer, S. (2002). From ear to cortex: A perspective on what clinicians need to understand about speech perception and language processing. *Language, Speech, and Hearing Services in Schools, 33,* 237-252.

Norris, J. A. (1997). Functional language intervention in the classroom: Avoiding the tutoring trap. *Topics in Language Disorders, 17,* 49-68.

Ogle, D., & Blachowicz, C. (2005). *Tools for teaching literacy series.* New York: Guilford Press.

Ogle, D. M. (1986). K-W-L: A teaching model that develops active reading of expository text. *Reading Teacher, 39,* 564-570.

Ogle, D. M. (1989). The know, want to know, learn strategy. In K. D. Muth (Ed.), *Children's comprehension of text* (pp. 205-223). Newark, DE: International Reading Association.

Ohlhausen, M., & Roller, C. (1988). The operation of text structure and content schemata in isolation and interaction. *Reading Research Quarterly, 23,* 70-88.

Osborn, S. (Producer), & Templeton, G. (Director). (1994). *Frog where are you?* [Video]. Available from the Phoenix Learning Group, 2349 Chaffee Drive, St. Louis, MO 63146; 314-569-0211.

Owens, R. E. (2001). School-age and adult pragmatic and semantic development. In R. E. Owens, *Language development: An introduction* (pp. 348-379). Boston: Allyn & Bacon.

Owens, R. E. (2004). *Language disorders: A functional approach to assessment and intervention* (4th edition). Boston: Allyn & Bacon.

Owens, R. E. (2005). Language-learning processes in young children. In R. E. Owens, *Language development: An introduction* (6th edition). (pp. 184-221). Boston: Allyn & Bacon.

Palincsar, A. S., & Brown, A. L. (1984). Reciprocal teaching of comprehension-fostering and comprehension-monitoring activities. *Cognition and Instruction, 1,* 117-175.

Palincsar, A. S., Collins, K. M., Marano, N. L., & Magnusson, S. J. (2000). Investigating the engagement and learning of students with learning disabilities in guided inquiry science teaching. *Language, Speech, and Hearing Services in Schools, 31,* 240-251.

Palincsar, A. S., & Duke, N. K. (2004). The role of text and text-reader interactions in young children's reading development and achievement. *Elementary School Journal, 105,* 183-197.

Palincsar, A. S., & Magnusson, S. J. (2001). The interplay of first-hand and second-hand investigators to model and support the development of scientific knowledge and reasoning. In S. Carver & D. Klahr (Eds.), *Cognition and instruction: Twenty-five years of progress* (pp. 151-194). Mahwah, NJ: Lawrence Erlbaum.

Palincsar, A. S., & Magnusson, S. J. (2002, October). Attending to the nature of subject matter in text comprehension assessment. Paper prepared for the CIERA Conference on Comprehension and Assessment, Ann Arbor, MI.

Pantaleo, S. (2004). Exploring Grade 1 students' textual connections. *Journal of Research in Childhood Education, 18,* 211-225.

Pappas, C. C. (2006). The information book genre: Its role in integrated science literacy research and practice. *Reading Research Quarterly, 41,* 226-250.

Parish, P. (1986). *Merry Christmas, Amelia Bedelia.* New York: Avon Books.

Pearson, P. D., & Spiro, R. J. (1982). Toward a theory of reading comprehension instruction. In K. G. Butler & G. P. Wallach (Eds.), *Language disorders and learning disabilities* (pp. 71-88). Rockville, MD: Aspen Publications.

Pena, E. D. (2000). Management of modifiability in children from culturally and linguistically diverse backgrounds. *Communication Disorders Quarterly, 21,* 87-97.

Peshkin, A. (1978). *Growing up in America: Schooling and the survival of the community.* Chicago: University of Chicago Press.

Peterson, C., & McCabe, A. (1983). *Developmental psycholinguistics: Three ways of looking at a child's narrative.* New York: Plenum.

Prelock, P., Miller, B., & Reed, N. (1993). *Working with the classroom curriculum: A guide for analysis and use in speech therapy.* San Antonio, TX: Communication Skill Builders.

Pressley, M. (2002). Comprehension strategies instruction. In C. C. Block & M. Pressley (Eds.), *Comprehension instruction: Research based best practices* (pp. 11-27). New York: Guilford Press.

Pressley, M., & Afflerbach, P. (1995). *Verbal protocols of reading: The nature of constructively responsive reading.* Hillsdale, NJ: Lawrence Erlbaum.

Pressley, M., Borkowski, J. G., & Schneider, W. (1987). Cognitive strategies: Good strategy users coordinate metacognition and knowledge. *Annals of Child Development, 14,* 89-129.

Pressley, M., Borkowski, J. G., & Sullivan, J. (1985). Children's metamemory and the teaching of memory strategies. In D. L. Forrest-Pressley, G. E. MacKinnon, & T. G. Waller (Eds.), *Metacognition, cognition, and human performance: Theoretical perspectives* (pp. 111-153). Orlando, FL: Harcourt Brace Jovanovich.

Pressley, M., & Hilden, K. (2004). Toward more ambitious comprehension instruction. In E. R. Silliman & L. C. Wilkinson (Eds.), *Language and literacy learning in schools* (pp. 151-174). New York: Guilford Press.

Proctor, B., & Prevatt, F. (2003). Agreement among four models used for the diagnosis of learning disabilities. *Journal of Learning Disabilities, 36,* 459-466.

Purcell-Gates, V., & Duke, N. K. (2001, August). Explicit explanation and teaching of information text genres: A model for research. Paper presented at Crossing Borders: Connecting Science and Literature, a conference sponsored by the National Science Foundation, Baltimore.

Raphael, T. E., & Au, K. H. (2001). *Super QAR for test use for students: Teacher resource guide*, Grade 6. Chicago: McGraw-Hill/Wright.

Raphael, T. E., & Au, K. H. (2005). QAR: Enhancing comprehension and test taking across grades and content areas. *Reading Teacher, 59*, 206-221.

Resnick, L. (1987). *Education and learning to think.* Washington, DC: National Academy Press.

Roth, F. P., & Troia, G. A. (2006). Collaborative efforts to promoting emergent literacy and efficient word recognition. *Topics in Language Disorders, 26*, 24-41.

Rubin, H., & Liberman, I. (1983). Exploring the oral and written language errors made by language disabled children. *Annals of Dyslexia, 33*, 11-20.

Sawyer, D. J. (2006). Dyslexia: A generation of inquiry. *Topics in Language Disorders, 26*, 95-109.

Scarborough, H. S. (2001). Connecting early language and literacy to later reading (dis)abilities: Theory and practice. In S. Neuman & D. Dickinson (Eds.), *Hand-book for research in early literacy* (pp. 97-110). New York: Guilford Press.

Schleppegrell, M., & Achugar, M. (2005). Learning language and learning history: A functional linguistic approach. *TESOL Journal, 12*(2), 21-27.

Science Discovery Works Series (2003). Grade 4. Boston: Houghton Mifflin.

Science Discovery Works Series (2003). Grade 6. Boston: Houghton Mifflin.

Scott, C. M. (1988). Spoken and written syntax. In M. A. Nippold (Ed.), *Later language development: Ages 9 to 19* (pp. 41-91). Austin, TX: Pro-Ed.

Scott, C. M. (1989). Problem writers: Nature, assessment, and intervention. In A. G. Kamhi & H. W. Catts (Eds.), *Reading disabilities: A developmental language perspective* (pp. 303-344). Austin, TX: Pro-Ed.

Scott, C. M. (1994). A discourse continuum for school-age students: Impact of modality and genre. In G. P. Wallach & K. G. Butler (Eds.), *Language learning disabilities in school-age children and adolescents: Some principles and applications* (pp. 219-252). Boston: Allyn & Bacon.

Scott, C. M. (2005). Learning to write. In H. W. Catts & A. G. Kamhi, *Language and reading disabilities* (pp. 233-273). Boston: Allyn & Bacon.

Scott, C. M., & Windsor, J. (2000). General language performance measures in spoken and written narratives and expository discourse of school-age children with language learning disabilities. *Journal of Speech, Language, and Hearing Research, 43*, 324-339.

Scruggs, T. E., & Mastropieri, M. A. (2003). Content area learning in inclusive middle school science and social studies classes. Grant proposal funded by the U.S. Department of Education, award number H324C020085.

Scruggs, T. E., & Mastropieri, M. A. (2004). Recent research in secondary content areas for students with learning and behavioral disabilities. In T. E. Scruggs & M. A. Mastropieri (Eds.), *Research in secondary schools: Advances in learning and behavioral disabilities* (Vol. 17, pp. 243-264). Oxford, UK: Elsevier Science.

Silliman, E. R., Butler, K. G., & Wallach, G. P. (2002). The time has come to talk of many things. In E. R. Silliman & K. G. Butler (Eds.), *Speaking, reading, and writing in children with language learning disabilities: New paradigms for research and practice* (pp. 3-24). Mahwah, NJ: Lawrence Erlbaum.

Silliman, E. R., & Wallach, G. P. (1991, November). The communication process model for LLD children: Making it work. Short course presented at the American Speech-Language-Hearing Association convention, Atlanta, GA.

Silliman, E. R., & Wilkinson, L. C. (1994). Discourse scaffolds for classroom intervention. In G. P. Wallach & K. G. Butler (Eds.), *Language learning disabilities in school-age children and adolescents: Some principles and applications* (pp. 27-52). Boston: Allyn & Bacon.

Silliman, E. R., & Wilkinson, L. C. (Eds.) (2004a). *Language and literacy learning in schools.* New York: Guilford Press.

Silliman, E. R., & Wilkinson, L. C. (2004b). Collaboration for language and literacy learning: Three challenges. In E. R. Silliman & L. C. Wilkinson (Eds.), *Language and literacy learning in schools* (pp. 3-38). New York: Guilford Press.

Silliman, E. R., Wilkinson, L. C., & Danzak, R. L. (2004). Putting Humpty Dumpty together again: What's right with Betsy. In E. R. Silliman & L. C. Wilkinson (Eds.), *Language and literacy learning in schools* (pp. 319-355). New York: Guilford Press.

Simon, C. (1987). Out of the broom closet and into the classroom: The emerging speech-language pathologist. *Journal of Childhood Communication Disorders, 11*(1), 41-66.

Singer, B. D., & Bashir, A. S. (2004). EmPOWER: A strategy for teaching students with language learning disabilities how to write expository text. In E. R. Silliman & L. C. Wilkinson (Eds.), *Language and literacy learning in schools* (pp. 239-272). New York: Guilford Press.

Snow, C. (2002). *Reading for understanding: Toward an R & D program in reading comprehension.* Santa Monica, CA. Rand.

Snow, C., & Goldfield, B. (1981). Building stories: The emergence of information structures from conversation. In D. Tannen (Ed.), *Analyzing discourse: Text and talk.* Washington, DC: Georgetown University Press.

Snowling, M. J., & Hayiou-Thomas, M. E. (2006). The dyslexia spectrum: Continuities between reading, speech, and language impairments. *Topics in Language Disorders, 26,* 110-126.

Snyder, L. E., Dabasinskas, C., & O'Connor, E. (2002). An information processing perspective on language impairment in children: Looking at both sides of the coin. *Topics in Language Disorders, 22,* 1-14.

Snyder, L. E., & Downey, D. M. (1997). Developmental differences in the relationship between oral language deficits and reading. *Topics in Language Disorders, 17,* 27-40.

Social Studies: The Early United States (Grade 5) (2000). New York: Harcourt Brace.

Stahl, S. A. (1986). Three principles of effective vocabulary instruction. *Journal of Reading, 29,* 662-668.

Stanovich, K. E. (1986). Matthew effects in reading: Some consequences of individual differences in the acquisition of literacy. *Reading Research Quarterly, 86,* 360-406.

Staskowski, M., & Rivera, E. A. (2005). Speech-language pathologists' involvement in responsiveness to intervention activities: A complement to curriculum-relevant practice. *Topics in Language Disorders, 25,* 13-147.

Stein, N. L., & Glenn, C. G. (1979). An analysis of story comprehension in elementary school children. In R. Freedle (Ed.), *New directions in discourse processing* (Vol. 2, pp. 53-120). Norwood, NJ: Ablex.

Steinhauer, J. (2005, May 22). Maybe preschool is the problem. *New York Times,* pp. 1, 4.

Stephens, M. I., & Montgomery, A. A. (1985). A critique of recent relevant standardized tests. *Topics in Language Disorders, 5,* 21-45.

Sternberg, R. (1987). Most vocabulary is learned from context. In M. McKeown & M. Curtis (Eds.), *The nature of vocabulary acquisition* (pp. 89-106). Hillsdale, NJ: Erlbaum.

Stothard, S. E., Snowling, M. J., Bishop, D. V. M., Chipchase, B. B., & Kaplan, C. A. (1998). Language-impaired preschoolers: A follow-up into adolescence. *Journal of Speech, Language, and Hearing Research, 41,* 407-418.

Straits, W. (2005). Mystery box writing. *Science and Children, 43,* 33-37.

Sutton-Smith, B. (1986). The development of fictional narrative performance. *Topics in Language Disorders, 7,* 1-10.

Swanson, L. (1999). Reading research for students with LD: A meta-analysis of intervention outcomes. *Journal of Learning Disabilities, 32,* 504-532.

Tabors, P. O. (2001). Supporting language and literacy development in the home. In D. K. Dickinson & P. O. Tabors, *Beginning literacy with language* (pp. 27-51). Baltimore: Paul H. Brookes.

Tabors, P. O., Beals, D. E., & Weizman, Z. (2001). "You know what oxygen is?" Learning new words at home. In D. K. Dickinson & P. O. Tabors, *Beginning literacy with language* (pp. 93-110). Baltimore: Paul H. Brookes.

Temple, C., Nathan, R., Temple, F., & Burris, N. (1993). *The beginnings of writing.* Boston: Allyn & Bacon.

Thelen, J. N. (1986). Vocabulary instruction and meaningful learning. *Journal of Reading, 29,* 603-609.

Tomblin, J. B., Records, N. L., Buckwalter, P., Zhang, X., Smith, E., & O'Brien, M. (1997). The prevalence of specific language impairment in kindergarten children. *Journal of Speech, Language, and Hearing Research, 40,* 1245-1260.

Torgeson, J. K., Al Otaiba, S., & Grek, M. L. (2005). Assessment and instruction for phonemic awareness and word recognition skills. In H. W. Catts & A. G. Kamhi, *Language and reading disabilities* (2nd edition, pp. 127-156). Boston: Allyn & Bacon.

Troia, G. A. (2004). Building word recognition skills through empirically validated instructional practices: Collaborative efforts of speech-language pathologists and teachers. In E. R. Silliman & L. C. Wilkinson (Eds.), *Language and literacy learning in schools* (pp. 98-129). New York: Guilford Press.

Troia, G. A. (2005). Responsiveness to intervention: Roles for speech-language pathologists in the prevention and identification of learning disabilities. *Topics in Language Disorders, 25,* 106-119.

Tyree, R. B., Firore, T. A., & Cook, R. A. (1994). Instructional materials for diverse learners: Features and considerations for textbook design. *Remedial and Special Education, 15,* 363-377.

Ukrainetz, T. A. (2006a). Scaffolding young students into phonemic awareness. In T. A. Ukrainetz, *Contextualized language intervention* (pp. 429-467). Eau Claire, WI: Thinking Publications.

Ukrainetz, T. A. (2006b). Teaching narrative structure: Coherence, cohesion, and captivation. In T. A. Ukrainetz, *Contextualized language intervention* (pp. 195-246). Eau Claire, WI: Thinking Publications.

Ukrainetz, T. A. (2006c). The many ways of exposition: A focus on discourse structure. In T. A. Unkrainetz, *Contextualized language intervention* (pp. 247-288). Eau Claire: WI: Thinking Publications.

Ukrainetz, T. A., & Ross, C.L. (2006). Text comprehension: facilitating active and strategic engagement. In T. A. Ukrainetz, *Contextual language intervention* (pp. 503-563). Eau Claie, WI; Thinking Publications.

Unsworth, L. (1999). Developing critical understanding of the specialized language of school science and history texts: A functional grammatical perspective. *Journal of Adolescent and Adult Literacy, 42,* 508-520.

U.S. Department of Education (2001). *Twenty-third annual report to Congress on the Implementation of Individuals with Disabilities Education Act.* Washington, DC: Author.

van Kleeck, A. (1984). Assessment and intervention: Does "meta" matter? In G. P. Wallach & K. G. Butler (Eds.), *Language learning disabilities in school-age children* (pp. 179-198). Baltimore: Williams & Wilkins.

van Kleeck, A. (1994). Metalinguistic development. In G. P. Wallach & K. G. Butler (Eds.), *Language learning disabilities in school-age children and adolescents: Some principles and applications* (pp. 53-98). Boston: Allyn & Bacon.

van Kleeck, A. (1998). Preliteracy domains and stages: Laying the foundations for beginning reading. *Journal of Childhood Communication Development, 20,* 33-51.

van Kleeck, A., & Vander Woude, J. (2003). Book sharing with preschoolers with language delays. In A. van Kleeck, S. A. Stahl, & E. B. Bauer (Eds.), *On reading books to children: Parents and teachers* (pp. 58-92). Mahwah, NJ: Lawrence Erlbaum.

van Kleeck, A., Vander Woude, J., & Hammett, L. (2006). Fostering literal and inferential language skills in Head Start preschoolers with language impairment using scripted book-sharing discussions. *American Journal of Speech-Language Pathology, 15,* 85-95.

VanSledright, B. A. (2002a). Fifth graders investigating history in the classroom: Results from a researcher-practitioner design experiment. *Elementary School Journal, 103,* 131-160.

VanSledright, B. A. (2002b). *In search of America's past: Learning to read history in elementary school.* New York: Teachers College Press.

VanSledright, B. A. (2004). What does it mean to read history? Fertile ground for cross-disciplinary collaborations? *Reading Research Quarterly, 39,* 342-346.

VanSledright, B. A., & Kelly, C. (1998). Reading American history: The influence of using multiple sources on six fifth graders. *Elementary School Journal, 98,* 239-265.

Vellutino, F. R. (2003). Individual differences as sources of variability in reading comprehension in elementary school children. In A. P. Sweet & C. E. Snow (Eds.), *Rethinking reading comprehension* (pp. 51-81). New York: Guilford Press.

Vellutino, F. R., Pruzek, R., Steger, J. A., & Meshoulam, U. (1973). Immediate visual recall in poor and normal readers as a function of orthographic-linguistic familiarity. *Cortex, 9,* 368-384.

Vellutino, F. R., Scanlon, D. M., & Tanzman, M. S. (1994). Components of reading ability: Issues and problems in operationalizing word identification, phonological coding, and orthographic coding. In G. R. Lyon (Ed.), *Frames of reference for the assessment of learning disabilities: New views of measurement issues* (pp. 279-329). Baltimore: Paul H. Brookes.

Vellutino, F. R., Steger, J. A., DeSetto, L., & Phillips, F. (1975). Immediate and delayed recognition of visual stimuli in poor and normal readers. *Journal of Experimental Child Psychology, 19,* 223-232.

Villano, T. L. (2005). Should social studies textbooks become history? A look at alternative methods to activate schema in the intermediate classroom. *Reading Teacher, 59,* 122-130.

Wadlington, E. M., & Wadlington, P. L. (2005). What do teachers really believe about dyslexia? *Reading Improvement, 42,* 16-33.

Wagner, C. R., Nettelbladt, U., Sahlen, B., & Nilholm, C. (2000). Conversation versus narration in preschool children with language impairment. *International Journal of Language and Communication Disorders, 35,* 83-95.

Wallach, G. P. (2003, October). Central auditory processing disorders (CAPD): Cause or result of linguistic or metalinguistic factors. Short course presented at the Kansas Speech, Language, and Hearing Association Conference, Wichita, KS.

Wallach, G. P. (2004). Over the brink of the millennium: Have we said all we can say about language-based learning disabilities? *Communication Disorders Quarterly, 25,* 44-55.

Wallach, G. P. (Issue Ed.). (2005a). Topics in language disorders and learning disabilities: A look across twenty-five years. *Topics in Language Disorders, 25,* 287-336.

Wallach, G. P. (2005b). A conceptual framework in language learning disabilities: School-age language disorders. *Topics in Language Disorders, 25,* 292-301.

Wallach, G. P., & Butler, K. G. (1994a). Creating communication, literacy, and academic success. In G. P. Wallach & K. G. Butler (Eds.), *Language learning disabilities in school-age children and adolescents: Some principles and applications* (pp. 2-26). Boston: Allyn & Bacon.

Wallach, G. P., & Butler, K. G. (Eds.) (1994b) *Language learning disabilities in school-age children and adolescents: Some principles and applications.* Boston: Allyn & Bacon.

Wallach, G. P., & Ehren, B. J. (2004). Collaborative models of instruction and intervention: Choices, decisions, and implementation. In E. R. Silliman & L. C. Wilkinson (Eds.), *Language and literacy learning in schools* (pp. 39-59). New York: Guilford Press.

Wallach, G. P., & Madding, C. C. (2005, November). The top ten myths in language intervention. Miniseminar presented at the American Speech-Language-Hearing Association Convention, San Diego, CA.

Wallach, G. P., & Madding, C. C. (2006, November). Myth Busters return: Dispelling questionable practices in language intervention. Miniseminar presented at the American Speech-Language-Hearing Association Convention, Miami, FL.

Wallach, G. P., & Miller, L. (1988). *Language intervention and academic success.* Boston: College-Hill Press.

Wasowicz, J., Apel, K., & Masterson, J. J. (2003, April). Spelling assessment: Applying research in clinical practice. *ASHA Special Interest Division 1, School-based Issues Newsletter, 4*(1).

Weade, R., & Green, J. L. (1985). Talking to learn: Social and academic requirements of classroom participation. *Peabody Journal of Education, 62,* 6-19.

Weaver, C. (1996). *Teaching grammar in context.* Portsmouth, NH: Boyton/Cook.

Weismer Ellis, S., & Evans, J. L. (2002). The role of processing limitations in the early identification of specific language impairment. *Topics in Language Disorders, 22,* 15-29.

West, R. F., Stanovich, K. E., & Mitchell, H. R. (1993). Reading in the real world and its correlates. *Reading Research Quarterly, 28,* 35-50.

Westby, C. E. (1984). The development of narrative language ability. In G. P. Wallach & K. G. Butler (Eds.), *Language learning disabilities in school-age children* (pp. 103-127). Baltimore: Williams & Wilkins.

Westby, C. E. (1985). Oral/literate language differences: Learning to talk—Learning to learn. In C. Simon (Ed.), *Communication skills and classroom success.* San Diego, CA: College-Hill Press.

Westby, C. E. (1994). The effects of culture on genre, structure, and style of oral and written texts. In G. P. Wallach & K. G. Butler (Eds.), *Language learning disabilities in school-age children and adolescents* (pp. 180-218). Boston: Allyn & Bacon.

Westby, C. E. (2000a). Who are adults with learning disabilities and what do we do about them? *Topics in Language Disorders, 21,* 1-14.

Westby, C. E. (2000b). Multicultural issues in speech and language assessment. In J. B. Tomblin, H. L. Morris, & D. C. Spriestersbach (Eds.), *Diagnosis in speech-language pathology* (2nd edition, pp. 35-62). San Diego, CA: Singular Publishing Group.

Westby, C. E. (2005). Assessing and remediating text comprehension problems. In H. W. Catts & A. G. Kamhi, *Language and reading disabilities* (2nd edition, pp. 157- 232). Boston: Allyn & Bacon.

Westby, C. E. (2006). There's more to passing than knowing the answers: Learning to do school. In T. A. Ukrainetz (Ed.), *Contextualized language intervention* (pp. 319-387). Eau Claire, WI: Thinking Publications.

Westby, C. E., & Clauser, P. S. (2005). The right stuff for writing: Assessing and facilitating written language. In H. W. Catts & A. G. Kamhi, *Language and reading disabilities* (2nd edition, pp. 274-345). Boston: Allyn &Bacon.

Westby, C. E., & Torres-Velasquez, D. (2000). Developing scientific literacy: A socio-cultural approach. *Remedial and Special Education, 21,* 101-110.

Whitaker, C. P., Gambrell, L. B., & Morrow, L. M. (2004). Reading comprehension instruction for all students. In E. R. Silliman & L. C. Wilkinson (Eds.), *Language and literacy learning in schools* (pp. 130-150). New York: Guilford Press.

Whitmire, K. (2005). Understanding language disorders: Can we see the future? Language and literacy, twenty-five years later. *Topics in Language Disorders, 25,* 302-309.

Williams, A. L., & Elbert, M. (2003). A perspective longitudinal study of phonological development in late talkers. *Language, Speech, and Hearing Services in Schools, 34,* 138-153.

Windsor, J. (2002). Contrasting general and process-specific slowing in language impairment. *Topics in Language Disorders, 22,* 62-86.

Windsor, J., Milbrath, R., Carney, E., & Rakowski, S. (2001). General slowing in language impairment: Methodological considerations in testing the hypothesis. *Journal of Speech, Language, and Hearing Research, 44,* 446-461.

Yore, L. D., Hand, B., Goldman, S. R., Hildebrand, G. M., Osborne, J. F., Treagust, D. F., & Wallace, C. S. (2004). New directions in language and science education research. *Reading Research Quarterly, 39,* 347-352.

Index

A

Abbreviated episode within narrative, 200b, 201f
ABONE mnemonic, 85
Abstract words, persuasive writing and, 284
Academic success, early reading routines connected to, 138–147
Accessible text to create content knowledge, 237–238
Action sequence, 199b, 200, 201f
Active sentence comprehension, 68–69
ADD. *See* Attention-deficit disorder
Adjective phrases, 255b
Adverbial construction, 255b
After sentence, 261, 262b
Agent focus, 196
American Speech-Language-Hearing Association, language defined by, 6
Analogies, teacher's use of, 57
Antonyms, 281, 282b
APD. *See* Auditory processing disorder
Argument, science and, 216
Argumentative text, 193f, 240–242, 240t, 241b
Articulation difficulties as meme, 125
ASHA. *See* American Speech-Language-Hearing Association
Asperger's as meme, 124
Assessment
    too much time spent on, 31
    Westby's framework for, 64–66, 65f
Attempts in narrative structure, 192f, 194
Attention-deficit disorder, 23
    too much time testing for, 31
Auditory discrimination, 320–321
    new vocabulary and, 111–112
Auditory figure ground problem, 113
Auditory learner, 18–19
Auditory memory problems, 322–323
    second language learning experiences and, 109–110
Auditory processing disorder, 114–116, 114b, 328–329
    as meme, 124
Authentic intervention activities, 236–237
Author & Me strategy, 231–232, 233
Authoritativeness of scientific text, 208, 208b
Automaticity, 126b, 128

B

B for *n* substitution, 112
Baby boomer generation, 286
Background knowledge
    as mental model, 126, 126b
    connected text and, 189–190, 190b, 210
    history and, 218
    narrative retelling and, 186–187
    narratives and, 123

Bashir and Singer EmPOWER strategy, 225–227, 226b, 227f, 228f
BEFORE, DURING, AFTER reading format, 315–316
Before-after sentence, 261, 262b
Blending activities, 115
Book-sharing intervention, 145–146, 337–338
Books
    selection of to read to preschooler, 142
    writing like, 36–37, 36b
Bottom-up processing, 122, 195
Brainstorming discussion
    as goal-specific strategy, 221
    for vocabulary intervention, 294, 296–297, 296f

C

California State Department of Education standards
    for English/language arts, 275–278, 275b–278b
    for history and social studies, 273, 274b–275b
    for science, 271–272, 272b
CAPD. *See* Central auditory processing disorder
Cause in scaffolding questions, 144b
Cause-effect text, 188, 191, 193f
Central auditory processing disorder, 23
    missteps in interventions for, 114–116
    second language learning experiences and, 109–110
    too much time spent on assessment of, 31
Central nervous system involvement in language disability and dyslexia, 28
Checklist
    curriculum-based intervention, 87–89, 88f
    self-evaluation vocabulary knowledge, 297–298, 297f
Cirrin's five basic curricula demand concepts, 86–87, 86b
Claim in argumentative text, 240t
Classification in Cirrin's five basic curricula demand concepts, 86, 86b
Classroom
    casual conversation *versus* language in, 108–109
    connecting language intervention to, 16–17
    connection of test results to, 15
    guidelines for observation in, 60, 61b
Cognitive referencing, 25, 32
Collaboration among professionals, 89–91, 91f
Comments in classroom setting, 58–59, 59t
Compare-contrast diagram for learning about expository text
    using grade 5 social studies, 167
    using sports topic, 165

Compare-contrast text, 164–169, 191, 193f
  in fourth grade, 188, 188b
  state standards for science and, 272–273
Competing resources, 15–16, 63,
  126–128, 126b
Complement clauses, 255b
Complementary services in curriculum-
  based therapy, 85
Complete episode within narrative, 199b,
  200b, 201f
Complex episode within narrative,
  199b, 200b
Complex sentence construction, 255b–256b,
  259–264, 262b
Complication in episodic narrative, 200, 201
Comprehension
  factors contributing to effective and
    efficient, 110, 111b
  inferential, 323–324
    versus literal in preschooler, 144–145
  missteps in interventions for,
    121–123, 121b
  on curriculum-based intervention
    checklist, 88f
  state standards for, 275b–277b
  strategies for, 219–223, 220b
    goal-specific, 220–221
    in history, 217
    language underpinnings of, 224–225
    monitoring and repair, 220b, 221
    packaging, 220b, 221
    titles and, 122
Computer literacy, 7
Concept formation, 281, 282b
Conceptual frameworks, 1–41
Conflict in episodic narrative, 200, 201
Conjunctions, 255b, 260
Connected discourse, 122, 170–265
  analysis of narratives in, 198–203
  comprehension strategies for, 219–223
    goal-specific, 220–221
    monitoring and repair, 220b, 221
    packaging, 220b, 221
  content and structure knowledge in,
    189–190, 190b
  content-area subjects and, 215–218, 215b
  evolving concepts in literacy and, 228–235
  expository text in fourth grade
    and, 188, 188b
  fundamental literacy and, 218–223
  Geddes and Fukumoto protocol
    for, 177–187, 178t
    conversational discourse and personal
      narratives in, 177–180, 178t, 182–183
    expository text in, 177–178, 178t, 181–183
    narrative retelling in, 177–178, 178t,
      183–186
  grammatical skills and, 254–264,
    255b–256b
  integration of literacy's in, 234–235
  interview format sampling for, 175–176,
    342–343

Connected discourse—cont'd
  introductory thoughts concerning,
    171–173, 172f
  K-W-L outline for, 174
  language underpinnings and, 224–224
  microstructure *versus* macrostructure
    aspects of, 173, 211–212
  narrative-expository text connection in,
    190–198, 192f, 192t, 193f
  putting "out-of-order" text in order,
    250–251
  QAR framework and, 230–234, 230f, 232b
  reciprocal teaching strategies for, 245–246
  retelling/generation format sampling for,
    175, 176–177, 344–346
  science text and, 171–172, 172f, 203–209,
    205f, 206f, 208b, 235–243
    accessible, 237–238
    authentic communication situations
      and, 236–237
    matching text activities to, 238–243,
      239f, 240t, 241b
  sentence-chunking strategies for, 247–250,
    248f, 249f
  stoplight organization in, 246–247
  teacher as audience for, 174–175
  titles and, 189
  variables related to, 173–174
  vocabulary and, 290–291
  writing strategies for, 225–227,
    226b, 227f, 228f
Connecting words, 259–261, 347–348
  persuasive writing and, 284–285
  sentence-building activity using,
    305–306
Consequences
  in episodic narrative, 200, 201
  in narrative structure, 192f, 194
Conservation in Cirrin's five basic curricula
  demand concepts, 86, 86b
Construction of meaning, 122
Constructively responsive reading, 221
Content knowledge
  connected text and, 189, 190b
  in scientific text, 207–208, 208b
  using accessible text to create, 237–238
Content words, 281, 282b
Content-area subjects, 215–218, 215b
  matching text activities to, 238–243,
    239f, 240t, 241b
Context
  creation of, 121
  inferential comprehension and, 324
  language comprehension and, 107–108
  reduction of dependency on, 109
  sentence comprehension and, 68
  vocabulary and, 291, 292b, 294–295
Contextual support
  competing resources and, 16–17
  in classroom, 108–109
Contextualized *versus* decontextualized
  language, 108

Conventional literacy, 150
Conversation
  eliciting, 341–346
  in Geddes and Fukumoto protocol,
    177–180, 182–183
  planning required for, 174
Coordinating conjunction, 255b
Correlative conjunction, 255b
Cover sheet, 70–71, 71f
  phonemic segmentation, 71–72, 72f
Critical literacy, 7
Critical stance, 216
Culture
  memes and, 124–125
  school
    home *versus*, 38–39
    teachers and, 56–62, 58b, 59t, 61b, 62b
Curriculum
  connecting language intervention to,
    16–17
  connection of test results to, 15
  mastery of connected text connected to
    mastery of, 187
  watering up, 73–77, 73t, 74t
Curriculum-based intervention, 79–101
  checklist for, 87–89, 88f
  Cirrin's five basic curricula demand
    concepts in, 86–87, 86b
  historical, 97–100, 98b, 100f
  language teaching continuum in,
    89–91, 90f
  mathematical, 80–83, 80b–81b, 83f
  responsiveness to intervention and,
    91–97, 93t–94t
  roles and responsibilities in, 84–89,
    86b, 88f
  self-evaluation questions for speech-
    language pathologists in, 93–96, 95b
  teaching of curriculum in, 84

D

Data in argumentative text, 240t
Decontextualized *versus* contextualized
  language, 108
Definition diagram, 308–309, 308f
Definitions, interlocking, in scientific text,
  208–209, 208b
Density of scientific text, 207–208, 208b
Derived literacy, 215–216, 215b
Descriptive sequence, 199–200, 199b, 201f
Diagram
  compare-contrast
    for learning about expository
      text, 165, 167
  definition, 308–309, 308f
  science report, 239, 239f, 306–307, 307f
Dictionary skills, 292b
Discourse
  connected, 122, 170–265
    analysis of narratives in, 198–203
    content and structure knowledge in,
      189–190, 190b

Discourse—cont'd
    content-area subjects and, 215–218, 215b
    evolving concepts in literacy and,
      228–235
    fundamental literacy and, 218–223
    Geddes and Fukumoto protocol for,
      177–187, 178t
    grammatical skills and, 254–264,
      255b–256b
    interview format sampling for,
      175–176, 342–343
    introductory thoughts, 171–173, 172f
    K-W-L outline for, 174
    language underpinnings and,
      224–224
    microstructure *versus* macrostructure
      aspects of, 173
    narrative-expository text connection in,
      190–198, 192f, 192t, 193f
    putting "out-of-order" text in order,
      250–251
    QAR framework and, 230–234,
      230f, 232b
    reciprocal teaching strategies for, 245–246
    science text and, 171–172, 172f, 203–209,
      205f, 206f, 208b, 235–243
    sentence-chunking strategies for,
      247–250, 248f, 249f
    stoplight organization in, 246–247
    strategies for, 219–223, 220b
    teacher as audience for, 174–175
    titles and, 189
    variables related to, 173–174
  conversational
    in Geddes and Fukumoto protocol,
      177–180, 178t, 182–183
    planning required for, 174
  in teacher-student interaction
    levels of, 57, 58b
    obliges and comments in, 58–59, 59t
  size of, 173, 174
  text-level, 174
Dynamic literacy, 7
Dyslexia
  as meme, 124
  defined by International Dyslexia
    Association, 28
  language disability *versus*, 31
  misperceptions about, 32

E

Early literacy, 150
Early reading routines and intervention,
  138–147, 142b, 144b, 145b, 157–158
  literature-based frameworks in,
    150–157, 155b–156b
  print awareness in, 147–150, 151f
  Westby framework for, 162
Education, mother's, 27, 27b
Elaborated question, 157
Ellis's concept of watering up curriculum,
  73–77, 73t, 74t

Emergent literacy, 150
EmPOWER strategy, 225–227, 226b, 227f, 228f
  for vocabulary intervention, 302–303, 302f
English
  scientific, 207–209, 208b
  state standards for, 275–278, 275b–278b
Evaluation in EmPOWER strategy, 225, 226b
  for vocabulary intervention, 302–303, 302f
Event description in scaffolding questions, 144b
Expectations, language abilities and, 110
Experience. *See* Background knowledge
Expository text, 164–169
  bottom-up processing in, 195
  challenges of, 195, 196b
  in fourth grade, 188, 188b
  in Geddes and Fukumoto protocol, 177–178, 178t, 181–183
  narrative text *versus*, 190–198, 192f, 192t, 193f
  planning required for, 174
  visual representation of components of, 192f
  word knowledge and, 283

F

Facilitation devices in storybook units, 154–155, 155b–156b
Familiarity, language comprehension and, 107–108
Fifth grade
  early literacy experiences' effect on learning in, 158–162, 159b
  English/language arts state standards for, 275–278, 275b–277b
  history in, 218
Figurative language, 312–313, 330–332
Finding of words, 285–290
Flipbook, science, 242
Forest-*versus*-tree metaphor, 11, 14b
Formal language
  language learning over time and, 30f, 35
  literacy and, 7
Fourth grade
  California State Department of Education standards
    for history and social studies, 273, 274b–275b
    for science, 271–273, 272b
  history in, 218
  science in, 204, 205f, 206f
  specific challenges of students in, 188, 188b
French as second language learning experiences, 106–111, 109b, 111b, 113
Fundamental literacy, 215–216, 215b, 218–223

G

Geddes and Fukumoto protocol, 177–187, 178t
  conversational discourse and personal narratives in, 177–180, 178t, 182–183
  expository text in, 177–178, 178t, 181–183
  narrative retelling in, 177–178, 178t, 183–186
Goal in narrative structure, 194, 200, 201, 202
Goal-specific strategies, 220–221
Grade 2, mathematics problems in, 80–82, 80b–81b
Grade 4
  California State Department of Education standards
    for history and social studies, 273, 274b–275b
    for science, 271–273, 272b
  history in, 218
  science in, 204, 205f, 206f
  specific challenges of students in, 188, 188b
Grade 5
  early literacy experiences' effect on learning in, 158–162, 159b
  English/language arts state standards for, 275–278, 275b–277b
  history in, 218
Grade 6, mathematics problems in, 80–83, 80b–81b
Grade 7, English/language arts state standards for, 275–278, 275b–278b
Grammar, story, 191–194, 192f
Grammatical skills, 254–264, 255b–256b
  poetry intervention, 301, 301f
Graphic organizers, 222b, 223, 224
  for organization of science report, 239, 239f, 306–307, 307f
  for sentence-chunking strategies, 248–250, 248f, 249f
  in EmPOWER strategy, 226–227, 227f, 228f

H

Hadley protocols, 175–177, 341–346
History, 158–162, 159b, 164–169
  conversion from expository to narrative text, 196–198
  curriculum-relevant therapy and, 97–100, 98b, 100f
  graphic organizer for comprehension of, 249f
  literacy and, 217–218
  state standards for, 273, 274b–275b

I

IDA. *See* International Dyslexia Association
Idioms, teacher's use of, 57
Immediate *versus* nonimmediate talk, 141–143, 142b
In My Head strategy, 231–234, 232b

In the Book strategy, 231–234, 232b
Incomplete episode within narrative, 200b
Individuals with Disabilities
　　Education Act, 32
Inferences, narratives and, 123
Inferential comprehension, 323–324
　　in preschooler, 144–145
Infinitive clause, 255b
Informal language
　　language learning over time
　　　　and, 30f, 35
　　literacy and, 7
Information processing theory,
　　125–128, 126b
　　questions for self-reflection
　　　　associated with, 133b–134b
Informational density of scientific text,
　　207–208, 208b
Inherent abilities, competing resources
　　and, 15
Initiating event in narrative structure,
　　192f, 194
Instruction
　　in language teaching continuum
　　　　of service therapy, 90–91, 90f
　　intervention *versus*, 89, 293–294
　　vocabulary, 294
Interactive episode within narrative, 200b
Interlocking definitions in scientific text,
　　208–209, 208b
International Dyslexia Association, 28
Intertextual ability, 216
Intervention. *See* Language intervention
Interview format sampling, 175–176,
　　342–343
IQ-achievement discrepancy model,
　　25, 32
It's in the kids head phenomenon, 14–16
Item elaboration, 144b

J

Journals, language learning over time
　　and, 30f, 35

K

K-W-L technique, 174, 210, 221, 222,
　　222b, 245
　　modification of, 246
Keeping your eyes on the horizon metaphor,
　　20
Kindergarten
　　assumed language abilities and, 51
　　sentence comprehension in, 68
Knowledge
　　background
　　　　activation of as goal-specific
　　　　　　strategy, 220, 220b
　　　　as mental model, 126, 126b
　　　　connected text and, 189–190, 190b, 210
　　　　history and, 218
　　　　narrative retelling and, 186–187
　　　　narratives and, 123

Knowledge—cont'd
　　content
　　　　structure and, 189–190, 190b
　　　　using accessible text to create,
　　　　　　237–238
　　language intervention and, 53–54, 54b

L

Labeling
　　in scaffolding questions, 144b
　　of students with language learning
　　　　disability, 23–25
　　changing of over time, 29, 30f
Language
　　abilities needed to succeed in
　　　　school, 52, 54
　　as meme, 124
　　awareness of, 129 (*See Also*
　　　　Metalinguistics)
　　contextualized *versus*
　　　　decontextualized, 108
　　definitions of, 5–6
　　judgments about, 115
　　learning disabilities and dyslexia
　　　　and, 28–29
　　mathematics, 81–82, 83
　　nonliteral, teacher's use of, 57
　　of history, 218
　　of science, 207–209, 208b
　　regular *versus* school, 37–39
　　spontaneous use of, 9
　　two layers of, 8–10
　　underpinnings of, 224–224
Language arts, state standards
　　for, 275–278, 275b–278b
Language intervention, 5, 45–78,
　　105–135, 318–320
　　assumed language abilities and, 50–52
　　auditory discrimination and new
　　　　vocabulary and, 111–112
　　auditory figure ground problems and, 113
　　authentic activities for, 236–237
　　automaticity in, 128
　　broader view of, 18–19, 18b
　　choosing focus and sequence for, 66–67
　　classroom observation in, 60, 61b
　　competing resources in, 15–16, 126–128
　　connection of to real world, 16–17
　　cover sheet in, 70–71, 71f
　　curriculum-based, 79–101
　　　　checklist for, 87–89, 88f
　　　　Cirrin's five basic curricula demand
　　　　　　concepts in, 86–87, 86b
　　　　historical, 97–100, 98b, 100f
　　　　language teaching continuum
　　　　　　in, 89–91, 90f
　　　　mathematical, 80–83, 80b–81b, 83f
　　　　responsiveness to intervention and,
　　　　　　91–97, 93t–94t
　　　　roles and responsibilities in,
　　　　　　84–89, 86b, 88f
　　　　teaching of curriculum in, 84

Language intervention—cont'd
early, 138–141
example of, 73–78, 73t–74t, 75b–77b
factors to consider in creation of goals
for, 107–110, 109b, 111b
for sentence comprehension, 67–73
future of, 40–41
in responsiveness to intervention
approach, 32–35, 33b, 34f
instruction *versus*, 89
knowledge, skills and strategies
in, 53–55, 54b
language and literacy definitions
and perceptions in, 5–7, 28–29
literature-based, 147–150, 151f,
157–158, 339–340
long-term view of, 20–21, 26
mental models in, 125–126
metalinguistic abilities and,
10, 129–132, 129b
metaphors in
forest-*versus*-tree, 11–14, 14b
it's in the kid's head phenomenon,
14–16
keeping your eyes on the horizon,
20–21
one-way mapping, 12–13
things are not always what they seem,
18–19, 18b
tip-of-the-iceberg phenomenon, 11–12
missteps in, 114–125
auditory processing disorders and,
114–116, 114b
meme theory and, 124–125
memory issues and, 120–123, 121b
narratives and, 118–120, 118b
quick and easy answers as, 123–125
working with 3 year old, 116–118
persistence-in-practice phenomenon
in, 124–125
print awareness/print referencing in,
147–150, 151f, 157–158
questions for self-reflection associated
with, 132–133, 133b–135b
questions that drive, 49–50, 50b, 61–62
second language learning experiences
and, 106–111, 113
self-talk in, 5
shared responsibilities in, 89–91, 90f
snapshots of language disorders in, 46–49
strategies for, 219–223, 220b
goal-specific, 220–221
monitoring and repair, 220b, 221
packaging, 220b, 221
teachers and, 56–62, 58b, 59t, 61b, 62b
ten scenarios, 320–334
theory-to-practice gap in, 4–5
traditions in, 8
variables in, 62–64
vocabulary, 293–294, 295–316
BEFORE, DURING, AFTER reading
format, 315–316

Language intervention—cont'd
brainstorming activity, 294,
296–297, 296f
completed science report frame,
306–307, 307f
definition diagram, 308–309, 308f
grammar-word practice using
poetry, 301, 301f
instruction *versus*, 293–295
literal and nonliteral translation
of sentences, 311–313
paraphrasing activity, 304–305
passive sentence activity, 303–304
persuasive writing game, 299f, 300
phonemic segmentation activities,
313–315, 314f
predict-o-gram, 298–300, 298f, 299f
self-evaluation vocabulary knowledge
checklist, 297–298, 297f
sentence-building activity using
connectors, 305–306
sentence-completion or paragraph-
completion task, 309–311
using EmPOWER strategy,
302–303, 302f
watering up curricula for, 73–77, 73t, 74t
Westby's framework for, 64–66, 65f
Language learning across time, 30f,
35–37, 36b
Language learning disability
auditory discrimination and new
vocabulary and, 111–112
changing and evolvement of,
25–26, 29–30, 30f
characteristics of children and
adolescents with, 109, 109b
competing resources and, 15–16
creation of, 55–56, 56b
dyslexia *versus*, 31
future of, 40–41
history of, 23–24
identifying children with, 24–25
labeling of students with, 23–25, 29, 30f
metaphors in
forest-*versus*-tree, 11–14, 14b
it's in the kid's head phenomenon,
14–16
keeping your eyes on the horizon,
20–21
one-way mapping, 12–13
things are not always what they seem,
18–19, 18b
tip-of-the-iceberg phenomenon, 11–12
neurological bases for, 14–16
reading disability and, 13
responsiveness to intervention
approach for, 32–35, 33b, 34f
snapshots of, 46–49
teachers and, 56–62, 58b, 59t,
61b, 62b
theory-to-practice gap and, 4–5
understanding of, 55–56, 56b

Language proficiency
  triple threat of, 50–51
  written language proficiency and, 53
Language rules as mental model, 126
Language teaching continuum, 89–91, 90f
Leaps of logic, 121b
Learning disability, 23, 24
  changing of over time, 29–32, 30f
  definition of provided by Joint Committee
    on Learning Disabilities, 28
  prevalence of, 32
Letter identification by preschooler and
    subsequent reading abilities in
    elementary grades, 27, 27b
Letters to friends, 30f, 35
Lexical knowledge and skills
  math problems and, 82
  vocabulary and, 280–281, 290–295,
    291b–292b
Linguistic "glue" words, 165, 167, 168
Linguistic cohesion in math problems, 81
Linguistic facilitations, 155, 155b–156b
Linguistic intrusion errors, 321
Linguistic layer of language, 8–9
Listening-to-learn, 159
Literacy
  content-area subjects and, 215–218, 215b
  definitions and perceptions of, 7
  emergent, early, and conventional, 150
  evolving concepts in, 228–235
  fundamental, 215–216, 215b, 218–223
  language learning over time and, 35–36
  transition from orality to, 36–37, 36b
Literal comprehension in preschooler,
    144–145
Literature-based frameworks, 150–157,
    155b–156b, 157–158, 339–340
LLD. *See* Language learning disability
Logic, leaps of, 121b

M

Macrolevels of discourse, 173, 210–211
Mapping, semantic, 120, 150–152, 153,
    329–330
Matching perception, 57, 58b
Mathematics problems, 80–83, 80b–81b, 83f
Meaning
  construction of, 122
  metalinguistics and, 130–131
Medical model format, 93b–94b
Memes, 124–125
  creation of new, 125–132
    information processing theory,
      125–128, 126b
    questions for self-reflection associated
      with, 135b
Memory activities, 120–123, 121b
Memory problems, 325–326
  auditory, 322–323
    second language learning experiences
      and, 109–110
    visual sequence problem with, 321

Memory, titles and, 122
Mental models, 125–126
  language performance and, 64
Metacognition, 130
Metalinguistics, 129–132, 129b
  as layer of language, 8–10
  missteps in language intervention
    and, 114–115
  print awareness/print referencing
    and, 150, 151f
  questions for self-reflection associated
    with, 134b–135b
  recognition of, 18, 18b
  vocabulary and, 290
Metaphors in language learning disabilities
  forest-*versus*-tree, 11–14, 14b
  it's in the kid's head phenomenon,
    14–16
  keeping your eyes on the horizon, 20–21
  one-way mapping, 12–13
  things are not always what they seem,
    18–19, 18b
  tip-of-the-iceberg phenomenon, 11–12
Metaverbs, persuasive writing and, 284
Microlevels of discourse, 173, 212
  in science text, 204, 205f
Memento, 194
Monitoring strategies, 220b, 221
  language underpinnings of, 224
Mother's education, 27, 27b
Multiple meanings, 282, 282b
Mushroom in the Rain, 153

N

Narrative retelling in Geddes and Fukumoto
    protocol, 177–178, 178t, 183–186
Narratives
  analysis of, 198–203
  challenges of, 195, 196b
  expository text *versus*, 190–198,
    192f, 192t, 193f
  in Geddes and Fukumoto protocol,
    177–180, 178t, 182–183
  intervention using, 327
    missteps in, 118–120, 118b
  language learning over time and, 35
  microstructures *versus*
    macrostructures in, 173
  planning required for, 174
  pre-episodic, 198–200, 199b
  titles and, 189
  top-down processing in, 195
  visual representation of components
    of, 192f
National Joint Committee on Learning
    Disabilities, 28
Neurologic system
  dyslexia and, 28
  language learning disability and, 14–16
NJCLD. *See* National Joint Committee on
    Learning Disabilities
Nominalization in scientific text, 208, 208b

Nonimmediate *versus* immediate talk, 141–143, 142b
Nonliteral language, teacher's use of, 57
Noun retrieval, 289
Noun-phrase expansion, 255b

O

Obliges in classroom setting, 58–59, 59t
Observation, classroom, 60, 61b
On My Own strategy, 231, 233
One-way mapping approach, 12–13, 14b
Oral-motor problem as meme, 125
Oral-motor training as meme, 124
Orality
    language learning over time and, 35–36
    on curriculum-based intervention checklist, 88f
    transition to literacy, 36–37, 36b
Order-of-mention, 19, 69–70
Organization
    in EmPOWER strategy, 225, 226b
    required for discourse, 173–174
    stoplight, 246–247
Organizer, graphic, 222b, 223, 224
    for organization of science report, 239, 239f, 306–307, 307f
    for sentence-chunking strategies, 248–250, 248f, 249f
    in EmPOWER strategy, 226–227, 227f, 228f
Out-of-order text, putting in order, 250–251

P

Packaging strategies, 220b, 221
Paragraph-completion activity, 309–311
Paraphrasing
    as goal-specific strategy, 220, 220b, 221
    language underpinnings of, 224
    state standards for, 279
    vocabulary intervention activity using, 304–305
    word knowledge and, 283
Participial clause, 255b
Passive sentence
    comprehension of, 68–69
    intervention activity involving, 303–304
Passive voice, 255b
Perception
    language abilities and, 110
    reordering of, 57, 58b
    math problems and, 82
Perfect aspect, 255b
Persistence-in-practice phenomenon, 124–125
Personal journal, 30f, 35
Personal narrative in Geddes and Fukumoto protocol, 177–180, 178t, 182–183
Personality, connected discourse sampling and, 177

Persuasive text and writing, 191, 193f
    word knowledge and, 283–285
Persuasive writing game, 299f, 300
Phoneme, 111
    missteps in language intervention and, 115
Phonemic segmentation activities, 313–315, 314f
Phonological awareness
    by preschooler and subsequent reading abilities in elementary grades, 27, 27b
    cover sheet for, 71–72, 72f
    vocabulary knowledge and, 287–288
Phonological impairment
    as meme, 124–125
    in preschooler, long-term outcomes for, 27, 27b
PLAI-2. *See* Preschooler Language Assessment Instrument-2
Plan in narrative structure, 194
Planning
    in EmPOWER strategy, 225, 226b
    required for discourse, 173–174
Poetry, grammar-word practice using, 301, 301f
Post-noun modifying phrases, 255b
Practical framework, 43–101
Practices, persistence of outdated, 124–125
Pre-episodic narratives, 198–200, 199b
Predicate expansion, 255b
Predict-o-gram for vocabulary intervention, 298–300, 298f, 299f
Preschool period
    assumed language abilities and, 51
    early reading routines during, 138, 141–142
    language disorders during, 26–27
        long-term outcomes for, 27, 27b
    language expectations during, 62b
    language intervention in, 20, 26, 138–141, 138–147
        grade 5 and, 158–162, 159b
        literature-based frameworks in, 150–157, 155b–156b
        print awareness in, 147–150, 151f
        Westby framework in, 162–163
    literacy development in, 7
    literacy-related activities during, success in school and, 138–147
    pre-episodic narratives in, 198–200, 199b
    print awareness/print referencing in, 147–150, 151f
    sentence comprehension in, 68
Preschooler Language Assessment Instrument-2, 144–145, 145b
Print awareness/print referencing, 147–150, 151f, 157–158
Print literacy, 7
Prior knowledge. *See* Background knowledge

Problem solving
  explain what is wrong in, 82, 83
  mathematical, 80–83, 80b–81b, 83f
  self-talk in, 5
Problem-solution text, 188, 191, 193f
Process grid, 242
Processes, bottom-up and top-down,
    122, 195
Processing
  factors contributing to effective and
    efficient, 110, 111b
  missteps in interventions for,
    121–123, 121b
Professionals, collaboration among,
    89–91, 91f
Prompting in narrative retelling, 186

Q

QAR framework, 230–234, 230f, 232b
Quality assurance, 334, 335b
Question-answer relationships format,
    230–234, 230f, 232b
Questions
  during preschool literacy activities,
    142–143
  elaborated, 157
  for self-evaluation/self-reflection, 93–96,
    95b, 132–133, 133b–135b
  from education side of fence, 96–97
  in Preschooler Language Assessment
    Instrument-2, 144–145, 145b
  reciprocal, 222–223, 222b
  scaffolding, 144, 145b
  that drive language intervention, 49–50,
    50b, 61–62

R

RAP format, 222, 222b
Rapid naming by preschooler and subsequent
    reading abilities in elementary grades,
    27, 27b
Reaction in scaffolding questions, 144b
Reactive sequence, 200, 201f
Reading
  constructively responsive, 221
  early language and literacy skills and
    subsequent abilities in, 27, 27b
  literacy and, 7
  shared book, 145–146, 337–338
Reading disability, 23
  changing of over time, 20f, 29–32
  language learning disability and, 13
Reading- to-learn, 159, 159b
Real-world
  language intervention connection
    to, 16–17
  scaffolding questioning related
    to, 144b
Reasoning
  about perception, 57, 58b
  in scaffolding questions, 144b
Reciprocal questioning, 222–223, 222b

Reciprocal teaching strategies, 245–246
Recounts, 120
Regulatory facilitations, 155, 156b
Reordering perception, 57, 58b
  math problems and, 82
Repair strategies, 220b, 221
  language underpinnings of, 224
Representation in mental models,
    125–126
Rereading of history text, 217
Resolution in narrative structure,
    192f, 194
Resources, competing, 15–16, 63,
    126–128, 126b
Response facilitations, 155, 156b
Responsiveness to intervention,
    32–35, 33b, 34f
  curriculum-relevant therapy and,
    91–97, 93t–94t
Retelling
  eliciting, 341–346
  in Geddes and Fukumoto protocol,
    177–178, 178t, 183–186
Retelling/generation format sampling,
    175, 176–177, 344–346
Retrieval of words, 285–290
Reversal errors, 321–322
Rework in EmPOWER strategy, 225, 226b
Rhyming activities, 115
Right There strategy, 231–232, 232f, 233
Routine, language comprehension and,
    107–108
RQ format, 222–223, 222b
RTI. *See* Responsiveness to intervention

S

Sampling
  interview format, 175–176, 342–343
  retelling/generation format, 175,
    176–177, 344–346
Sarcasm, teacher's use of, 57
Scaffolding, 144, 145b, 186
  for sentence-completion and paragraph-
    completion activities, 309–311
School
  as unique language and culture, 37–39
    teachers and, 56–62, 58b, 59t, 61b, 62b
  quality assurance in, 334, 335b
Science flipbook, 242
Science report diagram, 239, 239f,
    306–307, 307f
Science text, 171–172, 172f, 203–209,
    205f, 206f, 208b, 235–243
  accessible, 237–238
  argument and, 216
  authentic communication situations
    and, 236–237
  critical stance and, 216
  literacy and, 215–217
  matching text activities to, 238–243,
    239f, 240t, 241b
  state standards for, 271–273, 272b

Scientific English, 207–209, 208b
Second grade, mathematics problems in, 80–82, 80b–81b
Second language learning experiences, 106–111, 109b, 111b, 113
Segmentation skills, 115, 131
Selective analysis of perception, 57, 58b
Self-evaluation vocabulary knowledge checklist, 297–298, 297f
Self-questioning/self-reflection, 93–96, 95b, 133b–135b
  as goal-specific strategy, 220, 220b
Self-talk, 5
Semantic mapping, 120, 150–152, 153, 329–330
Semantics
  interventions for, 290–295, 291b–292b
  math problems and, 82, 83
  word approximation and, 287–288
Sensory integration disorder as meme, 124
Sentence combining, 257–260
Sentence completion, 259–261
  activity for, 309–310
Sentence comprehension intervention, 67–73
Sentence construction, complex, 255b–256b, 259–264, 262b
Sentence imitation by preschooler and subsequent reading abilities in elementary grades, 27, 27b
Sentence-chunking strategies, 247–250, 248f, 249f
Sequence
  action, 199b, 200, 201f
  descriptive, 199–200, 199b, 201f
  reactive, 200, 201f
Sequencing activity, 118–120, 118b
Sequencing problems, 321–322, 325–328
Seriation in Cirrin's five basic curricula demand concepts, 86, 86b
Setting in narrative structure, 192f, 194
Seventh grade, English/language arts state standards for, 275–278, 275b–278b
Shared reading experiences, 138–147, 337–338
SID. *See* Sensory integration disorder
Similes, teacher's use of, 57
Sixth grade, mathematics problems in, 80–83, 80b–81b
Size of discourse, 173, 174
Skills
  for thinking historically, 99
  language intervention and, 53–54, 54b
SLI. *See Also* Specific language impairment
SLP. *See* Speech-language pathologist
Social studies, 158–162, 159b, 164–169
  conversion from expository to narrative text, 196–198
  curriculum-relevant therapy and, 97–100, 98b, 100f
  graphic organizer for comprehension of, 249f
  literacy and, 217–218
  state standards for, 273, 274b–275b

Social-information processing, 161
Socialization, language proficiency and, 107
Space in Cirrin's five basic curricula demand concepts, 86–87, 86b
Specific language impairment, 15, 25. *See Also* Language learning disability
Speech-language pathologist
  role in responsiveness to intervention approach, 33–34, 34f
  role of in curriculum-based intervention, 84–85, 90f, 91
  role of in language teaching continuum of service delivery, 90f, 91
  self-evaluation questions for, 93–96, 95b
Spoken language
  along oral-to-literate continuum, 36–37, 36b
  in mathematics, 83, 83f
  integration of with written language, 136–169
    case study, 164–169
    early reading routines and, 138–147
    in grade 5, 158–162, 159b
    literature-based frameworks in, 150–157, 155b–156b
    print awareness and, 147–150, 151f
    Westby framework for, 162–163
  literacy and, 7
Spontaneous use of language, 9
Sports model for learning about expository text, 165
State standards and benchmarks
  for English/language arts, 275–278, 275b–278b
  for science, 271–280
  for social studies and history, 273, 274b–275b
Stoplight organization, 246–247
Story grammar, 191–194, 192f
Story grammar decision tree, 201, 201f
Story retelling, 341–346
Storybook reading, 138–147, 150–157, 155b–156b
Strategies, 53–54, 54b, 219–223, 220b
  attending to tricky words and phrases and putting them back together again, 251–253
  emPOWER, 225–227, 226b, 227f, 228f
  for writing, 225–227, 226b, 227f, 228f
  goal-specific, 220–221
  history-specific, 98–99, 99–100, 100f, 217
  in sentence comprehension, 68, 69–70
  In the Book and *In My Head*, 231–234, 232b
  monitoring and repair, 220b, 221
  packaging, 220b, 221
  putting "out-of-order" text in order, 250–251
  reciprocal teaching, 245–246
  sentence-chunking, 247–250, 248f, 249f
  stoplight organization, 246–247
  underpinnings of, 224–225
  vocabulary, 292b, 293

Structure knowledge, connected text and, 189, 190b
Subordinate and superordinate categories, 282, 282b
Subordinating conjunction, 255b
Summarizing
  as goal-specific strategy, 220, 220b, 221
  history and, 217
  state standards for, 279
Superordinate and subordinate categories, 282, 282b
Synonyms, 282, 282b, 283
Syntax
  development of, 254–256
  math problems and, 82

T

Talk. *See Also* Spoken language
Talk, immediate *versus* nonimmediate, 141–143, 142b
Target forms, identifying/becoming familiar with, 257
Task complexity, competing resources and, 127
Taxonomies in scientific text, 208b, 209
Teachers
  as only audience for school work, 174–175
  classroom discourse and, 56–62, 58b, 59t, 61b, 62b
  role of in language teaching continuum of service delivery, 90f, 91
  versus speech-language pathologist in teaching curriculum, 84
Technical taxonomies in scientific text, 208b, 209
Technical vocabulary in scientific text, 208, 208b
Tensed verb clause, 255b
Test results, connection of to classroom and curricula demands, 15
Testing, too much time spent on, 31
Text
  analysis of as goal-specific strategy, 220, 220b
  argumentative, 240–242, 240t, 241b
  competing resources and, 127
  connected (*See* Connected discourse)
  expository
    bottom-up processing in, 195
    challenges of, 195, 196b
    in fourth grade, 188, 188b
    in Geddes and Fukumoto protocol, 177–178, 178t, 181–183
    interventions for, 164–169
    planning required for, 174
    visual representation of components of, 192f
    word knowledge and, 283
  history, graphic organizer for comprehension of, 249f
  mathematical, 82

Text—cont'd
  narrative (*See* Narratives)
  persuasive, 191, 193f
    word knowledge and, 283–285
  putting "out-of-order" text in order, 250–251
  science, 171–172, 172f, 203–209, 205f, 206f, 208b
    accessible, 237–238
    authentic communication situations and, 236–237
    matching text activities to, 238–243, 239f, 240t, 241b
  titles in comprehension of, 52–53
Text-level discourse, 174
The Very Hungry Caterpillar, 138–142
Theory-to-practice gap, 4–5
Therapy. *See Also* Language intervention
Therapy in language teaching continuum of service therapy, 90f, 91
Therapy talk game, 119
Think & Search strategy, 231–233, 232f
Thinness of evidence, term, 217
Tier I activities
  across three models of service delivery, 93t–94t
  in responsiveness to intervention, 32, 33b, 34f, 93t
Tier II activities
  across three models of service delivery, 94t
  in responsiveness to intervention, 32, 33b, 34f
Tier III activities
  across three models of service delivery, 94t
  in responsiveness to intervention, 32, 33b, 34f, 94t
  curriculum-relevant therapy and, 92, 94t
Time in Cirrin's five basic curricula demand concepts, 86, 86b
Tip-of-the-iceberg phenomenon, 11–12, 14b
Title
  comprehension facilitated by, 52–53
  connected discourse and, 189
  in comprehension and memory, 122
Top-down processing, 122, 195
Traditions in language intervention, 8
Tutor trap, term, 84
TWA approach, 222–223, 222b

U

Utterance level, 174

V

VanSledright, history-specific strategies from work of, 99–100, 100f
Verb-form expansion, 255b
Villano's class description, 243–245
Visual imagery as goal-specific strategy, 220, 220b

Visual learner, 18–19
Visual sequence/memory problem, 321
Vocabulary, 279–316
  auditory discrimination and new, 111–112
  elements of vocabulary knowledge,
      281–283, 282b
  in scientific text, 208, 208b
  interventions for, 295–316
    brainstorming activity, 294,
      296–297, 296f
    completed science report frame,
      306–307, 307f
    definition diagram, 308–309, 308f
    grammar-word practice using
      poetry, 301, 301f
    instruction *versus*, 293–295
    literal and nonliteral translation of
      sentences, 311–313
    paraphrasing activity, 304–305
    passive sentence activity, 303–304
    persuasive writing game, 299f, 300
    phonemic segmentation activities,
      313–315, 314f
    predict-o-gram, 298–300, 298f, 299f
    self-evaluation vocabulary knowledge
      checklist, 297–298, 297f
    sentence-building activity using
      connectors, 305–306
    sentence-completion or paragraph-
      completion task, 309–311
    using EmPOWER strategy,
      302–303, 302f
  lexical knowledge and, 280–281
  mathematics, 81–82, 83
  paraphrasing and, 283
  persuasive writing and, 283–285
  semantic and lexical acquisition and,
      290–293, 291b–292b
  teaching of
    checklist for, 87–89, 88f
    Cirrin's five basic curricular demand
      concepts and, 86–87, 86b

Vocabulary—cont'd
  teacher *versus* speech-language
      pathologist in, 84, 85
  word finding and word retrieval, 285–290

W

Warrant in argumentative text, 240t
Washing clothes paragraph, 120–122
Watering up curriculum for language
    intervention, 73–77, 73t, 74t
Weade and Green's guidelines for classroom
    observation, 60, 61b
Westby framework, 162–163
Wh clause, 255b
What in language teaching continuum
    of service delivery, 90, 90f
Word finding and retrieval, 285–290
Word recognition, 286
Word substitution, 287
Word, finding of, 285–290
Word-order strategy in sentence
    comprehension, 69
Writing
  integration of spoken language
      with, 136–169
    case study, 164–169
    early reading routines and, 138–147
    in grade 5, 158–162, 159b
    literature-based frameworks in,
      150–157, 155b–156b
    print awareness and, 147–150, 151f
    Westby framework for, 162–163
  language abilities and, 53
  literacy and, 7
  math problems and, 82, 83, 83f
  on curriculum-based intervention
      checklist, 88f
  persuasive, 283–284
  scientific, 207–209, 208b, 216
  strategies for, 225–227, 226b, 227f, 228f
  transition of from writing like talking to
      writing like books, 36–37, 36b

Printed and bound by CPI Group (UK) Ltd, Croydon, CR0 4YY

03/10/2024

01040364-0001